AIDS EDUCATION

AIDS EDUCATION

Mark Hochhauser, Ph.D.
Consultant
and
James H. Rothenberger, III, M.P.H.
University of Minnesota

 Wm. C. Brown Publishers

Book Team
Editor *Chris Rogers*
Production Coordinator *Peggy Selle*

 Wm. C. Brown Publishers
President *G. Franklin Lewis*
Vice President, Publisher *Thomas E. Doran*
Vice President, Operations and Production *Beverly Kolz*
National Sales Manager *Virginia S. Moffat*
Marketing Manager *George Chapin*
Executive Editor *Ed Laube*
Managing Editor, Production *Colleen A. Yonda*
Production Editorial Manager *Julie A. Kennedy*
Production Editorial Manager *Ann Fuerste*
Publishing Services Manager *Karen J. Slaght*
Manager of Visuals and Design *Faye M. Schilling*

WCB Group
President-Chief Executive Officer *Mark C. Falb*
Chairman of the Board *Wm. C. Brown*

Cover design by Kay D. Fulton

Library of Congress Catalog Card Number: 90–85166

ISBN 0–697–11166–0

Printed in the United States of America by Wm. C. Brown Publishers,
2460 Kerper Boulevard, Dubuque, IA 52001

10 9 8 7 6 5 4 3 2 1

To Leonard and Mervin
Mark Hochhauser

To those who donate of themselves
James H. Rothenberger, III

Contents

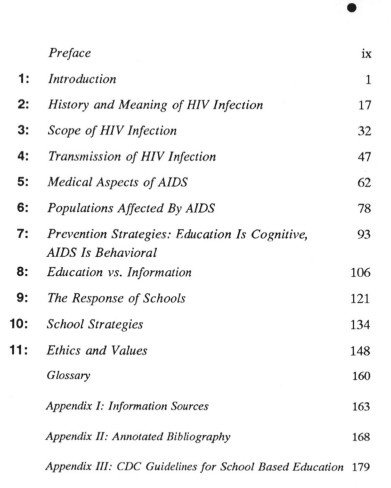

Preface

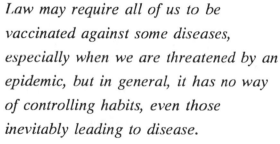

> *Law may require all of us to be*
> *vaccinated against some diseases,*
> *especially when we are threatened by an*
> *epidemic, but in general, it has no way*
> *of controlling habits, even those*
> *inevitably leading to disease.*
>
> EARL WARREN,
> Former Chief Justice, U.S. Supreme Court

Education, both as an institution and as a process, has been given the responsibility of "solving" a number of societal problems. Drug use, learning disabilities, racism, intolerance, lack of moral values, poverty, latchkey children, teenage pregnancy, sexually transmitted disease, child abuse, and scores of other dilemmas are to be addressed and resolved by our educational system. And now, the serious threat of HIV infection and the diagnosis of AIDS faces us in a context where we are told that "education" is the only solution for the moment.

Most of us in education recognize that we are being assigned tasks for which our system was never designed, for which we do not have adequate training, for which there is a lack of basic knowledge to guide us, and for which we are given less than necessary resources. HIV infection and AIDS present tremendous challenges and opportunities. These are issues that bring together many other issues, such as intoxication, sexuality, and racism, and demand that we work at changing behaviors.

The problem is that none of these issues is simplistically solved by only providing information—and that is what most people outside the educational process believe education is all about. Simply telling people about risks seldom changes behavior.

HIV infection and AIDS have challenged the medical community, and medical professionals have responded by discovering more basic knowledge about immunity in the last 10 years than the previous 100. The knowledge explosion from basic research in this area is comparable to the effort to put a person on the moon 20 years ago.

HIV infection and AIDS also are presenting a challenge to the educational community, and we need to respond in the same way. The opportunity exists to learn more about the relationship between education and behavior change than ever before. Like the medical research, the potential payoffs go far beyond this disease. We will learn to work with all behaviors that put people at risk.

This book is designed to provide a basic reference about HIV infection and AIDS to educators. It tries to be realistic and rational when basic fears about diseases and about the unknown cause us to become irrational. It tries to lay out the complexity of a serious problem when many around us want to simplify it for sound bites. It tries to point out that a great deal is known, on which we can build when many are paralyzed by the thought of having to start from scratch. Above all, the book concentrates on documentation and research instead of on impressions and impassioned warnings of doom.

People who work with HIV infection and AIDS deal in sensitivity. One cannot deal with mortality—one's own or that of someone else—without being fundamentally changed. A large part of sensitivity focuses on the words we use. Wherever possible, we differentiate between HIV infection, which means that a virus is active in the individual, and AIDS, which is a diagnosis of illness that often results from HIV infection, but only after a period of time. All people who have AIDS are HIV infected, but only a fraction of those who have HIV infection have developed AIDS or even know that they are infected.

Likewise, we use terms such as persons with AIDS (PWAs) to focus attention on people *living with* AIDS as opposed to people *dying of* AIDS. We now view this disease as a serious chronic disease more than as a terminal condition.

As in any technical field, some terms have specific meanings. Even though the word *quarantine* is loosely used by the lay population, it refers to the separation of people from others for a period of time to determine whether those who were separated become ill. Once they are ill, they are then isolated. We have used *quarantine* and *isolation* to refer to both situations.

Another area of sensitivity concerns the terms *homosexual* and *gay*. Whenever possible, we use the term *gay* in recognition that it implies far more than homosexual activity. *Gay* simply has a less negative connotation than *homosexual.*

Finally, we are sensitive to the World Health Organization's request dating back to the 1950s that medical writers not use the terms *addict* and *addiction.* Calling someone a name with a negative implication seldom has resulted in positive behavior change. Therefore, we use the terms *dependency, chemical dependency,* and *intravenous drug user (IVDU)* rather than *intravenous drug abuser (IVDA).* These may seem like small changes, but we feel that they are important in focusing on a problem that involves "us" as opposed to "them." However, when quoting other sources, we have used the terminology of the original report.

A careful study of HIV infection and all of the issues involved is, in many respects, a study of the modern human condition in microcosm. A hundred years ago, it was said that the doctor who knew syphilis knew all of medicine. Today we say that those who know HIV infection know all of public health. Maybe tomorrow we will say that those who know HIV infection know all of education.

Acknowledgments

This text has been strengthened by the suggestions and encouragements provided by the expert panel of reviewers: Dr. Matthew Adeyanju (University of Kansas), Dr. David Corbin (University of Nebraska, Omaha), Chris George (California State Polytechnic U., Pomona), William Hemmer (SUNY College, Brockport), Robin Sawyer (University of Maryland), and Dr. Sherman Sowby (California State University, Fresno).

We wish to thank Chris Rogers and Peggy Selle of Wm. C. Brown Publishers for all their help with our text.

Mark Hochhauser, Ph.D.
James H. Rothenberger, M.P.H.
November, 1990

Introduction

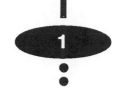

1

> *Nothing in life is to be feared. It is only to be understood.*
>
> MARIE CURIE

THE AIDS "PLAGUE"

What was to become known as Acquired Immune Deficiency Syndrome (AIDS) was first reported in the June 5, 1981, edition of *Morbidity and Mortality Weekly Report,* a publication of the Centers for Disease Control (CDC). A relatively unusual illness, *Pneumocystis carinii pneumonia* (PCP), was described in five young homosexual men from California. Because these immune deficiency cases were first identified in gay men, the disease was originally described by some federal researchers as *GRID*—gay related immune deficiency. Later, in 1981, the term *acquired immunodeficiency syndrome* was used to describe the collection of opportunistic diseases that were being seen in otherwise healthy young men. Unfortunately, the association of AIDS with homosexuality had some

unfortunate consequences for public health funding, health education programs, and, most importantly, the people who were diagnosed with AIDS.

As the reported cases of this new disease began to increase, the term *gay plague* was increasingly used to describe the phenomenon; it appeared as if being gay was the cause of AIDS, a concept that was reinforced by CDC in their description of risk groups for AIDS (homosexual or bisexual men, intravenous drug users, etc.). Unfortunately, the initial association of AIDS with "risk groups" may have been a consequence of some problems in the way the data were collected and reported.

In the early 1980s, a cause of AIDS had not yet been identified; some researchers implicated contaminated inhalants such as amyl nitrites, which were used by some gay men to heighten sexual experiences. Later research (Haverkos, 1988) did suggest the possibility that such nitrite inhalants might play a role in the development of Kaposi's sarcoma, a relatively rare cancer, in gay men with AIDS. However, the exact role of such nitrites is still unknown. Others believed that a yet unknown virus was the cause of the disease. The basic facts about AIDS were simply not known at that time.

There is no doubt that the vast majority of AIDS cases were found in gay men in New York and San Francisco. However, these cases may have been reported simply because many of these gay men had medical coverage and access to the health-care system. Despite the identification of AIDS with gay men, it should be noted that blood samples from the mid- to late 1970s of intravenous drug users in New York had antibodies to the AIDS virus (DesJarlais et al., 1989). Many intravenous drug users may have died of AIDS in the late 1970s and early 1980s, but the cause of their deaths was probably not investigated in much detail. Many IV drug users simply did not have insurance coverage or access to the health-care system; if they had, AIDS may have become known as a disease of IV drug users. This also suggests that the total number of reported AIDS cases may well be an underestimate of actual AIDS cases, as many AIDS cases were probably undiagnosed, uncounted, and unreported.

As the number of AIDS cases began to increase rapidly, many public health officials, writers, and scientists continued to discuss the "gay plague." Indeed, it was assumed in the early 1980s that the AIDS epidemic would be worse than the bubonic plague that wiped out a quarter of Europe's population in the fourteenth century. That comparison seems overblown at best and hysterical at worst. Politically, however, the description of AIDS as a plague did marshal some government support for research and prevention activities, although, as pointed out by Shilts (1987), these efforts were relatively small.

Unfortunately, the description of AIDS as a modern plague inaccurately used the terminology of plagues without making it clear what plagues were—and what they were not.

AIDS: A MODERN PLAGUE?

A dictionary defines a plague as "a pestilence, affliction, or calamity, originally one of divine retribution," or a "highly infectious, usually fatal, epidemic disease, especially the bubonic plague" (*American Heritage Dictionary,* 1970). AIDS clearly met some of these criteria, while not meeting others. There was—and is—no doubt that AIDS is infectious and highly fatal. As of mid-1990, there are an estimated 1 million Americans thought to be carrying the Human Immunodeficiency Virus (HIV) that causes AIDS; worldwide there are probably 5 to 10 million people carrying the virus. How many of these people will later develop AIDS is not known precisely, although current estimates are that perhaps 99 percent of those infected will develop full-blown AIDS within 10 to 20 years after infection. Neither is it known how many new infections will occur each year, although the Centers for Disease Control have estimated that there were probably about 80,000 new infections per year from 1986 to 1989, and a minimum of 40,000 new infections per year in adults and adolescents (CDC, 1990d).

It is important to point out some of the factors of the bubonic plague that may, or may not, be related to AIDS issues. As described by McNeill (1976), the bubonic plague killed about one-fourth of the population in Europe in only four years—from 1346 to 1350. Death from bubonic plague often took only 24 hours. Moreover, the religious implications of the bubonic plague were not to be overlooked; Jews were blamed for spreading the plague, and many were killed. Likewise, violence toward gays has been on the increase; some people justify "gay bashing" by saying that gays are to blame for the spread of AIDS. The influenza epidemic of 1918 killed 25 million people worldwide, and 650,000 (out of a population of slightly more than 100 million) in the United States alone. Both of these diseases killed quickly. When or whether AIDS deaths will equal these totals is not yet known.

A very important difference between AIDS, other infectious diseases, and plagues is the relatively long incubation period of the Human Immunodeficiency Virus. Despite the fact that AIDS has been studied intensively for about a decade, and that more has been learned about HIV and AIDS in that short period of time than probably any other disease in history, researchers still do not have all of the necessary information about the disease. The lack of early symptoms and long incubation period make AIDS different from many other diseases.

Asymptomatic decade

Recent estimates suggest that it may take 10 years or more for someone infected with the Human Immunodeficiency Virus to develop AIDS symptoms. In a study of gay men, Bacchetti and Moss (1989) calculated that the median incubation period from HIV infection to development of full-blown AIDS is 9.8 years, with 45 percent of the infected men having developed AIDS within nine years of being infected. A study of gay and bisexual men in San Francisco who were infected with HIV (Lemp et al., 1990) found a median incubation period from time of infection until onset of AIDS of about 11 years. During this "asymptomatic decade," the infected individual may feel perfectly healthy, have no symptoms whatsoever, and yet still carry the HIV in his or her immune system. The infected person is capable of infecting others throughout life if he or she engages in risky sexual or drug-using behaviors.

Once symptoms develop, the person may live from 18 to 36 months, or more in some cases. Some people with AIDS (PWAs) have survived for several years after being diagnosed as having AIDS, especially since the drug AZT was approved by the Food and Drug Administration as a treatment for AIDS. Thus, the time period from in-

fection to death may be 10, 15, or 20 years or more. This means that HIV and AIDS will be with us for decades; AIDS will not burn itself out in just a few years, as did the bubonic plague, or in one or two years, as did the 1918 worldwide influenza epidemic.

MORALITY AND MEDICINE

Some people have believed that the "gay plague" is God's way of punishing gay men. Some religious and political leaders have seemed happy that AIDS has arrived to rid the country of gay men, IV drug users, minorities, and others whom they did not consider to be part of the general population. Much media coverage of AIDS has addressed the issue of when AIDS will "spread" into the general population. As long as AIDS is viewed as a disease of "them" rather than of "us," behavioral change and public health efforts are likely to have minimal impact.

The attitude "they're getting what they deserve" was, and is, not uncommon. Public health efforts were remarkably slow to develop, as morality became a substitute for public health. This attitude was expressed concisely in a letter to one of the authors:

> August 12th, 1987
> Dear Sir:
> Don't you think its [sic] high time we obey God's orders and put gays to death? We haven't obeyed Him so He struck them down with aids [sic] and they still continue that filthy, foul life style. Leviticus 20 – 13 says gays should be put to death and we dont [sic] even puts aids [sic] patents to death. Just take them into hospitals to infect employees and cost the country billions.
> If we don't obey God we will have a plague worse than the black plague one doctor said.
> Fetuses are killed by the millions why not gays and aids [sic] patients?

Leviticus 18– 22 and Romans 1– 27 to 32 has more to say.

Prison guards, police and young boys are very vulnerable. They want to pass aids [sic] on to others.

Hopefully,

In contrast, Surgeon General Koop stated in his influential brochure on AIDS (1986):

At the beginning of the AIDS epidemic many Americans had little sympathy for people with AIDS. The feeling was that somehow people from certain groups "deserved" their illness. Let us put those feelings behind us. We are fighting a disease, not people. Those who are already afflicted are sick people and need our care as do all sick patients. The country must face this epidemic as a unified society. We must prevent the spread of AIDS while at the same time preserving our humanity and intimacy. (p. 6)

The impact of Surgeon General Koop cannot be overemphasized. At a time when the federal government was moving slowly to deal with the public health implications of AIDS Dr. Koop's leadership as Surgeon General of the United States was vital. His statement "I am the Surgeon General, not the chaplain, of all the people, and that includes homosexuals" (Carlson, 1989) summarizes the need for a public health perspective on AIDS.

WHERE DID AIDS COME FROM?

Why is the source of a disease important? In virtually every epidemic, someone else, or some other country, is blamed for this disease. Hence, many still "blame" Central Africa generally and blacks more specifically for the origin of AIDS. Some Americans have "blamed" Africa for the disease; some Africans have "blamed" Americans for the disease, insisting that it was brought to the African continent by Americans; some have "blamed" the U.S. Defense Department and the CIA for developing the virus in a laboratory and either letting it inadvertently escape or putting it deliberately into the environment to kill off certain segments of the population. Assigning blame will do nothing to slow the spread of the disease, but it may do quite a bit to harm international relations.

Some early data suggested that the virus migrated from the green monkey to human beings at some point early in its history, either through monkeys biting human beings, or through human beings eating monkey meat that was not properly cooked. Unfortunately, such hypotheses may have led some people to erroneously conclude that there is a strong animal-human linkage in transmission of HIV—hence the belief that HIV can be spread by household pets. A national survey of knowledge and attitudes about AIDS in December 1987 (Dawson and Thornberry, 1988) found that 11 percent of the general population believed that they could get the AIDS virus from pets or other animals, while 22 percent simply did not know!

Omitted from much of this discussion is the recognition that HIV apparently existed in the United States as early as 1968; a sexually active teenager who died in 1969 was probably infected with HIV or a virus very similar to it (Garry et al., 1988). In many respects, it is fortunate that AIDS was discovered in a portion of the population that exhibited common behavior patterns. If it had been randomly spread throughout the entire population, it might not have been identified as a disease syndrome for many more years. The public health reporting system may simply not have been sophisticated enough to identify the virus, especially in people with little or no access to health care.

In an attempt to minimize blame, in 1987, the World Health Assembly concluded that HIV is a "naturally occurring retrovirus of undetermined geographic origin" (Mann et al., 1988). Even if we knew exactly how and where this disease started, what would we do that would be different from what we are currently doing?

The religious implications of AIDS cannot be overlooked. Because most cases occur in gay men, many religious leaders described AIDS as God's punishment for an unacceptable lifestyle. (Interestingly, AIDS was not a disease of lesbians; did that mean that lesbianism was acceptable but that male homosexuality was unacceptable?) Interpreting AIDS within the context of divine retribution has several important implications, most of which were not addressed by those who viewed the disease from that perspective.

First, if AIDS were, in fact, a punishment from God, then it follows that nothing should be done to halt the spread of this disease. If, as some conservative religious leaders stated, AIDS was God's punishment of gay men, then any efforts to prevent or cure AIDS would be an attempt to contradict God's will. Disease as retribution essentially means that the virus should run its course without human intervention. However, the disease was not limited to gay men; hemophiliacs and children born of mothers with the disease became the ''innocent victims'' of the virus, while gay men were the ''deserving victims.'' For some, the fact that this disease affected groups other than gay men meant that some treatment and prevention efforts had to be taken. None of the religious leaders asked why God would be so unselective in choosing who would get AIDS.

Second, because the disease seemed primarily limited to gay men, relatively few federal public officials were willing to view AIDS as a public health problem. Considerable discussion ensued over whether the disease would spread to the ''general population'' (as if gays and others with AIDS are not a part of the general population). As long as AIDS was viewed as a disease of gay men, a disease that they ''brought on themselves,'' a disease that they ''deserved'' and was ''God-given,'' then federal, state, and local governments

really didn't have to do much in the way of prevention or treatment.

Third, the myopia about AIDS in the United States was based on an interpretation of AIDS cases in the United States alone, not on what was happening in other parts of the world. By the mid-1980s, it had become clear that AIDS was largely a heterosexual disease in other parts of the world, particularly in some Central African countries. In the United States, there were about 13 AIDS cases in men for every AIDS case in women; in some African countries, the ratio was closer to one male case to one female case. It became clear that the political and religious perspective overwhelmed public health responsibility.

THE CHANGING FACE OF AIDS

Characteristics of people with AIDS have changed during the past decade. Many people still view AIDS as primarily a disease of gay men; it is, but not to the extent that it was in the early 1980s. The table following gives the percentage of AIDS cases by transmission category and year of report from 1981 through 1989.

In August, 1982, about 15 to 20 new AIDS cases were being reported each week (Marx, 1982). By late 1990, AIDS cases were being reported at the rate of approximately 820 per week; in 1993, there will be between 1,200 and 1,900 AIDS cases per week (CDC, 1990d). Thus, weekly AIDS cases will have increased 100-fold in about 10 years. It took approximately eight years to record the first 120,000 cases; it will take only 18 months (beginning in January 1990) to record the next 120,000 cases. Since AIDS cases began to be reported in the early 1980s, several significant trends have evolved. As shown in Table 1.1, the percentage of AIDS cases in homosexual males decreased from 69 percent (prior to 1985) to 63 percent (in 1989), while the percentage of cases in IV drug users increased from 15 to 20 percent during the same period. In females, the percentage of cases arising from IV drug use dropped from 58

TABLE 1.1   Percent Distribution of AIDS Cases in the United States, from 1981 Through 1989.

Transmission Category	AIDS Cases (%)					
	Before 1985	1985	1986	1987	1988	1989
Adult Male (over 13 years old)						
Homosexual/bisexual only	69	72	71	70	64	63
IV drug user	15	15	15	14	21	20
Homosexual and IV drug user	10	8	8	8	8	7
Hemophiliac	1	1	1	1	1	1
Heterosexual						
Heterosexual contact	<1	<1	1	1	2	3
Born in Pattern II Country[a]	3	1	1	1	1	1
Transfusion	1	1	2	2	2	2
Undetermined[b]	2	2	2	2	3	5
Adult Female (over 13 years old)						
IV drug user	58	53	49	49	53	50
Coagulation disorder	<1	<1	<1	<1	<1	<1
Heterosexual						
Heterosexual contact	16	21	28	27	27	29
Born in Pattern II Country[a]	8	6	6	4	3	4
Transfusion	8	11	10	13	11	8
Undetermined[b]	10	9	6	6	6	9
Pediatric (less than 13 years old)						
Coagulation disorder	4	6	6	7	7	4
Transfusion	11	14	13	14	11	6
Mother with/at risk for AIDS/HIV Infection						
IV drug user	45	47	44	41	41	39
Sex with person at risk	11	17	24	21	21	27
Born in Pattern II Country[a]	22	14	6	7	7	8
Other	0	2	5	8	9	12
Undetermined[b]	6	0	2	3	4	4

[a] Pattern II countries are World Health Organization designated countries with predominantly heterosexual transmission of HIV.
[b] Of patients initially reported with an undetermined risk category, 75 percent are subsequently reclassified into known risk categories following investigation. Increases in the percentage of undetermined cases in more recent reporting periods reflect a higher percentage of patients who have not been investigated.
Sources: CDC (1989).
        CDC (1990a).

percent (before 1985) to 50 percent (in 1989), while cases due to heterosexual transmission nearly doubled from 16 percent to 29 percent during the same time.

Despite such large increases in the number of people diagnosed with AIDS, an early description of AIDS (Marx, 1983) is still remarkably accurate in its description of how the virus is spread:

"The disease was first diagnosed in adults, principally in male homosexuals who had been extremely active sexually, users of intravenous drugs, and Haitians. The disease is apparently spread by sexual contact among homosexuals and by contaminated needles in the drug users. The reason for its prevalence in Haitians is unclear."

The connection to Haiti requires some analysis. Early in the epidemic, several AIDS cases were identified in Haitian residents and citizens of the United States. Demographically, it appeared as though merely being Haitian put one at risk for AIDS. Part of the association of AIDS with Haiti may have been an attempt to explain AIDS as a disease from "somewhere else," a strategy common when epidemics strike. The influenza epidemic of 1918 was known as the "Spanish influenza," and the influenza of 1957 as the "Hong Kong flu."

Analysis of the Haitian link to AIDS (Moore and LeBaron, 1986) identified several factors that might account for both the origin and the spread of the disease in Haiti:

1. Haitians are predisposed to immunosuppression because of malnutrition, parasitic infections, recreational drug use, and multiple infections.
2. Homosexuality among Haitians might be responsible for spreading the virus to gay American tourists; conversely, gay American tourists might have spread the virus to Haiti.
3. Haitians infected with the virus may have taken it to African countries such as Zaire, where they have worked in the government for decades.
4. Haitians may have brought the virus back to Haiti from other African countries.
5. Voodoo practitioners may have ingested infected animal blood during voodoo rituals. Chickens, bulls, goats, pigs, and pigeons are sacrificed, and blood is rubbed on the body or swallowed. There is no evidence, however, that any of these animals carry the Human Immunodeficiency Virus.

Despite the appearance of blaming Haiti for the international outbreak of AIDS, Moore and LeBaron (1986) do suggest research strategies for testing the above hypotheses. However, they do not address the question of whether it really matters where AIDS came from, nor do they discuss the political implications of identifying any country as the "home of AIDS."

Haitians protested the ethnic association with AIDS and, in response, the CDC dropped Haitians as a risk group in its statistical reports. As more information about AIDS became available, it became increasingly clear that one's behavior, not one's ethnic background or sexual preference, put one at risk for AIDS. However, in the early 1980s, it still seemed possible that the cause of AIDS might be related to geography. Indeed, early reports of AIDS cases relied heavily, if not exclusively, on data collected in San Francisco and New York City. During the early and mid-1980s, these two cities formed the epicenters of the AIDS epidemic. Much of what was known about AIDS was based on data collected from those two cities.

San Francisco model

In San Francisco, in 1990, AIDS was still primarily a disease of gay men. More than 80 percent of all AIDS cases reported are in gay men; only a very small percentage (less than 5%) has occurred in intravenous drug users. However, the number of AIDS cases in gay and bisexual men has apparently leveled off. (There were 1,368 cases in 1987, 1,356 in 1988, and 1,301 in 1989). The number of AIDS cases in IV drug users increased from 12 cases in 1985 to 71 cases in 1989. Through June, 1990, the city reported 8,754 AIDS cases, with 5,798 deaths—a case fatality ratio of 66 percent (San Francisco Department of Public Health, 1990). However, Lemp, et al. (1990) have projected that by June, 1993, San Francisco will have a cumulative total of 12,500 to 17,000 AIDS cases, with about 10,000 to 13,000 deaths.

The gay community in San Francisco has some unique characteristics. First, San Francisco has a relatively large gay population. Some of these men have been involved in health studies for a decade or more. Second, the gay lifestyle has a degree of acceptance in San Francisco that probably does not exist in many other American cities,

Box 1

afrAIDS

The irrational fear of AIDS (*afrAIDS*) has had, and will continue to have, a major impact on American society, particularly the U.S. educational system. Such irrational fears about AIDS have several sources.

Do you believe the government?

Many people do not believe the information about AIDS that federal public health officials have provided. A recent national survey (Hardy, 1990) found that about 27 percent of the American public said that they did not believe the AIDS information provided by federal public health officials, while 6 percent said that they "didn't know"; overall, 60 million people have some doubt about federally distributed AIDS information. The reasons for such disbelief are not clear. Perhaps there is a general mistrust of government agencies. Perhaps it is a result of prior errors in government health judgment (e.g., the potential swine flu epidemic of the 1970s, which never occurred). Perhaps it is caused by the belief that the government has conspired to withhold the truth about AIDS. Whatever the reasons, people's irrational fears about AIDS are not likely to be calmed by government proclamation alone.

What if . . .

The impact of "hypothetical" transmission routes cannot be overestimated. Despite considerable evidence to the contrary, many people still believe that HIV can be spread not only by mosquitoes, but by household pets as well. The latter misconception might be the result of findings regarding a feline leukemia virus that is somewhat similar in structure to the Human Immunodeficiency Virus. Without any supporting evidence, Masters, Johnson, and Kolodny (1988) state the following:

> Is it possible to become infected with the AIDS virus in a touch football game, on the soccer field, while sliding into second base, or on the basketball court? In a word, yes . . . There is no way of quantifying the magnitude of this risk at present. But even if it is now very small, as the prevalence of HIV infection in the general population mounts, the risk of infection from nonsexual, non-drug abuse, nontransfusion contact with blood will mount too. (p. 32)

Fear and hatred of homosexuality

The association of AIDS with homosexual behavior cannot be ignored as a contributing factor of afrAIDS. For many people, the real fear is homophobia (an irrational fear of homosexuals and homosexuality); that is, if a man is diagnosed with AIDS, his family and friends will assume that he is gay. Moreover, such fear often is expressed through violence against gays and lesbians—known as gay bashing. Some gays have been killed simply because they are gay. If AIDS were more of an equal opportunity disease, as it is in some parts of Central Africa, the association of AIDS with homosexuality would not be nearly so significant.

Because AIDS has been associated with homosexuality, drug abuse, and death, the perception of the disease has been less a public health problem and more a religious or moral issue. In a survey of 54 home-health aides (Thompson, 1990), six (11%) identified homosexuality as a mental illness, despite the fact that neither the American Psychiatric Association nor the

Psychological Association considers homosexuality to be a mental illness. Twelve (24%) classified homosexuality as a sin. It should not be surprising, then, that some health-care providers have a difficult time providing quality care to patients who are thought to be mentally ill or sinners.

Education versus fear

Information alone will not necessarily reduce the irrational fear of AIDS, nor will reliance upon federal "experts." A survey of American adults (Hardy, 1990) found that when asked, "When federal public officials give advice about how to help keep from getting AIDS, do you believe their advice or are you doubtful about what they say?" 81 percent believed the officials, 15 percent were doubtful, and 3 percent did not know.

AfrAIDS exists in the medical as well as the nonmedical professions. Gerbert and co-workers (1988) have identified three reasons for the continuing fear of AIDS by health-care professionals:

1. Occupational exposure poses real risks. Although the statistical risk for health-care workers is low, many providers, when exposed to HIV-infected blood, do not think of themselves at low risk. (How would you feel if you stuck yourself with a needle after drawing blood from an infected patient? How would you feel if an infected student came to you with a cut hand and dripped blood on you?)

2. Infection-control procedures cannot be guaranteed. Accidents still occur with scalpel and needlestick injuries, even when appropriate infection-control procedures are followed. (Do you know how to protect yourself from infection where you work?)

3. Communication between health-care authorities and health-care professionals is essential. Health-care authorities may send mixed messages. They ask why extraordinary, inconvenient, and expensive infection control procedures are advocated for a disease that is fragile and not easily transmitted (p. 3482). (Do you believe the experts? Why or why not?)

They don't know everything, so they must know nothing . . .

Revision of AIDS-related information has tended to make health-care authorities lose some of their credibility with the professionals who work with patients. Moreover, scientists, administrators, and health-care professionals may have different values and goals (e.g., quality of research findings, reduction of employee fear, quality of patient care, moral judgments), thus causing conflict and mistrust. Unfortunately, some people have erroneously assumed that because health-care professionals do not know everything about AIDS, they know nothing about AIDS.

The recommendations suggested for health-care professionals are equally relevant to educational professionals who must deal with some of the same issues with students, faculty, staff, parents, and administrators.

First, the risks should be acknowledged and discussed, then minimized where appropriate. Some fears may be irrational, but they should not be dismissed out of hand; people do not become rational simply by being labeled irrational.

Second, the strengths and limitations of infection-control procedures should be conveyed. Not all risks can be eliminated, but they can be reduced; a risk-free environment is not feasible, but a less risky environment is attainable.

Third, scientific and administrative authorities should develop their credibility as experts. Advanced degrees alone do not confer expertise about AIDS; an M.D. or Ph.D. may be necessary, but it is not sufficient.

Fourth, small discussion groups should be used to address concerns and fears, because such groups allow people to express their fears. Simply handing out brochures on the facts about AIDS is not AIDS education. Group discussions can identify both problems and solutions if given proper leadership.

Finally, acknowledging differences in professional domains and perspectives can help improve communication. Conflicting perceptions can be shaped into a consensus that will reduce the irrational fear of AIDS.

where gay men are likely to remain "in the closet." Third, some of these gay men have had hundreds or even thousands of sexual partners over the past decade. These observations suggest that much of what is known about AIDS based on gay men in San Francisco may not generalize to other cities, where there may be proportionately fewer gay men whose sexual orientation remains largely hidden, who have had fewer sexual partners, who did not get the early safer sex educational material that was distributed to the gay community in San Francisco, and who may be less likely to participate in gay-related health-care studies.

New York City model

In New York City, about 55 percent of the new AIDS cases have been reported in IV drug users and about 45 percent in gay men, as reported by the New York City Department of Health (*New York Times,* June 6, 1988). In New York City, new AIDS cases in gay men have decreased by more than 40 percent. Unfortunately, this decrease has been offset by an increase in AIDS cases among IV drug users of almost 300 percent since 1982. One major difference between AIDS cases in San Francisco and New York City is in the number of pediatric AIDS cases reported. Because the spread of HIV in San Francisco is closely associated with homosexual transmission, (through June, 1990), San Francisco reported only 17 AIDS cases in children under the age of 13. By contrast, New York City reported 635 pediatric cases (CDC, 1990b), due to the spread of the virus from mother (IV drug user) to child or from an HIV-infected male partner to his uninfected female partner.

Thus, in San Francisco, AIDS has become primarily a male-to-male sexually transmitted disease, but in New York City it is primarily a disease spread by the sharing of needles. Such differences have profound implications for both treatment and prevention. Unfortunately, it is not possible to accurately estimate how these percentages will change in the future.

MEASURING THE PROBLEM

Geographically, most early AIDS cases were reported in New York City and San Francisco. Since 1981, however, AIDS cases have been reported in every state. Despite the tendency to view AIDS as a serious health problem restricted primarily to the east and west coasts, a state-by-state comparison of reported cases based on population (rather than on the absolute number of reported cases) shows a different picture of the disease.

Figure 1.1 shows the incidence of AIDS per 100,000 population from July 1989 through June 1990 (CDC, 1990b). The District of Columbia had the highest incidence of cases (about 86 cases per 100,000), followed by Puerto Rico (45 per 100,000), New York (43 per 100,000), Florida (31 per 100,000), New Jersey (29 per 100,000), and California (24 per 100,000). Thus, although most people think of California when they think of AIDS, the District of Columbia had almost 3.5 times as many cases as California on a per capita basis, and twice as many cases as New York!

Even a state-by-state summary does not provide a complete picture of reported AIDS cases, because most cases are concentrated in urban metropolitan areas. About 85 percent of the reported AIDS cases have come from metropolitan areas with populations of 500,000 or more. However, recent trends suggest that many future cases will occur in smaller cities: From 1988 to 1989, reported cases increased by only 5 percent in metropolitan areas with more than 1 million people, but they increased by 35 percent in metropolitan areas with less than 100,000 people, and by 32 percent in metropolitan areas with populations of 100,000 to 500,000 (CDC, 1990c).

Table 1.2 shows the AIDS cases and annual incidence rates per 100,000 population by metropolitan area. Within the same state, different metropolitan areas may have very different rates of disease; in New York State, for example, the rate per 100,000 population was 8.4 in Syracuse, 9.0 in

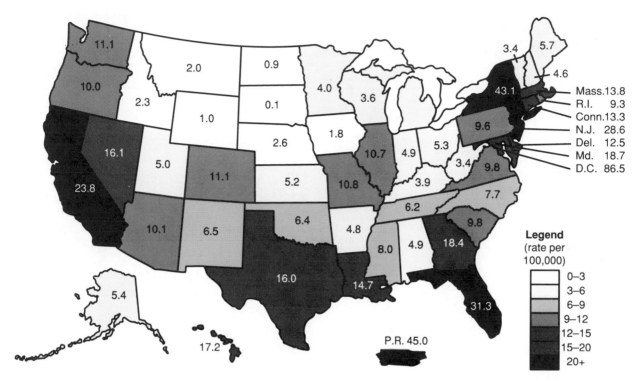

Mass.13.8
R.I.   9.3
Conn.13.3
N.J. 28.6
Del. 12.5
Md. 18.7
D.C. 86.5

Legend
(rate per
100,000)

	0–3
	3–6
	6–9
	9–12
	12–15
	15–20
	20+

° FIGURE 1.1   AIDS annual incidence rates per 100,000 population, for causes reported July 1989–June 1990 United States. Source: Centers for Disease Control, HIV/AIDS Surveillance Report, July 1990.

Rochester, 10.6 in Buffalo, 10.8 in Albany-Schenectady, 15.7 in Nassau-Suffolk, and 75.3 in New York City.

By comparison, other cities with high rates include San Francisco (119 cases per 100,000), Ft. Lauderdale (73 cases per 100,000), San Juan (60 cases per 100,000), Miami (59 cases per 100,000), Jersey City (52 cases per 100,000), Newark (51 cases per 100,000), and West Palm Beach (40 cases per 100,000).

These AIDS cases represent HIV infections that probably occurred 7 to 10 years before an AIDS diagnosis was made. Thus, AIDS cases that were reported in 1982 may well have been contracted between 1975 and 1978; AIDS cases reported in 1991 may have been contracted in the mid-1980s. Therefore, relying on AIDS cases as a measure of the prevalence of the disease may tell

us who became infected a decade ago, but not who will be infected a decade from now.

Finally, such cases probably represent somewhat of an underestimate of the total number of AIDS cases. A review (Conway et al., 1989) of the completeness and accuracy of AIDS cases in South Carolina for an 18-month period found that only 60 percent of probable AIDS cases were reported to the South Carolina AIDS registry at the time of diagnosis, with such reports being poorer for blacks (53 percent of likely cases) than for whites (72 percent of likely cases). While such findings cannot be generalized to the rest of the United States, they do suggest that in some areas, the number of AIDS cases "officially" reported may seriously underrepresent the "actual" number of such cases. In their estimates of future AIDS cases, the Centers for Disease Control add 18 percent to their projec-

....
TABLE 1.2   AIDS Cases and Annual Rates per 100,000 Population, by metropolitan area with 500,000 or More Population, Reported July 1988 Through June 1989, July 1989 Through June 1990; and Cumulative Totals, by Area and Age Group, Through June 1990

Metropolitan Area of Residence	July 1988–June 1989		July 1989–June 1990		Cumulative Totals		
	Number	Rate	Number	Rate	Adults/Adolescents	Children <13 years old	Total
Akron, Ohio	32	5.0	22	3.4	90	—	90
Albany-Schenectady, N.Y.	58	6.8	92	10.8	287	3	290
Albuquerque, N.M.	42	8.2	54	10.4	154	1	155
Allentown, Pa.	31	4.6	54	7.9	135	4	139
Anaheim, Calif.	264	11.5	332	14.2	1,151	8	1,159
Atlanta, Ga.	772	27.3	931	32.0	2,781	25	2,806
Austin, Tex.	151	19.1	224	27.3	601	5	606
Bakersfield, Calif.	17	3.2	44	8.1	98	—	98
Baltimore, Md.	397	16.9	580	24.6	1,524	46	1,570
Baton Rouge, La.	47	8.6	66	11.9	174	2	176
Bergen-Passaic, N.J.	243	18.7	280	21.6	1,166	25	1,191
Birmingham, Ala.	81	8.7	61	6.5	234	6	240
Boston, Mass.	613	16.3	613	16.3	2,278	48	2,326
Bridgeport, Conn.	135	16.5	115	14.0	485	17	502
Charleston, S.C.	56	10.7	83	15.6	204	—	204
Charlotte, N.C.	76	6.7	95	8.3	283	5	288
Chicago, Ill.	890	14.3	1,036	16.6	3,427	44	3,471
Cincinnati, Ohio	65	4.5	112	7.7	298	6	304
Cleveland, Ohio	137	7.4	117	6.4	499	7	506
Columbus, Ohio	128	9.5	122	9.0	431	3	434
Dallas, Tex.	546	21.0	635	23.7	2,349	11	2,360
Dayton, Ohio	61	6.5	54	5.7	192	3	195
Denver, Colo.	284	16.7	310	18.0	1,129	5	1,134
Detroit, Mich.	357	8.2	377	8.7	1,186	19	1,205
El Paso, Tex.	10	1.7	40	6.5	85	1	86
Fort Lauderdale, Fla.	473	39.4	883	72.5	2,175	42	2,217
Fort Worth, Tex.	139	10.2	167	11.9	527	7	534
Fresno, Calif.	51	8.3	56	8.9	165	2	167
Gary, Ind.	17	2.9	28	4.8	75	—	75
Grand Rapids, Mich.	31	4.6	19	2.8	77	1	78
Greensboro, N.C.	62	6.6	82	8.7	214	4	218
Greenville, S.C.	28	4.5	38	6.0	104	—	104
Harrisburg, Pa.	46	7.8	41	6.9	145	4	149
Hartford, Conn.	134	12.0	154	13.7	479	10	489
Honolulu, Hawaii	93	10.9	124	14.4	417	2	419
Houston, Tex.	852	25.7	1,149	34.0	4,106	31	4,137
Indianapolis, Ind.	117	9.4	137	10.9	399	3	402
Jacksonville, Fla.	149	16.2	242	25.7	592	12	604
Jersey City, N.J.	412	75.9	282	52.1	1,503	34	1,537
Kansas City, Mo.	204	12.9	322	20.1	862	3	865
Knoxville, Tenn.	28	4.7	28	4.6	98	—	98
Lake County, Ill.	16	3.1	18	3.5	64	2	66
Las Vegas, Nev.	98	15.4	132	20.2	380	5	385
Little Rock, Ark.	30	5.7	52	9.8	139	3	142
Los Angeles, Calif.	1,778	20.2	2,294	25.7	9,118	81	9,199
Louisville, Ky.	46	4.7	62	6.4	174	2	176
Memphis, Tenn.	78	7.9	109	10.9	305	5	310
Miami, Fla.	959	52.6	1,077	58.6	3,541	145	3,686
Middlesex, N.J.	198	19.9	173	17.1	709	22	731
Milwaukee, Wis.	68	4.9	96	6.9	308	1	309
Minneapolis-Saint Paul, Minn.	155	6.5	158	6.5	629	6	635
Mobile, Ala.	42	8.5	34	6.8	157	—	157
Monmouth-Ocean City, N.J.	165	16.6	170	16.8	543	20	563
Nashville, Tenn.	106	10.7	87	8.6	296	6	302
Nassau-Suffolk, N.Y.	329	12.5	413	15.7	1,438	37	1,475
New Haven, Conn.	116	14.5	130	16.2	519	26	545

TABLE 1.2 Continued

Metropolitan Area of Redidence	July 1988–June 1989		July 1989–June 1990		Cumulative Totals		
	Number	Rate	Number	Rate	Adults/Adolescents	Children <13 years old	Total
New Orleans, La.	264	19.8	390	29.0	1,244	18	1,262
New York, N.Y.	5,571	65.0	6,474	75.3	26,140	635	26,775
Newark, N.J.	1,012	53.3	964	50.7	3,782	103	3,885
Norfolk, Va.	86	6.2	153	10.8	382	7	389
Oakland, Calif.	319	15.8	507	24.8	1,676	10	1,686
Oklahoma City, Okla.	78	7.8	113	11.2	318	—	318
Omaha, Neb.	29	4.6	34	5.4	109	1	110
Orlando, Fla.	186	18.7	187	18.2	562	7	569
Oxnard-Ventura, Calif.	38	5.8	39	5.8	129	—	129
Philadelphia, Pa.	760	15.5	830	16.8	2,914	46	2,960
Phoenix, Ariz.	183	8.7	285	13.1	859	4	863
Pittsburgh, Pa.	135	6.5	143	7.0	492	2	494
Portland, Oreg.	157	13.2	213	17.8	664	2	666
Providence, R.I.	77	8.5	88	9.7	307	6	313
Raleigh-Durham, N.C.	73	10.4	123	17.2	308	8	316
Richmond, Va.	83	9.8	128	15.0	336	7	343
Riverside-San Bernardino, Calif.	216	9.4	260	11.0	866	14	880
Rochester, N.Y.	71	7.3	88	9.0	317	2	319
Sacramento, Calif.	174	12.4	122	8.5	552	5	557
Saint Louis, Mo.	182	7.3	210	8.4	658	6	664
Salt Lake City, Utah	64	5.8	76	6.8	248	5	253
San Antonio, Tex.	352	25.5	202	14.3	689	9	698
San Diego, Calif.	453	18.8	724	29.3	2,067	17	2,084
San Francisco, Calif.	1,813	112.5	1,938	119.3	8,440	17	8,457
San Jose, Calif.	158	11.0	139	9.6	609	7	616
San Juan, P.R.	886	56.7	938	59.8	2,420	89	2,509
Scranton, Pa.	23	3.1	34	4.6	100	3	103
Seattle, Wash.	341	18.4	395	21.1	1,405	9	1,414
Springfield, Mass.	40	6.8	67	11.4	155	7	162
Syracuse, N.Y.	18	2.8	54	8.4	139	4	143
Tacoma, Wash.	29	5.2	37	6.5	119	1	120
Tampa, Fla.	445	21.7	387	18.4	1,326	22	1,348
Toledo, Ohio	21	3.4	40	6.6	96	3	99
Tucson, Ariz.	55	8.4	57	8.6	214	2	216
Tulsa, Okla.	52	7.0	55	7.3	176	3	179
Washington, D.C.	864	22.9	973	25.4	3,841	54	3,895
West Palm Beach, Fla.	324	38.2	348	39.7	1,174	50	1,224
Wilmington, Del.	70	12.3	74	12.8	221	3	224
Worcester, Mass.	37	5.5	37	5.5	138	3	141
Metropolitan area subtotal[a]	28,294	19.3	33,231	22.5	117,918	2,003	119,921
All other areas	5,218	5.1	6,775	6.5	19,467	377	19,844
Total	33,512	13.3	40,006	15.7	137,385	2,380	139,765

[a]Includes data from metropolitan areas that have populations of 500,000 or more.

tions, which are obtained from reported cases to account for unreported cases (CDC, 1990b).

BEHAVIORAL CONTROL OF AIDS

Disease can be spread via a number of different routes, some of which can be controlled, some of which cannot be. There is very little that can be done to protect oneself from the common cold; the virus is everywhere and one cannot avoid contact with it. Similarly, for diseases that are food-borne or waterborne, there may be relatively little that one can do to protect oneself from infection.

Superficially, at least, AIDS appears to be a disease that is amendable to personal control, especially since the major modes of transmission can be controlled. Changes in sexual behavior should reduce the spread of the virus to sexual partners; similarly, changes in needle-using behavior should reduce the spread of the virus to one's needle-using or sexual partners. AIDS prevention should be relatively simple: Don't engage in risky behaviors. Unfortunately, both history and psychology suggest that the behavioral changes necessary to prevent the further spread of AIDS are likely to be inadequate.

Several methods have been used in the past to deal with sexually transmitted diseases and they have had varying degrees of success. Brandt (1988) has compared AIDS to syphilis:

> By the time of World War I, concern about syphilis had reached unprecedented heights. The military draft and consequent physical examinations had revealed high rates of infection—13% of those drafted were found to be infected with either syphilis or gonorrhea. The war touched off the most vigorous antivenereal disease campaign in American history. (p. 377)

A major method for preventing syphilis in the military was to use education to promote sexual abstinence—a procedure that has done little to change behavior, either in the 1900s or the 1990s. Assuming that education alone can change complex human behaviors shows both a naivete about education and an ignorance about human behavior.

Human behavior is difficult to change. With all of the educational efforts, media coverage, and changes in laws aimed at reducing the incidence of smoking, in 1964 about 46 percent of the American public were smokers; by 1988, that percentage had decreased to about 26 percent. Twenty years of intensive public health education has produced a drop of about 20 percent in the percentage of smokers. One can be either optimistic or pessimistic about such changes. However, consider the implications for the spread of AIDS if we do no better than that in AIDS prevention over the next two decades.

Much of the emphasis on behavioral change has been directed toward getting "other people" (i.e., risk groups) to change their behaviors, rather than emphasizing the need for all of us to change our own behaviors. There is no doubt that persons who engage in risky sexual or drug-using behaviors need to modify their behaviors to protect both themselves and others. Considerable effort and money has been spent on providing educational materials and programs.

At some smaller risk, however, are health-care workers who come into direct contact with HIV-infected blood and body fluids. As a way of protecting themselves, the CDC has recommended "universal blood and body fluid precautions." That is, health-care workers must assume that every patient is HIV-infected and that all blood and certain body fluids are infected, and they must use the same precautions with everyone. Such universal precautions mean that health-care workers will have to change how they perform routine procedures, when they must wear protective gloves, gowns, and masks, and so on. Anecdotal reports suggest that many health-care workers still do not practice appropriate safety techniques. Human behavior is difficult to change, no matter what behavior is being changed, and no matter who is trying to change his or her behavior.

SUMMARY

AIDS was first identified among gay men in 1981, and while some referred to it as the "gay plague," researchers soon discovered that the disease was transmitted sexually, by sharing contaminated needles, and from pregnant women to their fetuses. The most recent data suggest that it may take 10 years for someone who is infected with the Human Immunodeficiency Virus to develop AIDS; once symptoms develop, the person may live from 18 to 36 months or more.

By the fall of 1982, about 15 or 20 new cases were reported to CDC each week; by the fall of 1990, that figure had risen to about 820 per week; and by 1993, there may be as many as 1,500 new AIDS cases per week. The first 50,000 AIDS cases were reported in the seven-year period from 1981 through 1987. It took only 18 months (January 1987–July 1989) for the second 50,000 cases to occur; 50,000 AIDS cases may be reported in the first eight or nine months of 1993.

While most of the early cases were seen in major cities such as New York and San Francisco, more recent data suggest that by the mid-1990s, the majority of new AIDS cases will be found outside these cities. Despite much public concern regarding the spread of this disease, history has shown that scare tactics and education may not be successful in changing human behavior. Attitudes about homosexuality, intravenous drug use, and death will play an important role in the public's understanding of AIDS and in its willingness to deal with AIDS in ways that are humane, compassionate, and effective.

REFERENCES

American Heritage Dictionary of the English Language (1970) New York: American Heritage Publishing Co.

Bacchetti, D., and Moss, A. R. (1989) Incubation period of AIDS in San Francisco. *Nature,* 338 (6212), 251–253.

Brandt, A. M. (1988) The syphilis epidemic and its relation to AIDS. *Science,* 239, 375–380.

Carlson, M. (1989) A doctor prescribes hard truth. *Time,* 133 (117) 82–84.

CDC (1989) *Morbidity and Mortality Weekly Report.* AIDS and human immunodeficiency virus infection in the United States: 1988 update. 38 (S–4), 1–38.

CDC (1990a) *HIV/AIDS Surveillance Report. Year-end edition.* January 1990, 1–22.

CDC (1990b) *HIV/AIDS Surveillance Report.* July 1990, 1–18.

CDC (1990c) *Morbidity and Mortality Weekly Report.* Update: Acquired Immunodeficiency Syndrome—United States, 1989. 39 (5), 81–86.

CDC (1990d) *Morbidity and Mortality Weekly Report.* Estimates of HIV prevalence and projected AIDS cases: Summary of a workshop. October 31–November 1, 1989. 39 (7), 110–112; 117–119.

Conway, G. A., Colley-Niemeyer, B., Pursley, C., et al. (1989) Underreporting of AIDS cases in South Carolina, 1986 and 1987. *Journal of the American Medical Association,* 262 (20), 2859–2863.

Dawson, D. A., and Thornberry, O. W. (1988) AIDS knowledge and attitudes for December 1987: Provisional data from the National Health Interview Survey. *Advance Data from Vital and Health Statistics,* No. 153. DHHS Pub. No. (PHS) 88–1250. Hyattsville, MD: Public Health Service.

DesJarlais, D. C., Friedman, S. R., Novick, D. M., et al. (1989) HIV-1 infection among intravenous drug users in Manhattan, New York City, from 1977 through 1987. *Journal of the American Medical Association,* 261 (7), 1008–1012.

Garry, R. F., Witte, M. H., Gottlieb, A. A. et al. (1988) Documentation of an AIDS virus infection in the United States in 1968. *Journal of the American Medical Association,* 260 (14), 2085–2087.

Gerbert, B. Maguire, B., Badner, V., et al. (1988) Why fear persists: Health care professionals and AIDS. *Journal of the American Medical Association,* 260 (23), 3481–3483.

Hardy, A. M. (1990) AIDS knowledge and attitudes for October–December 1989: Provisional data from the National Health Interview Survey. *Advance Data from Vital and Health Statistics,* No. 186, DHHS Pub. No. (PHS) 90–1250. Hyattsville, MD: Public Health Service.

Haverkos, H. W. (1988) Epidemiologic studies—Kaposi's sarcoma vs. opportunistic infections among homosexual men with AIDS. In H. W. Haverkos and J. A. Dougherty, eds. (1988) *Health hazards of nitrite inhalants. NIDA Research Monograph 83,* Rockville, MD: National Institute on Drug Abuse.

Koop, C. E. (1986) *Surgeon General's Report on Acquired Immune Deficiency Syndrome.* Washington, DC: U.S. Public Health Service.

Lemp, G. F., Payne, S. F., Rutherford, G. W., et al. (1990) Projections of AIDS morbidity and mortality in San Francisco. *Journal of the American Medical Association,* 263 (11), 1497–1501.

Mann, J. M., Chin, J., Piot, P. and Quinn, T. (1988). The international epidemiology of AIDS. *Scientific American,* 259 (4), 82–89.

Marx, J. (1982) New disease baffles medical community. *Science,* 217, 618–621.

Marx, J. (1983) Spread of AIDS sparks new health concern. *Science,* 219, 42–43.

Masters, W. H., Johnson, V. E., and Kolodny, R. C. (1988) *Crisis: Heterosexual behavior in the age of AIDS.* New York: Grove Press.

McNeill, W. H. (1976) *Plagues and peoples.* Garden City, New York: Anchor Books.

Moore, A., and LeBaron, R. D. (1986) The case for a Haitian origin of the AIDS epidemic. In D. A. Feldman and T. M. Johnson, eds. *The social dimensions of AIDS: Method and theory.* New York: Praeger Publishers.

San Francisco Department of Public Health. *AIDS Monthly Surveillance Report.* June 30, 1990.

Shilts, R. (1987) *And the band played on: Politics, people and the AIDS epidemic.* New York: St. Martin's Press.

Thompson, C. W. (1990) Home health aide willingness to care for patients with AIDS. *Home Healthcare Nurse,* 8 (2), 20–24.

History and Meaning of HIV Infection

2

> *The principal mark of genius is not perfection, but originality, the opening of new frontiers.*
>
> ARTHUR KOESTLER

Despite massive amounts of information directed at the general public, considerable misinformation still exists regarding important aspects of HIV infection. Such misinformation is important because it not only points out what students know and do not know about AIDS, but it has implications for the development of prevention programs. Far too often, AIDS education programs are based more on the knowledge of the educator than on the ignorance of the audience. As a result, many in the audience may be bored by yet another discussion of the "facts about AIDS" or a generic "AIDS 101" lecture.

The first part of this chapter briefly reviews the discovery of the virus, a few basic principles of HIV infection, and some of the historical facts about HIV infection. The last part of the chapter summarizes those areas of misinformation among young people that have been identified in knowledge and attitude surveys during the past few years.

SEARCH FOR THE "CAUSE" OF AIDS

As more and more cases of Pneumocystis carinii pneumonia (PCP) and Kaposi's sarcoma (KS) were reported to CDC, considerable effort went into the search for the cause of these diseases. Until a virus was implicated as the likely cause of AIDS, the world was being confronted by a new disease for which there was no identifiable cause. Without an identified cause, methods of transmission, treatment strategies, and prevention programs would amount to little more than guesswork. Ultimately, the virus that causes AIDS was almost simultaneously identified in 1985 by Luc Montagnier at the Pasteur Institute in Paris, and Robert Gallo at the National Institutes of Health in the United States. One or both researchers may receive the Nobel Prize for his work on the virus.

The French researchers named the virus LAV, the American researchers HTLV-III. In 1986 all researchers agreed on the term HIV (Human Immunodeficiency Virus) to replace all of the different terms that had been used to describe the virus that causes AIDS.

The search for the "cause" of AIDS was both scientific and political; Shilts (1987) provides an excellent summary of the scientific, political, and psychological factors at work both in the United States and in France. Despite their professional (and personal) conflicts, Gallo and Montagnier (1988) have collaborated on a comprehensive article, "AIDS in 1988." Excellent historical reviews on AIDS can be found in Kulstad (1986) and Cole and Lundberg (1986).

PRINCIPLES OF HIV INFECTION

An understanding of HIV infection and AIDS requires some discussion of the immune system and the ways in which the HIV compromises the immune system, thus leading to attack by opportunistic infections. As reviewed by Redfield and Burke (1988), in a normally functioning immune system, white blood cells (known as T4 lymphocytes or helper T cells) help coordinate the body's defenses by recognizing antigens (i.e., markers) on infected cells and helping to activate other defensive cells, including B lymphocytes and macrophages (which absorb infected cells or foreign particles). The T4

cells help fight off infections from some bacteria (including the bacteria that causes tuberculosis), fungi, parasites, and viruses.

Orchestration of the immune system

Anthony Fauci, the director of the National Institute of Allergy and Infectious Diseases, has described the T4 helper cells as the "orchestrator" of the immune system (Marwick, 1985). In this analogy, elimination of the T4 helper cells via HIV infection causes the most damage to the immune system, because the T4 cell is the focal cell of the entire immune system. It "orchestrates" the immune system through a variety of functions, including the involvement of T cells and killer cells in the fighting off of infection; the involvement of B cell antibody production, and the growth and differentiation in a variety of other lymph cells that help fight off infection. Destroy the T4 helper cells, and you destroy the immune system.

Thus, anyone whose T4 cells have been reduced is likely to suffer from a variety of infections, as the immune system simply has fewer and fewer defensive cells. In a healthy individual, the normal T4 cell count is about 800 cells per cubic millimeter of blood. In someone whose immune system has been affected by HIV, the cell count drops to 400 per cubic millimeter, and in the later stages of AIDS, to 100 or less. Such a reduction occurs in people with HIV infection because a protein (gp120) on the viral envelope of the HIV attaches itself to a protein (CD4) on the T4 cell surface, much as a key fits into a lock. The method by which HIV invades healthy T4 cells is crucial, because the virus itself is inert and cannot do any damage to the body until it enters and infects a host cell (Weber and Weiss, 1988). HIV infection is not the same as AIDS; this is an important biological and semantic issue that will be discussed later.

After the virus attaches itself to the T4 cell, it injects its genetic material (DNA) into the immune system cell, changing the T4 cell's own genetic material and causing it to produce defec-

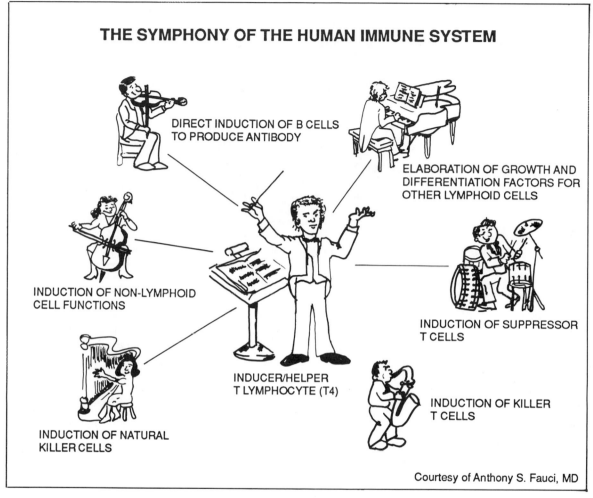

THE SYMPHONY OF THE HUMAN IMMUNE SYSTEM

DIRECT INDUCTION OF B CELLS
TO PRODUCE ANTIBODY

ELABORATION OF GROWTH AND
DIFFERENTIATION FACTORS FOR
OTHER LYMPHOID CELLS

INDUCTION OF NON-LYMPHOID
CELL FUNCTIONS

INDUCTION OF SUPPRESSOR
T CELLS

INDUCER/HELPER
T LYMPHOCYTE (T4)

INDUCTION OF KILLER
T CELLS

INDUCTION OF NATURAL
KILLER CELLS

Courtesy of Anthony S. Fauci, MD

• FIGURE 2.1 The symphony of the human immune system. Source: Journal of American Medical Assn., 1985, Volume 253, pp. 3371, 3375–3376, copyright © 1985, American Medical Association

tive cells when it reproduces. After the initial infection, the HIV in the blood slowly reproduces itself over a period of years and gradually attacks more and more T4 cells and macrophages within the immune system. Over time, diseases that had been successfully fought off in the past can no longer be fought off, and as the immune system continues to weaken, it becomes increasingly susceptible to such "opportunistic infections."

OPPORTUNISTIC INFECTIONS

A good example of an opportunistic infection is PCP (*Pneumocystic carinii pneumonia*). The or-

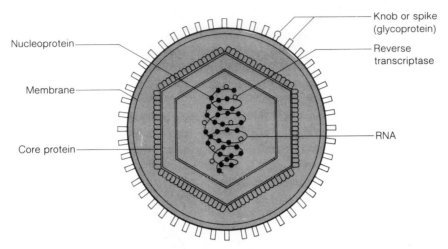

- FIGURE 2.2   Human Immunodeficiency Virus. From: Curtis O. Byer, Louis W. Shainberg, and Kenneth L. Jones, DIMENSIONS OF HUMAN SEXUALITY, 2d ed. Copyright © 1988 Wm. C. Brown Publishers, Dubuque, Iowa. All Rights Reserved. Reprinted by permission.

ganisms that cause PCP are quite common; many healthy people have them in their respiratory system; a healthy immune system keeps such organisms under control. However, if one's immune system becomes weakened (i.e., an "immune deficiency"), as occurs in HIV infection, the PCP organisms begin to multiply, eventually filling the lungs and causing death. Prior to 1981, PCP was a relatively rare medical phenomenon, seldom seen in healthy patients but occasionally seen in patients whose immune system had been damaged by other diseases.

A second disease that began to be seen in some homosexual patients with immune deficiencies was Kaposi's sarcoma (KS). Typically, KS was seen in elderly men of Mediterranean origin (Marx, 1982), so its appearance in young men in New York and California in the early 1980s was quite puzzling. The disease is characterized by the development of purple skin lesions either on internal organs or on the skin. Although it is often linked with PCP as an opportunistic infection, not all researchers are convinced that KS is truly an opportunistic disease, because it is often seen in homosexual men with AIDS (Institute of Medicine, 1988) but not as commonly in IV drug

users with AIDS or in children with AIDS. In contrast, more than half of the hemophiliacs with AIDS were diagnosed with *Pneumocystic carinii pneumonia,* but very rarely with Kaposi's sarcoma (Ragni, 1989). Although HIV attacks the immune system, not everyone is susceptible to the same opportunistic infections; why there is such a variety of opportunistic infections in HIV-infected individuals is not yet completely clear.

Thus, AIDS is diagnosed primarily on the basis of opportunistic infections, not on the basis of HIV infection alone. This is a particularly important distinction for those who seek HIV antibody testing, which is obviously not an "AIDS test." As described, KS was a disease primarily of older men; for example, the average age of KS patients at diagnosis at Memorial Sloan-Kettering Cancer Institute in New York City was 63. Thus, the diagnosis of KS in 26 relatively young homosexual men (average age of 39) was unexpected and unexplainable (CDC, 1981). Another major disorder related to AIDS is AIDS dementia complex (Price et al., 1988), a neurological syndrome characterized by abnormalities in cognition, motor performance, and behavior.

As of June 30, 1990, about 51 percent of the AIDS cases in San Francisco were due to *Pneumocystis carinii pneumonia,* 24 percent to Kaposi's sarcoma, and the rest to a wide variety of other diseases. Based on the new case definition of AIDS, almost 3 percent of the San Francisco cases were diagnosed on the basis of "HIV wasting syndrome," and another 2.5 percent due to "AIDS dementia" (San Francisco Department of Public Health, 1990).

In Uganda and Tanzania in early 1984, reports began to mount of many young people dying of a mysterious disease similar to "slim disease" in Uganda. Typical symptoms of this disease involved severe weight loss (hence the term *slim*), diarrhea, and prolonged fever. This wasting-away disease was the Central African version of AIDS (Hiza, 1988). Although "slim disease" was quite common in Central Africa, as used as a diagnosis for AIDS, the CDC did not include the "HIV wasting syndrome" as a diagnostic category for AIDS until 1987.

Although the opportunistic infections could be treated with drugs, the person carrying the virus was still infected—and infectious. The opportunistic infections that are characteristic of AIDS are really *only the symptoms* of AIDS, and treatment of the symptoms does not mean that AIDS itself is treatable or curable. Understanding the distinction between being infected with the virus and having an opportunistic infection is crucial in effectively preventing AIDS.

The particular opportunistic infection that develops is a function of many variables, including the integrity of the immune system, other bacteria or viruses in the environment, and use of alcohol or other drugs. As more information about opportunistic diseases was collected, the Centers for Disease Control changed the case definition for AIDS in 1985 and 1987. As a result, the statistics have changed; early AIDS cases may well have been underreported as a result.

WHO IS AT RISK? GROUPS VERSUS BEHAVIORS

As AIDS cases became more frequent in the early 1980s, they seemed to cluster in certain categories of people. Initially, almost all AIDS cases seemed to appear in gay men; somewhat later, AIDS began to show up in Haitians, hemophiliacs, intravenous drug users, and children. For data collection, it became convenient to categorize people with AIDS. Unfortunately, such categorizations often led to inaccurate labelings, as summarized by the Institute of Medicine (1986):

> Certain groups—for example, male homosexuals and intravenous drug users—have been designated as being at high risk for contracting the disease. However, the designation "at high risk" encompasses more people than is necessary, because not all members of these groups are at high risk for being infected with HIV. A more appropriate designation might be "persons who engage in high-risk behaviors," and references in this report to "high-risk groups" should be so interpreted. Furthermore, references to high-risk groups may lead persons outside of these groups to believe mistakenly that they are not susceptible to HIV infection even if they engage in high-risk activities. It may also lead individuals to consciously or unconsciously deny that they are at risk. (pp. viii–ix)

By so closely linking AIDS with homosexuality, homosexuality itself was seen by many as the "cause" of AIDS, rather than HIV. Many believed, and still believe, that if only gay men would give up homosexuality, AIDS would simply go away. For some, the disease became a conflict of "us" (heterosexuals) versus "them" (homosexuals), rather than "all of us" versus "the virus."

Table 2.1 depicts AIDS cases by age group, exposure category, and race or ethnicity through June 1990. To consider AIDS only as a gay disease does a considerable injustice to minority people with AIDS. Although 77 percent of the

TABLE 2.1   AIDS Cases by Age Group, Exposure Category, and Race/Ethnicity, Reported Through June 1990, United States

Adult/Adolescent Exposure Category	White, Not Hispanic Number (%)	Black, Not Hispanic Number (%)	Hispanic Number (%)	Asian/Pacific Islander Number (%)	American Indian/ Alaskan Native Number (%)	Total[a] Number (%)
Male homosexual/bisexual contact	59,000 (77)	13,717 (36)	8,673 (41)	633 (75)	101 (53)	82,304 (60)
Intravenous (IV) drug use (female and heterosexual male)	5,964 (8)	14,777 (39)	8,598 (40)	35 (4)	33 (17)	29,487 (21)
Male homosexual/bisexual contact and IV drug use	5,494 (7)	2,475 (7)	1,347 (6)	16 (2)	24 (13)	9,370 (7)
Hemophilia/coagulation disorder	1,032 (1)	82 (0)	93 (0)	15 (2)	8 (4)	1,234 (1)
Heterosexual contact:	1,445 (2)	4,273 (11)	1,177 (6)	31 (4)	8 (4)	6,952 (5)
Sex with IV drug user	802	1,857	941	13	5	3,627
Sex with bisexual male	225	132	50	6	1	415
Sex with person with hemophilia	57	7	1	1	—	66
Born in Pattern-II[b] country	5	1,836	11	4	—	1,861
Sex with person born in Pattern-II country	33	62	5	—	—	101
Sex with transfusion recipient with HIV infection	76	18	12	1	—	109
Sex with HIV-infected person, risk not specified	247	361	157	6	2	773
Recipient of blood transfusion, blood components, or tissue[c]	2,335 (3)	549 (1)	314 (1)	66 (8)	3 (2)	3,273 (2)
Other/undetermined[d]	1,815 (2)	1,809 (5)	1,035 (5)	52 (6)	12 (6)	4,765 (3)
Adult/adolescent subtotal	77,085(100)	37,682(100)	21,237(100)	848(100)	189(100)	137,385(100)
Pediatric (<13 years old) exposure category						
Hemophilia/coagulation disorder	83 (16)	16 (1)	16 (25)	3 (25)	—	119 (5)
Mother with/at risk for HIV infection:	303 (58)	1,128 (92)	521 (86)	4 (33)	5(100)	1,966 (83)
IV drug use	148	563	275	1	2	991
Sex with IV drug user	67	180	166	1	—	415
Sex with bisexual male	17	20	9	—	—	46
Sex with person with hemophilia	5	2	1	—	—	8
Born in Pattern-II country	2	194	1	—	—	197
Sex with person born in Pattern-II country	—	9	—	—	—	10
Sex with transfusion recipient with HIV infection	5	3	2	—	—	10
Sex with HIV-infected person, risk not specified	14	37	29	1	1	83
Receipt of blood transfusion, blood components, or tissue	14	15	11	—	—	40
Has HIV infection, risk not specified	31	105	27	1	2	166
Receipt of blood transfusion, blood components, or tissue	126 (24)	51 (4)	51 (8)	5 (42)	—	233 (10)
Undetermined	9 (2)	32 (3)	21 (3)	—	—	62 (3)
Pediatric subtotal	521(100)	1,227(100)	609(100)	12(100)	5(100)	2,380(100)
Total	**77,606**	**38,909**	**21,846**	**860**	**194**	**139,765**

[a]Includes 350 persons whose race/ethnicity is unknown.
[b]See technical notes.
[c]Includes 12 transfusion recipients who received blood screened for HIV antibody, and one tissue recipient.
[d]"Other" refers to three health-care workers who seroconverted to HIV and developed AIDS after occupational exposure to HIV-infected blood. "Undetermined" refers to patients whose mode of exposure to HIV is unknown. This includes patients under investigation; patients who died, were lost to follow-up or refused interview; and patients whose mode of exposure to HIV remains undetermined after investigation.

AIDS cases in white males have occurred in male homosexuals and bisexuals, only 36 percent of the AIDS cases in blacks and 41 percent of the cases in Hispanics have occurred as a result of exclusive homosexual or bisexual contact. Overemphasis on AIDS as a disease primarily of gay white males often made it difficult to reach women and people of color, many of whom simply believed that since they were not gay, white, or male, they were not at risk for HIV and did not need to take appropriate precautions. Many still do not realize that risk for HIV infection is based on behavior, not group affiliation.

Simply being a homosexual does not put one at risk for contracting HIV; the risk comes from engaging in risky behaviors such as unprotected anal intercourse. Simply being an IV drug user does not put one at risk for contracting HIV; the risk comes from sharing needles or syringes with someone who is infected with HIV. The confusion of risk groups and risky behaviors has simply added to the difficulty of developing effective AIDS prevention programs.

HOW OLD IS AIDS?

Although AIDS was "officially" identified in the United States in 1981, there may have been many deaths from AIDS before that time. Stored blood and tissue samples have made it possible to not only test blood samples stored many years after a patient has died, but new techniques such as polymerase chain reaction (PCR) have allowed researchers to identify a small amount of DNA from HIV in stored tissue samples and to "grow" HIV from that DNA. As this research expands, it may be possible to identify patients who died of HIV infection much earlier than 1981.

In a review entitled "AIDS in the Pre-AIDS Era," Huminer and coauthors (1987) identified 19 probable AIDS cases before 1981, the earliest of which may have occurred in 1952. Another case, that of a 34-year-old Haitian, may have occurred in 1978 (Noel, 1988). Although blood samples

from these potential AIDS cases were not available, the researchers were able to apply the CDC surveillance definition of AIDS to those published reports in which patients died of underlying immune deficiencies.

Their review focused only on published reports, there is no way of knowing how many other AIDS-related deaths occurred from 1950 to 1980, but were not reported in the professional literature. Huminer, and coauthors (1987) concluded: "The historical data presented in our review lead us to believe that AIDS is an old disease that has been unrecognized in the past because of its sporadic occurrence." (p. 1106)

AIDS-RELATED COMPLEX

Scientists were not sure exactly what it meant to be infected with HIV. Early on in the epidemic, estimates were that only 20 to 30 percent of those infected with the virus would go on to develop full-blown AIDS. Some even referred to having been "exposed" to the HIV, but not infected. However, between being relatively healthy with no symptoms (i.e., asymptomatic), and being symptomatic and having AIDS were those individuals who developed AIDS-Related Complex (ARC), sometimes referred to as pre-AIDS. Because ARC was not a reportable condition, there was no way of knowing how many people were suffering from it. Estimates were that 10 times the number of people with AIDS may have had ARC (Volberding, 1988). Many of these ARC patients were diagnosed with persistent generalized lymphadenopathy (PGL; swollen lymph nodes), an early precursor of AIDS. Others had some of the chronic symptoms of AIDS—fever, weight loss, night sweats, chronic diarrhea, fatigue, and so on—but did not fit the CDC definition for AIDS. (Although people with AIDS were considered to be handicapped or disabled, and therefore entitled to specific government protection, people with ARC were excluded from such legal protection.)

TABLE 2.2   AIDS Knowledge and Attitudes for Adults 18 and Over

Percent Responding			Question
Yes	No	Don't Know	
65%	17%	18%	To the best of your knowledge, is there a difference between having the AIDS virus and having the disease AIDS?
74%	22%	4%	Have you ever heard of a blood test that can detect the AIDS virus infection?
61%	39%	0%	Have you ever discussed AIDS with a friend or relative?
62%	38%	0%	Have you ever discussed AIDS with any of your children aged 10–17?
True[a]	False[a]	Don't Know	
86%	4%	9%	AIDS can reduce the body's natural protection against disease.
57%	19%	24%	AIDS can damage the brain.
82%	7%	11%	AIDS is an infectious disease caused by a virus.
78%	9%	13%	A person can be infected with the AIDS virus and not have the disease AIDS.
78%	11%	11%	A person who has the AIDS virus can look and feel healthy and well.

[a]"True" responses are comprised of those answering "definitely true" and "probably true." "False" responses are comprised of those responding "probably false" and "definitely false." Source: Hardy, 1990.

The Institute of Medicine (1988) recommended that the term *ARC* was no longer useful, and that HIV infection itself should be considered a disease. *HIV infection* included a continuum of symptoms, including acute symptoms that were associated with seroconversion, HIV infection without symptoms, HIV infection with symptoms, and AIDS itself.

MYTHS ABOUT AIDS

General Public

Having summarized some of the basic facts about HIV transmission and opportunistic infections, we now ask: How much does the general public know about HIV and AIDS? Despite all of the information that has been disseminated about AIDS in the last decade, there is still considerable ignorance about this disease, both in the population at large, and in adolescents and young adults. Because prevention programs will continue to focus on young people at risk, educators must be aware of areas of knowledge and ignorance in student populations, not only in K–12 students, but in college students as well. Table 2.2 is a brief summary of selected AIDS knowledge and attitudes among persons 18 years of age and over (Hardy, 1990).

The data reported are for the total population; there are differences in responses based on age, sex, race, and education. Nevertheless, the survey points out that from October through December of 1989, when the data were collected, there was still serious misinformation about AIDS in the general population. In particular, many people (35%) are not clear about the difference between having the AIDS virus and having the disease AIDS. Nearly half (43%) do not know that AIDS can damage the brain. A surprising 18 percent do not know that AIDS is an infectious disease caused by a virus. Roughly comparable data are available on blacks alone (Dawson and Hardy, 1989a) and Hispanics alone (Dawson and Hardy, 1989b).

These surveys have found that about 30 to 35 percent of the general public doubts the information that has been disseminated about AIDS by the U.S. Public Health Service. Such doubt has important implications for health educators who rely on federal information for classroom instruction. On the one hand, teachers may give students the latest CDC information; on the other hand, the students' parents may be telling them not to believe such information.

Box 2

How Expert Are The Experts?

Public health officials often suggest that you should talk to a physician if you have questions about AIDS. Many AIDS information brochures recommend "seeing your doctor" if you have a question or concern about AIDS. However, not all physicians are competent to deal with AIDS-related issues.

Lest one assume that only high school and college students are misinformed about AIDS, reports clearly indicate significant levels of misinformation among physicians, as well. A 1986 survey of California physicians (Lewis et al., 1987) concluded that ". . . on a statewide basis, a majority of those interviewed lack the AIDS-related knowledge and skills required to carry out their roles in dealing with AIDS." A physician's competence in dealing with AIDS cases was directly related to his or her discomfort in treating homosexuals. Nearly two-thirds of the physicians did not inquire about the sexual orientation of their patients; 18 percent did not know about antibody screening tests.

A survey of Minnesota physicians (Schultz et al., 1988) found similar limitations in physicians, particularly among those who had not yet seen any HIV-infected patients. Among this group, fewer than half would discuss the following health education and risk-reduction topics with HIV-infected patients: knowledge about the HIV antibody test, use of condoms, decreasing the number of sex partners, avoiding exchange of body fluids, and avoiding IV needle sharing. Among physicians who had seen 10 or more HIV-infected patients, 77 to 88 percent reported that they would discuss such topics.

Avoiding AIDS

More recently, an article by Lambert (1990) summarized how many physicians have simply avoided AIDS issues:

- Some physicians are not accepting new AIDS patients. New York City has about 25,000 physicians; one very large AIDS volunteer agency has a referral list of only 45 qualified private AIDS physicians for the borough of Manhattan who are willing to take patients. The other four New York City boroughs have only one or two AIDS specialists, despite the fact that some AIDS patients from Connecticut and New Jersey rely on Manhattan physicians.

  Nationally, there are about 600,000 physicians and 180,000 dentists. However, the Physicians Association for AIDS Care, based in Chicago, has only 600 member physicians nationally. These physicians treated 58,000 AIDS patients, an average of almost 100 patients per physician.

- Some physicians are not taking sexual and drug histories. A study for the California Medical Association found that 79 percent of all California residents had seen a physician, but AIDS was mentioned in only 6 percent of the visits.

- Relatively few physicians are testing their patients for HIV infection. For example, in New York City, with an estimated 200,000 HIV-infected residents and more confirmed AIDS cases than any other city in the world, data from the New York Health Department showed that 78 percent of local physicians and dentists have never ordered a single HIV antibody test. One patient, a New York businesswoman, became increasingly disabled over several months. Physicians in her county of residence were unable to diagnose her illness, although one suggested melancholia and another joked about AIDS. On her own, the patient took the HIV antibody test and found it to be positive. At that time, AIDS was positively diagnosed, and she began treatment with AZT.

- Many physicians seem to be avoiding not only AIDS patients, but AIDS education programs as well. Invitations sent to 1,300 medical practitioners in Albuquerque, New Mexico for a program on AIDS treatment produced only one respondent; a survey of 65 rural physicians in Georgia found only two who would treat an AIDS patient.

Many explanations have been offered for these findings. These include inadequate training about AIDS, especially because many physicians received their medical school training before AIDS became a problem; feeling uncomfortable about providing treatment to homosexuals and IV drug users or about discussing sexual practices and drug-using behaviors; difficulty in

coping with the deaths of many young patients; inexperience in the complexities of AIDS treatment; and fear of losing patients if they find out that their doctor is treating patients with AIDS.

Physicians As Educators

Physician limitations may have an impact beyond their patient care practices. In a survey of college students' preferences for AIDS education (Manning et al., 1989), physicians were the preferred source for AIDS education, perhaps because of students' comfort level when talking to a physician about sensitive issues or because of the perceived expertise that a physician would bring to a discussion of AIDS. However, educators who rely on physician expertise should carefully document the professional qualifications and experience on AIDS-related issues before bringing in a physician or someone else to conduct an AIDS education program. Questions about one's experience with HIV and AIDS patients, relevant presentations or publications, and recommendations from other programs should be reviewed before a speaker is selected.

Students

Numerous surveys have been conducted on adolescents and young adults to measure their knowledge, attitudes, and behaviors regarding sexuality and HIV infection. One difficulty with such data is that often the data were collected a year or more before publication of the journal article; where possible, mention of the time period of data collection will be made, since students' knowledge and behaviors may have changed significantly since the survey was done.

An early study (DiClemente, et al., 1986) measured knowledge, attitudes, and beliefs about AIDS in San Francisco among 1,326 adolescents in May 1985. Although more than 90 percent of the students knew that "sexual intercourse was one mode of contracting AIDS," only 60 percent knew

that "use of a condom during sexual intercourse may lower the risk of getting the disease."

Kegeles and coauthors (1988) surveyed 204 adolescents in San Francisco between February 1984 and October 1986. They found that, although the adolescents were aware that condoms could prevent sexually transmitted diseases (STDs) and the adolescents wanted to prevent STDs, their awareness and concern did not result in a greater intention to use condoms or in actual increased usage of condoms. Similar findings were reported by Katzman and co-workers (1988), who surveyed undergraduate students at Arizona State University; although the vast majority of students reported that they would like to practice "safer sex," only 44 percent reported that their behavior had changed as a result of AIDS issues.

Strunin and Hingson (1987) surveyed 860 Massachusetts adolescents in August through October 1986. They found that many adolescents were both misinformed and confused. Of the 70 percent of the adolescents who reported being sexually active, only 15 percent reported changing their sexual behavior because of AIDS fears, and, of those, only one-fifth used effective methods. Of those reporting drug use, 8 percent did not know that AIDS could be transmitted by contaminated needles. Twenty-two percent did not know that AIDS was transmitted via semen. More than half reported that AIDS had been discussed by a teacher, but not taught.

A survey of 161 students (McDermott et al., 1987) in a general university studies course (date of survey administration not reported) found that nearly 40 percent of the students were unclear about the lethal potential of AIDS, 35 percent did not recognize opportunistic diseases, and 31 percent did not relate risk of contracting AIDS to indiscriminate sexual behavior. When queried about their primary source of AIDS information, the vast majority identified television (44%), newspapers (36%), or magazines (10%); relatively few got their AIDS information from teachers or schools (3%), physicians (0%), or AIDS seminars and workshops (0%).

Many college campuses have relied on educational movies as a way of changing students' knowledge, attitudes, and behaviors. However, a recent assessment of the efficacy of such movies (Gilliam and Seltzer, 1989) found that the showing of a single movie produced only very slight changes in knowledge and attitudes. When several movies were compared (Rhodes and Wolitski, 1989), increases in knowledge were found and maintained for four to six weeks for three of the four videos. Knowledge and attitude changes were not related to the postvideo discussion.

Films and videos apparently have a minimal effect on students' knowledge and attitudes about AIDS. Although they can be useful as part of a more comprehensive educational program, movies should not be expected to produce significant behavioral change.

A survey of 495 undergraduates at a midwestern university was conducted in the fall of the 1985–1986 academic year (Goodwin and Roscoe, 1988). The students were generally very knowledgeable about the incidence, transmission, and symptoms of AIDS, although males were more homophobic than females in their desire to avoid people known or suspected to be homosexual, in avoiding places where homosexuals may be present, in fighting to have a child with AIDS removed from school, and in keeping their own child home from school if a classmate had AIDS.

AIDS has taken a disproportionate toll on blacks and Hispanics; while making up about 18 percent of the U.S. population, they account for about 40 percent of reported AIDS cases. The knowledge, attitudes, and behaviors of blacks and Hispanics regarding AIDS is critical, since they may be at increased risk given the relatively higher number of infected individuals within the black and Hispanic communities. DiClemente, Boyer, and Morales (1988) collected data from 261 white, 226 black, and 141 Latino adolescents in San Francisco in May 1985. While nearly 75 percent of the white adolescents believed that using condoms would lower the risk of disease transmission, only 60 percent of the blacks and 58 percent of the Latino adolescents believed in the protective value of condoms. Dealing with issues of sexuality, condoms, and AIDS must become a priority in minority populations; however, any such educational efforts must take into account the unique ethnic, cultural, and religious characteristics of those minority groups.

Experience on many college and university campuses has found that attendance at AIDS educational programs is relatively sparse, given the size of the student body and the seriousness of the disease. Homophobic attitudes as identified by Goodwin and Roscoe (1988) may be one reason for such attendance problems, if many male students want to avoid homosexuals or places where homosexuals might be present. Such attitudes are not likely to be modified easily, yet they must be considered when developing AIDS education programs. A survey at Tulane University (Manning et al., 1989) found that students generally preferred small-group discussions, movies, or panel discussions—all formats where they could remain anonymous.

Unfortunately, much of what is known about adolescents and AIDS is based on surveys done in states that have had a relatively large percentage of AIDS cases, such as California and New York. However, it is not clear how closely the knowledge, attitudes, and behaviors of adolescents in San Francisco resemble those of adolescents in other parts of the country. Moreover, as will be discussed in later chapters, much of what is known about behavior change in gay men is based on self-reported survey data in San Francisco, New York City, Boston, and other cities with large gay populations. How gay men in these cities are similar to or different from gay men in other cities or small towns is not as well known. Preliminary data (St. Lawrence et al., 1989) suggest that the most common sexual activity among gay men in a large city is mutual masturbation (a low risk behavior for transmitting HIV), while the most common sexual activity among gay men in smaller cities is unprotected anal intercourse (a very high risk behavior for transmitting HIV). Efforts to generalize findings of knowledge, attitudes, or behaviors must be done with considerable caution.

INTERNATIONAL IMPLICATIONS

Many people tend to view AIDS as primarily a disease of gay men living in San Francisco or of IV drug users living in New York City. Despite such media-derived images, the reality of AIDS is that it is an international disease, with international implications for economy, travel, and education.

Many diseases are spread by travelers; air travel makes the spread of diseases from country to country or continent to continent even more ef-

ficient. Shilts (1987) described the impact of "Patient Zero," a gay Canadian airline steward who may have been responsible for directly or indirectly infecting dozens of people with HIV. However, it is unlikely that the steward was the only international traveler who helped spread the HIV. For example, Clumeck and coauthors (1989) identified a cluster of 19 women in Belgium who had sexual intercourse with an HIV-infected civil engineer from a Central African country; 11 of the women became infected with HIV as a result of their sexual contact, some after only one sexual encounter with the infected man.

Such international issues will affect travel and education. Samuels and co-workers (1988) have described some of the international implications of AIDS, including its impact on tourism, foreign investment, reallocation of funds from other areas (such as education) to deal with AIDS treatment costs, and its effect on a country's blood supply.

Many countries do not have the capacity for testing the blood supply that is available in the United States. Consequently, travelers to foreign countries (such as exchange students or faculty) who need a blood transfusion as a result of an accident or injury may be putting themselves at considerable risk. For example, a 32-year-old American traveler presumably contracted the HIV following a motor vehicle accident in Rwanda; the traveler had multiple cuts resulting from the accident and was covered with blood from other passengers (Hill, 1989). Although the contraction of HIV in this way probably does not happen very often, any accident in which a person is exposed to the blood of another, possibly infected, person is a possible route for HIV infection. Some employees of the U.S. State Department in foreign countries have been banking their own blood in the event that they need surgery. (Use of one's own blood is called autologous banking.)

Travelers do not contract HIV via casual contact; they contract the virus through risky sex practices. Erlanger (1989) describes the possibility of an AIDS epidemic in Thailand as a result of Bangkok's "thriving sex industry." Other observers believe that such an epidemic is more of a reality than a mere possibility. In 1988, 4 million people visited Thailand, nearly two-thirds of them single males, many traveling from West Germany and Japan for specially planned sex tours. Safer sex is the exception rather than the norm.

Some countries, particularly those where the current rate of HIV infection is very low, have considered HIV screening of international travelers in an attempt to further slow the spread of HIV within the country (Chin, 1988). China, for example, requires anyone who will be visiting the country for more than six months to provide proof of being negative for HIV infection.

Many college and university campuses have large numbers of international students, and some high schools have foreign exchange students. Given recent worldwide political changes, many refugees and immigrants may be traveling to the United States for educational purposes. A few of these students may arrive on campus being HIV-positive; others may acquire the virus while living in the United States. Most campuses have not developed policies to deal with complex issues like the following:

1. Who will pay for the treatment of an HIV-infected international student, especially one who does not have health insurance? Most international students are generally *not* eligible for care in public hospitals.

2. What information is given to students and faculty who travel to foreign countries regarding potential HIV risks? Is the institution liable if the student or faculty member contracts HIV?

3. What kinds of AIDS educational programs are needed to reach international students, many of whom have limited knowledge of the English language? Are these students being missed by traditional campus health education programs? Have religious and cultural differences been taken into account in the development of such programs?

In the absence of a planned response, most organizations will be forced to respond to these issues through crisis-management policies. Under those conditions, there is a very real possibility that the situation will be made worse, rather than better, and that such crises will affect the organization locally, nationally, and perhaps even internationally.

SUMMARY

The virus (HIV) that causes AIDS was discovered almost simultaneously by Luc Montanier of the Pasteur Institute in Paris, and Robert Gallo, at the National Institutes of Health in the United States. Once the virus was identified, "high-risk groups" (male homosexuals, intravenous drug users, Haitians, hemophiliacs, and others) were designated as a way to categorize how the virus was transmitted. Later, the emphasis was shifted to "high-risk behaviors" instead, because behaviors are the true risk factors, not group affiliations.

Opportunistic diseases, especially *Pneumocystic carinii pneumonia* (PCP) and Kaposi's sarcoma (KS) developed in people who were infected with the HIV. The presence of these opportunistic diseases (and others) became the major criterion for an AIDS diagnosis. Although these diseases were seen more frequently in the 1980s than in the past, some researchers believe that AIDS may, in fact, be a relatively old disease occurring as early as the 1950s.

Despite major efforts at public education, national surveys have found that many people still harbor misconceptions about AIDS. In particular, although studies have shown that adolescents and young adults are reasonably knowledgeable about AIDS, such knowledge has not always been translated into appropriate behavioral change. Students may know about safer sex, but they don't necessarily practice it.

The ability of the virus to be carried across national and international boundaries has potentially serious implications both for international travel and international education programs. Many countries are struggling to develop appropriate policies for dealing with international travelers or students who carry HIV into their country or who contract the virus while visiting.

REFERENCES

CDC (1981) Kaposi's sarcoma and pneumocystis pneumonia among homosexual men—New York City and California. *Morbidity and Mortality Weekly Report.* 39 (25), 305–308.

Chin, J. (1988) HIV and international travel. In A. F. Fleming, M. Carballo, D. W. FitzSimons, M. R. Bailey, and J. Mann, eds. *The global impact of AIDS.* New York: Alan R. Liss, Inc.

Clumeck, N., Taelman, H., Hermans, et al. (1989) A cluster of HIV infection among heterosexual people without apparent risk factors. *New England Journal of Medicine,* 321 (21), 1460–1462.

Cole, H. M., and Lundberg, G. D., eds. (1986) *AIDS from the beginning.* Chicago, IL: American Medical Association.

Dawson, D. A., and Hardy, A. M. (1989a) AIDS knowledge and attitudes of Black Americans. Provisional data from the 1988 National Health Interview Survey. *Advance Data from Vital and Health Statistics.* No. 165. DHHS Pub. No. (PHS) 89–1250. Public Health Service. Hyattsville, MD.

Dawson, D. A., and Hardy, A. M. (1989b) AIDS knowledge and attitudes of Hispanic Americans. Provisional data from the 1988 National Health Interview Survey. *Advance Data from Vital and Health Statistics.* No. 166. DHHS Pub. No. (PHS) 89–1250. Public Health Service. Hyattsville, MD.

DiClemente, R. J., Boyer, C. B., and Morales, E. S. (1988) Minorities and AIDS: Knowledge, attitudes, and misconceptions among Black and Latino adolescents. *American Journal of Public Health,* 78 (1), 55–57.

DiClemente, R. J., Zorn, J., and Temoshok, L. (1986) Adolescents and AIDS: A survey of knowledge, attitudes and beliefs about AIDS in San Francisco. *American Journal of Public Health,* 76 (12), 1443–1445.

Erlanger, S. (1989) Thriving sex industry in Bangkok is raising fears of an AIDS epidemic. *New York Times,* March 30, 1989.

Gallo, R. C., and Montagnier, L. (1988) AIDS in 1988. *Scientific American,* 259 (4), 40–48.

Gilliam, A., and Seltzer, R. (1989) The efficacy of educational movies on AIDS knowledge and attitudes among college students. *Journal of American College Health,* 37, 261–265.

Goodwin, M., and Roscoe, B. (1988) AIDS: Students' knowledge and attitudes at a Midwestern University. *Journal of American College Health,* 36 (4), 214–222.

Hardy, A. M. (1990) AIDS knowledge and attitudes for October–December 1989: Provisional data from the National Health Interview Survey. *Advance Data from Vital and Health Statistics.* No. 186. DHHS Pub. No. (PHS) 90–1250. Public Health Service. Hyattsville, MD.

Hill, D. R. (1989) HIV infection following motor vehicle trauma in Central Africa. *Journal of the American Medical Association,* 261 (22), 3282–3283.

Hiza, P. R. (1988) International co-operation in the national AIDS control programme. In A. F. Fleming, M. Carballo, D. W. FitzSimons, M. R. Bailey, and J. Mann, eds. *The global impact of AIDS.* New York: Alan R. Liss, Inc.

Huminer, D., Rosenfeld, J. B., and Pitlik, S. D. (1987) AIDS in the pre-AIDS era. *Reviews of Infectious Diseases,* 9 (6), 1102–1108.

Institute of Medicine (1988) *Confronting AIDS: Update 1988.* Washington, DC: National Academy Press.

Katzman, E. M., Mulholland, M., and Sutherland, E. M. (1988) College students and AIDS: A preliminary survey of knowledge, attitudes and behavior. *Journal of American College Health,* 37, 127–130.

Kegeles, S. M., Adler, N. E., and Irwin, C. E. (1988) Sexually active adolescents and condoms: Changes over one year in knowledge, attitudes and use. *American Journal of Public Health,* 78 (4), 460–461.

Kulstad, R., ed. (1986) *AIDS: Papers from Science, 1982–1985.* Washington, DC: American Association for the Advancement of Science.

Lambert, B. (1990) AIDS war shunned by many doctors. *New York Times,* April 23, 1990, A1; C10.

Lewis, C. E., Freeman, H. W., and Corey, C. R. (1987) AIDS-related competence of California's primary care physicians. *American Journal of Public Health,* 77 (7), 795–799.

Manning, D. T., Barenberg, N., Gallese, L., and Rice, J. C. (1989) College students' knowledge and health beliefs about AIDS: Implications for education and prevention. *Journal of American College Health,* 37, 254–259.

Marwick, C. (1985) "Molecular level" view gives immune system clues. *Journal of the American Medical Association,* 253, 3371, 3375–3376.

Marx, J. (1982) New disease baffles medical community. *Science,* 217, 618–621.

McDermott, R. J., Hawkins, M. J., Moore, J. R., and Cittadino, S. K. (1987). AIDS awareness and information sources among selected university students. *Journal of American College Health,* 35 (5), 222–226.

Noel, G. E. (1988) Another case of AIDS in the pre-AIDS era. *Reviews of Infectious Diseases,* 10 (3), 668–669.

Price, R. W., Brew, B., Sidtis, J., et al. (1988) The brain in AIDS: Central nervous system HIV-1 infection and AIDS dementia complex. *Science,* 239, 586–591.

Ragni, M. W. (1989) Medical aspects of hemophilia and AIDS. *Focus: A Guide to AIDS Research,* 4 (5), 1–2.

Redfield, R. R., and Burke, D. S. (1988) HIV infection: The clinical picture. *Scientific American,* 259 (4), 90–98.

Rhodes, F., and Wolitsky, R. (1989) Effect of instructional videotapes on AIDS knowledge and attitudes. *Journal of American College Health,* 37, 266–271.

St. Lawrence, J. S., Hood, H. V., Brasfield, T., et al. (1989) Difference in gay men's AIDS risk knowledge and behavior patterns in high and low AIDS prevalence cities. *Public Health Reports,* 104 (4), 391–395.

Samuels, M. E., Mann, J., and Koop, C. E. (1988) Containing the spread of HIV infection: A world priority. *Public Health Reports,* 103 (3), 221–223.

San Francisco Department of Public Health (1990) S.F. AIDS incidence and mortality by months of diagnosis or death, 1980–90. June 30, 1990.

Schultz, J. M., MacDonald, K. L., Heckert, K. A., and Osterholm, M. T. (1988) A statewide survey of physician knowledge and clinical practice regarding AIDS. *Minnesota Medicine,* 71, 277–283.

Shilts, R. (1987) *And the band played on: Politics, people and the AIDS epidemic.* New York: St. Martin's Press.

Strunin, L., and Hingson, R. (1987) Acquired Immunodeficiency Syndrome and adolescents: Knowledge, beliefs, attitudes and behaviors. *Pediatrics,* 79 (5), 825–828.

Volberding, P. A. (1988) AIDS overview. In I. B. Corless and M. N. Pittman-Lindeman (1988) *AIDS: Principles, practices & politics.* New York: Hemisphere Publishing Corp.

Weber, J. N., and Weis, R. A. (1988) HIV infection: The cellular picture. *Scientific American,* 259 (4), 100–109.

3
Scope of HIV Infection

A single death is a tragedy, a million deaths is a statistic.

JOSEPH STALIN

Although much emphasis has focused on AIDS cases since mid-1981, only a small fraction of those infected have yet to be diagnosed with full-blown AIDS. As of July 1990, approximately 140,000 AIDS cases had been reported to the Centers for Disease Control. Using the 1989 CDC estimate of 1 million Americans infected with the virus, these 140,000 cases represent perhaps 14 percent of those currently carrying the virus. If the vast majority of people infected with HIV develop AIDS, then the United States has seen only a very small part of the total number of AIDS cases and AIDS-related deaths.

One way to represent the scope of HIV infection is to use the "iceberg" analogy. Although most of the media attention has been directed to those individuals who have been diagnosed as having AIDS (14%—the tip of the iceberg), most people who are carrying HIV (86%) are asymptomatic, representing the base of the iceberg.

ESTIMATING AIDS AND HIV INFECTION

Over time, as more and more HIV-infected people are diagnosed as having AIDS, the percentages will probably change, although the rate of new infections is still poorly understood. In late 1987, the CDC estimated that there were 945,000 to 1.4 million HIV-infected individuals; in late 1989 (CDC, 1990c) they revised that estimate to 1 million.

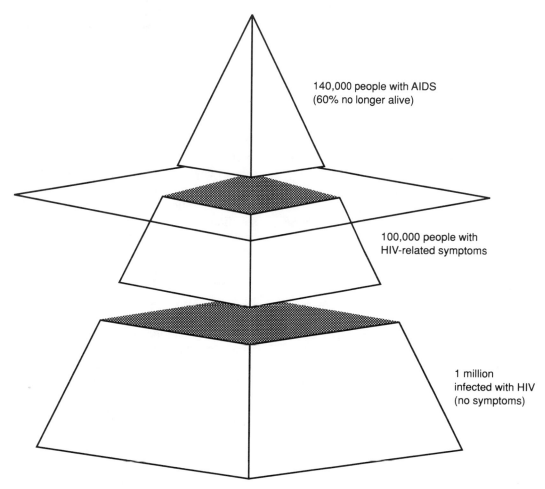

140,000 people with AIDS
(60% no longer alive)

100,000 people with
HIV-related symptoms

1 million
infected with HIV
(no symptoms)

• FIGURE 3.1 AIDS Iceberg

Other estimates of the number of HIV-infected Americans have ranged from 650,000 (Osmond and Moss, 1989) to more than 3 million (Masters, Johnson, and Kolodny, 1988). Unfortunately, methodological differences make a precise estimate difficult, if not impossible. A General Accounting Office (1989) government report reviewed 13 national forecasts of the cumulative number of AIDS cases through the end of 1991 and concluded that these 13 forecasts seriously underestimated the extent of the epidemic. While the best estimates from the 13 models ranged from 120,000 to 400,000 cases by the end of 1991, the GAO estimated 300,000 to 480,000 cumulative cases by that time. Virtually all researchers have used somewhat different methods for estimating the current and future number of AIDS cases.

Using a rather obscure statistical procedure—Farr's Law of Epidemics—Bregman and Langmuir (1990) concluded that the U.S. AIDS epidemic actually peaked in 1988, and that by the year 2000 the cumulative number of AIDS cases would be about 200,000—in stark contrast to the CDC estimate of 390,000 to 480,000 cases by the end of 1993. Morgan, Curran, and Berkelman (1990) argued strongly that the Bregman and Langmuir statistical procedures and conclusions were simply wrong. It should be noted that Langmuir (1989) earlier forecasted that the AIDS epidemic would peak in the middle of 1986, and somewhat later estimated that it would peak in 1988, with a total number of 150,000 cases.

Any projections are subject to change. If AZT or other treatments achieve success, fewer people who are HIV infected may develop AIDS, thus reducing the number of AIDS cases. To the extent that such AIDS cases are reduced, AIDS deaths will be reduced. Recently, some researchers have observed that the rate of increase of reported AIDS cases began to slow in mid-1987, suggesting the possibility that there may be 15 percent fewer AIDS cases over the next three years than had been projected (Palco, 1989.) In an assessment of this "AIDS deficit," Gail, Rosenberg, and Goedert (1990) found that there were fewer AIDS cases than projected among all homosexual and bisexual men, but especially among homosexual and bisexual men in New York City, San Francisco, and Los Angeles. IV drug users did not show such reductions, however. The researchers concluded that the major contribution to this reduction was the use of AZT to treat those with AIDS, and that other explanations for this deficit (e.g., a slower spread of HIV infection in the mid-1980s, increasing delays in reporting AIDS cases, changes in the definition of AIDS in 1987) were unlikely to account for such a deficit.

A few researchers have attempted to estimate the number of HIV-infected individuals; Salzberg and Dolins (1989) have projected that by the end of 1991, there will be about 2.75 million HIV-infected Americans. If that figure turns out to be accurate, about 1 percent of the American population would be infected with HIV. That may be somewhat on the high side, since about 1 percent of the population of San Francisco is currently thought to be HIV positive; it seems unlikely that the rest of the United States would have an infection rate equal to that of San Francisco in 1989.

A major difficulty in constructing such estimates is that because of the lengthy and highly variable incubation period of HIV, reported AIDS cases reflect those individuals who most likely contracted the virus 2 to 10 years ago, or perhaps longer. Thus, AIDS cases in 1990 may reflect people who were HIV infected in the early 1980s. Increased testing of the population would be necessary to develop a more accurate estimate of future HIV infections and future AIDS cases.

In addition, AZT, if given early, when a person finds out that he or she is HIV positive, may help slow down the progression to AIDS, so that HIV infected individuals will take more time to develop AIDS, as noted by Gail, Rosenberg, and Goedert (1990). If that trend continues, there will be fewer AIDS cases than had been projected, but the number of people who are HIV positive would remain high. Moreover, despite the continuing interest in knowing the precise number of people who are infected, the value of that number must be questioned on several grounds.

IMPLICATIONS OF HIV/AIDS STATISTICS

What would be done differently if the number of people infected with HIV were significantly higher or lower than the current official estimates? If there are actually more people infected with HIV than we expect, what implications does that have for federal, state, and local government policy; for educational programs; for health-care facilities? If the number of AIDS cases turns out to be substantially smaller than had been estimated, future heath-care costs will be less than has been estimated, and federal funding for AIDS projects will probably be reduced. If the number of AIDS cases turns out to be substantially higher than had been estimated, future health-care costs will probably be more than had been estimated, and both state and federal governments will have to develop innovative ways to pay for such increased heath-care costs. All estimates of AIDS cases are based on probabilities, and no one will know for sure how many AIDS cases there will be in 1993 until the year 1993.

One country that will have a fairly accurate number of identified HIV infected individuals is Cuba, which is planning to test every Cuban citizen for the presence of HIV antibodies, and then send those who are infected to a sanatorium outside Havana. By mid-1989, after about 3 million people had been tested (nearly 25 percent of the population), about 260 HIV infected people had been identified, not including 140 seropositive foreign students. However, between 21 and 53 of those 260 may be false positives (Bayer and Healton, 1989).

Nevertheless, with international travel, the long incubation period of the virus, and occasional false negative results, it is unlikely that *all* HIV infected individuals will or can ever be precisely identified. To reach all HIV infected people, national testing programs will have to be virtually continuous; one testing cycle simply will not identify every HIV infected Cuban citizen.

Would federal agencies respond differently, allocating more or less money to AIDS issues? As described by Shilts (1987) and Panem (1988), federal agencies are simply not equipped to respond quickly to health-care emergencies such as AIDS. Although AIDS cases first became known in 1981, the federal government (as well as national political leaders) was slow to respond. Bureaucratic organizations tend to respond slowly, rather than quickly, and political ramifications may play a significant role in affecting not only the funds that an agency is given for dealing with a particular problem, but the speed with which that agency is expected to respond.

Organizations such as the Food and Drug Administration (FDA), which developed lengthy protocols for testing and approving new drug treatments (often taking more than a decade to approve a new drug), have been pressured by AIDS groups and by politicians to speed up the drug review process. The likely result is that, not only will

some AIDS drugs be brought to market sooner, but drugs for other diseases will be as well. Although some of the recent decisions made by the FDA have been criticized by scientists because they speed up the drug review process and have possibly compromised the quality of the research data, those same decisions have been criticized by AIDS patients—who may be dying—as being far too slow to meet their immediate survival needs.

More important than knowing the actual number of HIV infected individuals is knowing how the virus is spreading—or not spreading—throughout various segments of the population. Knowing the number of HIV infected persons at a given time is a little like knowing the temperature of your city at noon on July 1: That number will tell you very little about the climate of your city for the rest of the year. Precision is not the same as accuracy. The number of people carrying the virus is changing every day, probably every hour, given the number of unprotected sexual contacts that occur and the sharing of needles and syringes throughout the United States.

To understand AIDS, we must understand where it was, where it is, and where it will be in the future. The changes that have been identified in AIDS and HIV have unfortunately led many people to assume that we know very little about the virus and how it is spread. In fact, *the major modes of HIV transmission have not changed since 1981.* What has changed are the percentages of different types of individuals who have contracted the virus and some of the characteristics of the virus itself.

COSTS OF NATIONAL HIV ANTIBODY TESTING

Californians who planned to vote on Proposition 102 in November 1988 had to consider the financial costs of implementing a proposal that ordered heath authorities to take "all measures reasonably necessary to prevent transmission" of the Human Immunodeficiency Virus (HIV). Such measures could presumably have included the isolation or quarantine of some or all HIV positive individuals, as well as people with AIDS.

Some writers and politicians have suggested that people who have been diagnosed with AIDS or who have tested HIV positive be quarantined or isolated as a way of halting the further spread of this disease. They point to the fatal nature of AIDS and the historical use of quarantine as a traditional public health measure to justify such a program. Historically, public health officials have quarantined those who might have been exposed to a disease to determine whether they will develop the disease. Once a person was diagnosed, he or she was isolated until no longer infectious or until he or she died. However, such proposals seldom offer sufficient detail for public discussion.

How long would the quarantine or isolation last: one week, one month, one year, a lifetime? How will it be enforced? How much will it cost? Who will pay for it—the state or federal government?

There is no question that a massive quarantine program would have significant legal, ethical, medical, and political implications as did the quarantine of more than 100,000 Americans of Japanese descent during World War II. Almost 50 years later, the federal government is still dealing with issues of financial reparation for those Americans whose property was taken away from them because they were of Japanese ancestry. Quarantining hundreds of thousands of Americans would probably have political implications well into the next century—and beyond.

Equally important, but seldom discussed, is the feasibility of such a quarantine program, especially with respect to the costs of implementing a statewide or national quarantine or isolation. Only rough estimates are available, but they provide a glimpse into the consequences of dealing with AIDS from a political rather than a public health perspective.

Testing and counseling costs for California

There are an estimated 250,000 Californians carrying HIV, out of a total state population of about 26.5 million people. In 1987, the Centers for Disease Control estimated that testing and counseling for HIV ranged between $22 and $75 per person. To test and counsel the entire population of California just once would cost between $583 million and $2.0 billion, averaging about $1.2 billion.

One testing of the state population would probably not identify everyone who is HIV positive, because some people may have been exposed to the virus just before the test. Other HIV infected individuals may have moved into the state after the testing program began; some people may take many months to develop antibodies to the virus.

To identify every HIV carrier, repeated statewide testing would be necessary; two statewide tests in a year could cost the state about $2.4 billion. The logistics of such a program—such as drawing 26.5 million blood samples, ensuring quality control to reduce false positives, and providing administrative and management controls—would be enormous.

To put this into perspective, in fiscal year 1988, California had allocated about $58 million for all AIDS-related activities (Rowe and Ryan, 1988). This would have to be increased 20-fold to do statewide testing only once, and all other AIDS-related projects would probably come to a complete halt.

Advocates for populationwide testing and quarantine-isolation should specify the source of such funds. Will state taxes be increased, or will existing programs be reduced or eliminated? Where will the extra $1.2 to $2.5 billion come from to test the population? If only certain segments of the population were to be tested (i.e., gay men or intravenous drug users), how would those individuals be reliably identified? Would many move "underground" to avoid testing and possible subsequent quarantine?

National testing and counseling costs

On a national level, the CDC has estimated that about 1 million Americans are carrying HIV. To identify them all by testing the entire population would cost between $5.5 billion and $19 billion, with an average cost of $12 billion per national test. The total of all state expenditures for AIDS-related projects in fiscal year 1988 has been estimated to be about $156 million (Rowe and Ryan, 1988). If the states were required to pay for testing costs, they would have to increase their AIDS budgets 80-fold.

If the federal government were to pay the cost of testing all 250 million Americans one time, the $12 billion cost would be a significant part of the federal budget. In 1987, the combined budgets of the U.S. State Department, the Justice Department, and the Commerce Department equaled about $10.5 billion. The 1989 budget for the entire U.S. Public Health Service is about $11 billion. Where would the federal funds come from to pay for national testing?

Medical costs

Medical care must be provided for the quarantined. California would be responsible for providing medical care for 250,000 people. If all of those who are quarantined went on to develop AIDS, at an average cost of $40,000 per case, the medical treatment would cost the state billions of dollars.

Legal costs

A person deprived of his or her liberty because of AIDS would no doubt have some legal recourse. In 1986, about 250,000 civil cases were heard in the U.S. district courts; legal action by all of the 250,000 HIV-labeled residents of California could equal the national civil case load.

Numerical comparisons are helpful to put this issue into perspective. Quarantining or isolating 1 million Americans should be compared to other quarantined populations. For example, there are about 600,000 inmates in the entire federal and state prison system. Any sort of official AIDS quarantine-isolation program would have to be twice the size of the current federal and state prison system.

Transportation and housing costs

Compare an AIDS quarantine-isolation program to the size of the U.S. military. There are about 200,000 Marines on active duty, about 600,000 Air Force personnel, 580,000 Navy personnel, and 780,000 Army personnel. Quarantining-isolating 1 million HIV positive Americans would be equivalent to the U.S. Army and Marines. Quarantining-isolating 1 million HIV positive Americans would be equivalent to quarantining of the 972,000 secondary school teachers in this country. Or compare 1 million quarantined to the population of American cities: 1 million people is equivalent to the population of Detroit, Dallas, or San Diego; 1 million people is equivalent to the entire population of Hawaii, Idaho, Maine, or Rhode Island.

Many of the 1 million quarantined-isolated HIV positive Americans will need medical care, because a large percentage will probably develop AIDS. In 1985, for every 100,000 people there were 237 physicians, 57 dentists, and 641 nurses. If 1 million were quarantined or isolated, there would need to be a minimum of 2,370 physicians, 570 dentists, and 6,410 nurses—not to mention auxiliary personnel—and perhaps another $500 million to $1 billion in costs. Current estimates for the treatment of AIDS are about $40,000 during the lifetime of the individual. If 1 million people are quarantined or isolated, they would lose all health-care benefits, and their medical treatment would have to be paid for in its entirety by the federal or state government. If all 1 million of the quarantined-isolated went on to develop AIDS, their medical treatment could cost the federal government up to $40 billion.

Costs of transportation, food, clothing, shelter, and so on cannot be estimated, since the proponents of quarantine-isolation have not offered any detailed programs. It would probably take about 500,000 persons to test all Americans, build quarantine-isolation facilities, transport the sick to quarantine-isolation facilities, and enforce the quarantine-isolation. At an average of $20,000 per year for salary and fringe benefits, this would add about $10 billion to the costs of a national quarantine-isolation.

In 1986, the average per capita federal tax bill was about $3,233. The 1 million quarantine-isolated would not pay $3.2 billion in federal income tax, thus increasing state and federal deficits.

In summary, estimated costs for quarantining or isolating 1 million people include the following:

• Identification: $12 billion per national test
• Lost federal tax: $3.2 billion per year
• Medical costs: $1 billion (personnel)
• Personnel: $10 billion per year
• Meals: $1–2 billion per year
• Transportation: $250 –$500 million
• Housing: $10 billion

Total estimated costs for the first year or two are $40 billion.

THE HIV CONTINUUM

Although the media coverage has focused on the disease of AIDS and the death that often accompanies it, we must remember that AIDS is only the final stage in a relatively lengthy disease process. The process begins with the initial infection, progresses through an asymptomatic period (lasting perhaps a decade or more), advances to a period of illness with opportunistic infections (lasting perhaps one to five years), and ultimately ends in death.

Although AIDS cases were reported in the medical literature in mid-1981, the virus that causes AIDS was not isolated until 1984, and an antibody test for the virus was not developed until the spring of 1985. Although originally known as HTLV-III in the United States, and LAV in France, the research community agreed on the term *HIV* in 1986. However, as late as 1989, not all researchers agreed that HIV is the cause of AIDS. Peter Duesberg, a well-known professor of microbiology at the University of California at Berkeley has argued that ''HIV is not the cause of AIDS'' (Duesberg, 1989). His views have not been widely accepted by the medical community, but they have met with some support from members of the gay community who believe that the federal government has been misleading the public as to the true nature of AIDS.

Much of what is known about AIDS is a result of the Multicenter AIDS Cohort Study (MACS) of gay and bisexual men. Begun in 1983, several thousand gay and bisexual men in Baltimore, Chicago, Los Angeles, and Pittsburgh volunteered to provide blood samples, answer questionnaires, and participate in a continuing study. Key findings from this group (Ginzburg, Fleming, and Miller, 1988) include (1) identifying the most risky behavior in HIV transmission (being the receptive partner in anal intercourse); and (2) pointing out the importance of personally knowing someone with AIDS as a motivation for behavior change.

Incubation period and blood samples

Early in the epidemic, researchers believed that the incubation period from the time of infection until the development of full-blown AIDS was two to three years. More recent studies (Lui, Darrow, and Rutherford, 1988), based on a sample of homosexual men, suggested that the average incubation period was 7.8 years, with a range of 4.2 to 15.0 years, very close to the 8.2 years for adults developing transfusion-associated AIDS. As noted in Chapter 1, Bacchetti and Moss (1989) found an incubation period for the virus of about 11 years. As time goes by, researchers seem to be finding an increasingly lengthy incubation period; of course, an 11-year incubation period could not be determined in the first years of the epidemic. But, if present trends continue, the actual incubation period may turn out to be even longer than is now known.

It is not clear whether this incubation period holds for other groups at risk for AIDS. The populations upon which such data are collected are rather limited. Much has been gathered from a relatively small sample of gay men in San Francisco who agreed to participate in health studies in the late 1970s and early 1980s, and from intravenous drug users in New York City. Although some researchers have collected data from other populations at risk (e.g., military recruits, patients at clinics for sexually transmitted diseases, people with hemophilia), all of these groups are based on samples that may or may not represent the broader population.

Blood samples have been taken from patients entering key hospitals throughout the country in an attempt to collect more data, but even hospital patients are only a small segment of the entire population, and they tend to be overrepresented by women and the elderly. It will be some time before a more complete picture is available of HIV infection and AIDS throughout the United States, and that image may change over time. Constant monitoring will be essential, especially if HIV changes its molecular structure.

COMPARING AIDS AND OTHER DISEASES

To understand the broader impact of AIDS, it is valuable to compare AIDS with other notifiable diseases. In 1989, the 34,340 reported AIDS cases

Table 3.1   Notifiable diseases: 1989

Disease	Number of Cases
Gonorrhea (civilian)	689,922
Syphilis (civilian)	42,600
Hepatitis (type A)	35,165
AIDS	34,340
Hepatitis (type B)	22,963
Tuberculosis	21,520
Measles	16,236
Gonorrhea (military)	10,829
Aseptic meningitis	9,983
Mumps	5,611
Rabies (animal)	4,460
Pertussis	3,745
Meningococcal infections	2,595
Hepatitis (non-A, non-B)	2,323
Hepatitis (unspecified)	2,304
Malaria	1,232
Legionellosis	1,128
Encephalitis	916
Typhus fever, tick-borne (RMSF)	619
Typhoid fever	478
Rubella (German measles)	373
Toxic shock syndrome	376
Leprosy	169
Tularemia	144

Source: CDC, 1989.

were exceeded by gonorrhea, syphilis, and hepatitis A, all of which are related in some ways to AIDS (gonorrhea and syphilis because they are sexually transmitted diseases, and Hepatitis A because it is sometimes associated with oral anal contact. Despite the oft-heard concern that AIDS is getting far too much attention in the media, AIDS is being reported at a significantly higher rate than other diseases thought to be more common. For example, there were about 5,600 cases of mumps in 1989, (one-sixth the number of AIDS cases) and about 16,000 measles cases (one-half the number of AIDS cases).

In the 50-year period from 1938 to 1988, there were about 447,000 polio cases, and in the 20-year period from 1968 to 1988, there were 875,000 cases of mumps. Table 3.1 shows the comparison of notifiable AIDS cases to other notifiable diseases in 1989 (CDC, 1990a).

PROJECTIONS AND COSTS

United States

Any projections for HIV or AIDS will be affected by several factors, including the ability to diagnose AIDS or HIV infection, the willingness to report cases, time lags in reporting cases to appropriate health organizations, and political considerations. Consequently, all projections should be taken as rough estimates, particularly the worldwide estimates. Table 3.2 presents the 1989 projections from the Centers for Disease Control.

National projections are helpful, but HIV and AIDS are likely to have significant regional variations. Through June 1990, New York State had reported about 31,000 AIDS cases, the vast majority of those (27,000) occurring in New York City. By 1993, estimates are that New York City will be dealing with 60,000 AIDS cases; what that means for the city is that the 1,800 current hospital beds will have to be increased to 4,000 (Lambert, 1989). The number of nursing home beds will have to increase from 128 to 1,200. City, state, and federal governments, along with insurers and patients, are spending about $700 million on AIDS in New York City. By 1993, the city will need $1.9 billion, an increase of almost 300 percent.

Direct health care costs

Most of the emphasis on the economic costs of AIDS has focused on the health-care costs. The first study of health-care costs (Hardy et al., 1986) estimated the lifetime hospital costs of the first 10,000 people with AIDS at $147,000 per person, an estimate that was later considered to be far too high. More recent estimates (Bloom and Carliner, 1988) suggest a lifetime cost of $80,000, with cities such as San Francisco and New York bearing a disproportionate case load. Bloom and Carliner suggest that the lifetime costs of treating AIDS patients in 1991 are $350 per resident in San Francisco and $100 per resident in New York City. Despite such regional concerns, Bloom and Carliner concluded that the overall treatment costs for AIDS will be small relative to total national health-care expenditures.

Hay, Osmond, and Jacobson (1988) have estimated the average 1990s total medical costs per AIDS patient at about $28,000–$40,000, with total AIDS medical costs for the nation at $2–$4 billion

Table 3.2   Projected Numbers of AIDS Cases, Deaths Attributable to AIDS, and Living Persons with AIDS, After Adjustments for Underreporting[a]—United States, 1989–1993

	AIDS Cases		
Year	New cases[b]	Alive[c]	Deaths
1989	44,000–50,000	92,000– 98,000	31,000–34,000
1990	52,000–57,000	101,000–122,000	37,000–42,000
1991	56,000–71,000	127,000–153,000	43,000–52,000
1992	58,000–85,000	139,000–188,000	49,000–64,000
1993	61,000–98,000	151,000–225,000	53,000–76,000
Total through 1993[d]:	390,000–480,000		285,000–340,000

Source: CDC (1990d).
[a] Projections are adjusted for underreported diagnoses of AIDS by adding 18 percent to projections obtained from reported cases (corresponding to 85% of all diagnosed cases being reported and rounded to the nearest 1,000).
[b] Number of cases diagnosed during the year.
[c] Person alive with AIDS during the year.
[d] Rounded to the nearest 5,000. Includes an estimated 120,000 AIDS cases diagnosed through 1988, 48,000 persons alive with AIDS at the end of 1988, and 72,000 deaths in diagnosed patients through 1988.

Box 3

The Hidden Costs of AIDS

Although most economists have focused on the direct costs associated with the delivery of health-care services to people with AIDS, the hidden (indirect) costs associated with AIDS have not been so well analyzed. Indirect costs arise from lost productivity as a result of illness and premature death. Such costs are measured by wages lost because of illness and disability (morbidity costs) and the present value of future earnings lost (mortality costs) by people who die before age 65. Scitovsky (1988) estimated indirect costs at $3.9 billion in 1985, $7.0 billion in 1986, and $55.6 billion in 1991—about seven times the direct medical care costs.

Similar estimates have been made by Carwein and Ray (1989), who calculated past and future lost income for all AIDS cases reported in Nevada in 1987 and 1988, and determined that the total economic losses to Nevada and to the United States would total more than $300 million. They suggest that if the CDC estimates are correct for future AIDS cases, the income lost because of AIDS deaths from 1993 to the end of the work life expectancy for the youngest person

could exceed $150 billion. However, because these losses will be spread out over several decades, such losses may not become readily apparent.

Some have tried to estimate costs of dying. For example, Kiker and Birkelli (1972) estimated that all losses (both deaths and disabilities) due to the Vietnam War cost between $5.8 and $11.6 billion. However, as noted by Mishan (1979), there seems to be no universally agreed upon method for evaluating the economic costs associated with death or the saving of lives. Nevertheless, AIDS deaths will have important economic implications beyond those associated with health-care costs.

Another type of indirect costs are those economic losses that will occur because of the premature deaths of millions of people worldwide (Hochhauser, 1988). The World Health Organization has estimated that 5 to 10 million people worldwide are carrying the Human Immunodeficiency Virus. If most develop full-blown AIDS and die within a year or two of diagnosis, there will be 5 to 10 million fewer consumers.

by 1991. Other researchers have estimated total medical costs to be $9–$100 billion.

Demographics of AIDS deaths

In the United States, the average male with AIDS was diagnosed at age 37, and the average female with AIDS at about age 36. Thus, the vast majority

of AIDS cases have been diagnosed in the 30-to-39 year-old age range, at a time when these people would be approaching their peak earning (and purchasing) potential.

Data on persons dying from AIDS (Kapantais and Powell-Griner, 1989) show that AIDS deaths occur in people who are younger than those who die of other causes. About 90 percent of the AIDS

Table 3.3   Estimated Years of Potential Life Lost in 1988

Cause of Death	Years of Potential Life Lost (1988)
All causes	12,281,741
Unintentional injuries	2,319,400
Malignant neoplasms	1,809,289
AIDS (1993 estimate; 64,500 deaths)	1,612,000
Heart disease	1,466,629
Suicide/Homicide	1,361,473
Congenital anomalies	671,709
Human Immunodeficiency Virus infection	472,800
Prematurity	432,342
Sudden Infant Death Syndrome	296,304
Cerebrovascular disease	245,722
Chronic liver diseases/Cirrhosis	236,944
Pneumonia/Influenza	172,712
Diabetes mellitus	130,666
Chronic Obstructive Pulmonary Diseases	128,126

Source: CDC, (1990b).

Table 3.4   Estimated Economic Losses Due to AIDS Deaths: 1981–1993 (in 1985 dollars)

Item	Estimated Cumulative Losses
Personal income	$196 billion
Shelter	$30 billion
Food	$26 billion
Personal taxes	$17 billion
Fuel/Utilities	$13 billion
Apparel/Services	$9 billion
Gasoline/Motor oil	$8 billion
Health care	$8 billion
Household furnishings	$7 billion
Life insurance	$2 billion

Sources
Statistical abstract of the United States: 1988 Washington, D.C.: U.S. Department of Commerce, 1987. Average annual income and expenditures of all consumer units: 1985 (No. 688). CDC, (1990d) (312,000 estimated deaths, 1981 through 1993 = estimated 7,800,000 YPLL) Calculations: Estimated economic losses = YPLL x average annual expenditures.

deaths in 1986 occurred in those aged 25 to 54, in contrast to 11 percent of the deaths from other causes. Moreover, those dying from AIDS tended to be better educated (33% with four or more years of college) than those who died from other causes (8% with four or more years of college) and more likely to be in managerial or professional occupations (39% of the AIDS deaths) than those who died of all other causes (16%).

Years of potential life lost (YPLL)

One way to analyze the business lost to AIDS is through "years of potential life lost" (YPLL). Each year not lived before age 65 is a year of potential life lost. Someone who dies at age 40 has lost 25 years of potential life; this person has also lost 25 years of economic, or consumer, purchases. The CDC estimates about 312,000 AIDS deaths by the end of 1993. At roughly 25 YPLL per death, that is the equivalent of 7,800,000 YPLL.

In 1988, there were about 473,000 YPLL from AIDS. The 64,000 estimated AIDS deaths in

1993 may cause about 1.6 million YPLL and may surpass both heart disease and cancer in terms of YPLL! Table 3.3 shows the estimated YPLL in 1988 (CDC, 1990b) with AIDS projections for 1993.

Multiplying each YPLL lost by the average annual income and average annual expenditures gives some idea of the total economic losses due to these 7,800,000 YPLL, as shown in Table 3.4. Of course, new developments, such as more effective treatments, could have an impact on the number of deaths and subsequent YPLL among people with AIDS. However, given the lengthy incubation period of the virus, most, if not all, of the people who will die of AIDS by the end of 1993 have already been infected. Although the economic losses seem high (and they are), the perception of economic loss will probably not be very apparent, because the losses will occur over many years.

INTERNATIONAL PROJECTIONS

The World Health Organization (WHO) has estimated that more than 250,000 cases of AIDS have occurred worldwide, that 5 to 10 million people are infected with HIV, and that there will be 1 million AIDS cases within the next five years (Mann et al., 1988). Because of political and economic concerns, WHO has estimated that in some countries as many as 90 percent of the AIDS cases are not being reported. Some countries simply do not want to admit that AIDS is a problem, perhaps because the tourist trade might evaporate, perhaps because they don't want to be judged by other countries that may make assumptions about the morality or immorality of their citizens.

More than 70 percent of the worldwide reported AIDS cases have come from the Western Hemisphere, and of the estimated 5 to 10 million people infected worldwide, as many as 2.5 million reside in North and South America (Quinn, Zacarias, and St. John, 1989). In some Latin American countries, specifically Brazil, Haiti, Mexico, and the Dominican Republic, these researchers found that HIV transmission has been occurring via bisexual men (15%–25% of AIDS patients) and heterosexual IV drug users, and an increasing number of women are being infected via heterosexual transmission.

Researchers have identified two AIDS-related viruses: HIV-1, which was the virus identified in the early 1980s as the cause of AIDS: and HIV-2, a virus similar to HIV-1 that has been seen in some parts of Western Africa and Latin America. Although one case of HIV-2 has been found in a West African visiting the United States (CDC, 1988), it is not yet known whether HIV-2 will be as infectious as HIV-1, or whether HIV-2 will actually cause AIDS.

Some patients in Brazil have been diagnosed as carriers of both HIV-1 and HIV-2 (Cortes, et al., 1989). In Brazil, HIV-1 infection is established among homosexuals, bisexuals, and female prostitutes from lower socioeconomic classes, with bisexual men acting as the bridge between the homosexual and heterosexual communities. HIV (both 1 and 2) is likely to increase among Latin American heterosexuals.

Worldwide, three infection patterns of HIV have been identified (Piot et al., 1988):

Pattern 1—Includes North and South America, Western Europe, Scandinavia, Australia, and New Zealand. In Pattern 1 countries, the vast majority (90%) of the AIDS cases are in homosexual or bisexual males or intravenous drug users, with limited heterosexual transmission at the present time. Spread of HIV probably began in the mid-1970s or early 1980s.

San Francisco has been hit very hard by the AIDS epidemic. As noted earlier, by June 30, 1990, San Francisco had reported 8,754 AIDS cases, with 5,798 deaths (San Francisco Department of Public Health, 1990). The number of San Franciscans who have died from AIDS is higher than the number of soldiers who died in World War I, World War II, the Korean War, and the Vietnam War combined.

Pattern 2—Includes Africa, the Caribbean and some areas of South America. In these countries, the virus began to spread in the early to late 1970s, and the primary method of HIV transmission is heterosexual. The number of infected males and females is approximately equal. Homosexual transmission is not a major factor in these areas.

In many urban areas of Central and Eastern Africa, from 5 to 20 percent of the sexually active age group has already been infected with HIV. Close to half of all hospital patients in some cities are HIV infected. Child mortality may increase by 25 percent during the next few years, since 10 to 25 percent of women of childbearing age are HIV infected.

Pattern 3—Includes Eastern Europe, North Africa, the Middle East, Asia, and the Pacific. In these areas, there are relatively few AIDS cases. Most of the documented AIDS cases have been a result of people having contact with infected individuals from pattern 1 or pattern 2 countries. HIV transmission began in the early to mid-1980s, and homosexual and heterosexual transmission is only now being documented.

Worldwide economic costs

AIDS is having a devastating impact on some Third World developing countries. In 1988, in Tanzania, for example, the per capita health budget was about $1. The cost of treating a Tanzanian AIDS patient ranges from about $100 to $600 (Perlez, 1988). The Harvard Institute of Economic Development has estimated that by 1995, the annual financial loss to Zaire will be $350 million—8 percent of the country's 1984 Gross National Product (Mann et al., 1988).

The millions of deaths that will come from AIDS will affect the economies of many countries: food production in East and Central Africa (Abel et al., 1988); copper mining in Zambia (Nkowane, 1988); the financial burden on families caring for children with AIDS in Zaire (Davachi et al., 1988).

Poorer countries, including many in warmer climates, simply do not have the funds for disposable needles and syringes or for refrigeration units to store donated blood. As a result, it is pos-sible that HIV is being spread through medical procedures such as childhood inoculations, because the same syringe may be used over and over again. Similarly, testing donated blood for HIV infection may be difficult, if not impossible. Blood from a donor to a recipient may be given almost immediately after donation, so that the likelihood of transfusion-related cases become significantly higher than in the United States.

As devastating as AIDS may become in the United States, other countries may have a significantly higher death rate. The lack of condoms, the absence of disposable needles and syringes (as well as inadequate supplies of bleach), and a potentially contaminated blood supply may literally wipe out some communities. Finally, the presence of other diseases that affect the immune system, such as malaria, will create additional health problems both for persons who suffer from multiple diseases and for health agencies that must struggle to cope with such diseases.

SUMMARY

Although 1 million Americans may be carrying HIV, only 14 percent have actually been diagnosed with AIDS, suggesting that the major impact of AIDS has yet to hit the United States. Internationally, the World Health Organization has estimated that between 5 and 10 million people are carrying the virus, a number that may grow to 100 million by the beginning of the twenty-first century.

Some have argued that quarantine-isolation would be an effective public health measure for slowing the rate of HIV infection. However, state and national costs for testing and counseling, medical care, transportation, housing, and other services could cost as much as $40 billion for the first two years.

The average period of time from HIV infection to development of AIDS is now thought to be eight years or more, with some persons taking even longer to become ill. As more and more HIV infected people become ill in the 1990s, researchers have suggested that treatment for people with AIDS could cost several billion dollars per year or more. Such costs will have devastating effects on poorer countries as they struggle to provide treatment while providing for other economic needs at the same time.

REFERENCES

Abel, N., Barnett, T., Bell, S., Blaikie, P., and Cross, S. (1988) The impact of AIDS on food production systems in East and Central Africa over the next ten years: A programmatic paper. In A. F. Fleming, M. Carballo, D. W. FitzSimons, M. R. Bailey, and J. Mann., eds. *The global impact of AIDS*. New York: Alan R. Liss, Inc.

Bacchetti, D., and Moss, A. R. (1989) Incubation period of AIDS in San Francisco. *Nature,* 338 (6212), 251–253.

Bayer, R., and Healton, C. (1989) Controlling AIDS in Cuba: The logic of quarantine. *New England Journal of Medicine,* 320 (15), 1022–1024.

Bloom, D., and Carliner, G. (1988) The economic impact of AIDS in the United States. *Science,* 239, 604–610.

Bregman, D. J., and Langmuir, A. D. (1990) Farr's Law applied to AIDS projections. *Journal of the American Medical Association,* 263 (11), 1522–1525.

Carwein, V. L., and Ray, C. G. (1989) AIDS-related income losses and implications for policy making. *AIDS & Public Policy Journal.* 4 (2), 106–111.

CDC (1988) *Morbidity and Mortality Weekly Report.* AIDS due to HIV-2 infection—New Jersey. 37 (3), 33.

CDC (1989) *Morbidity and Mortality Weekly Report,* 38 (51, 52), 891.

CDC (1990a) *Morbidity and Mortality Weekly Report,* 39 (2), 21.

CDC (1990b) *Morbidity and Mortality Weekly Report.* YPPL before Ages 65 and 85—U.S., 1987, 1988. 39 (2), 20–21.

CDC (1990d) *Morbidity and Mortality Weekly Report.* Estimates of HIV prevalence and projected AIDS cases: Summary of a workshop, October 31–November 1, 1989. 39 (7), 110–112; 117–119.

Cortes, E., Detels, R., Aboulafia, D., et al. (1989) HIV-1, HIV-2 and HTLV-1 infection in high-risk groups in Brazil. *New England Journal of Medicine,* 320 (15), 953–958.

Curran, J. W., Jaffe, H. W., Hardy, A. M., et al. (1988) Epidemiology of HIV infection and AIDS in the United States. *Science* 239, 610–616.

Davachi, F., Baudoux, P., Ndoko, K., N'Galy, B., and Mann, J. (1988). The economic impact on families of children with AIDS in Kinshasa, Zaire. In A. F. Fleming, M. Carballo, D. W. FitzSimons, M. R. Bailey, and J. Mann., eds. *The global impact of AIDS.* New York: Alan R. Liss, Inc.

Duesberg, P. (1989) HIV is not the cause of AIDS. *Science,* 241, 516.

Gail, M. H., Rosenberg, P. S., and Goedert, J. J. (1990) Therapy may explain recent deficits in AIDS incidence. *Journal of Acquired Immune Deficiency Syndromes,* 3 (4), 296–306.

General Accounting Office (1989) *AIDS forecasting: Undercount of cases and lack of key data weaken existing estimates.* Washington, DC: United States General Accounting Office.

Ginzburg, H. M., Fleming, P. L., and Miller, K. D. (1988) Selected public health observations derived from the Multicenter AIDS Cohort Study. *Journal of Acquired Immune Deficiency Syndromes,* 1 (1), 2–7.

Hardy, A. M., Rauch K., Echenberg, D., Morgan, W., and Curran, J. (1986) The economic impact of the first 10,000 cases of acquired immunodeficiency syndrome in the United States. *Journal of the American Medical Association,* 255, 209–215.

Hay, J. W., Osmond, D. H., and Jacobson, M. A. (1988). Projecting the medical costs of AIDS and ARC in the United States. *Journal of the Acquired Immune Deficiency Syndromes,* 1, 466–485.

Hochhauser, M. (1988) AIDS to impact business' bottom line. *The Meeting Manager,* 8 (12), 16–17.

Kapantais, G., and Powell-Griner, E. (1989) Characteristics of persons dying from AIDS. Preliminary data from the 1986 National Mortality Followback Survey. *Advance Data from Vital and Health Statistics of the National Center for Health Statistics.* DHHS Publication No. (PHS) 89–1250. Hyattsville, MD: National Center for Health Statistics.

Kiker, B. F., and Birkelli, J. (1972) Human capital losses resulting from U.S. casualties of the war in Vietnam. *Journal of Political Economy,* 1023–1030.

Lambert, B. (1989) AIDS in a deficit year: More plans than money. *New York Times,* April 23, 1989.

Langmuir, A. D. (1989) Round table. AIDS projections are too high. In *AIDS. Profile of an epidemic. Scientific Publication No. 514.* Washington, DC: Pan American Health Organization.

Lui, K. G., Darrow, W. W., and Rutherford, G. W. (1988) A model-based estimate of the mean incubation period for AIDS in homosexual men. *Science,* 240, 1333–1335.

Mann, J., Chin, J., Piot, P., and Quinn, T. (1988) The international epidemiology of AIDS. *Scientific American,* 259 (4), 82–89.

Masters, W. H., Johnson, V. E., and Kolodny, R. C. (1988) *Crisis: Heterosexual behaviors in the age of AIDS.* New York: Grove Press.

Mishan, E. J. (1979) Evaluation of life and limb: A theoretical approach. *Journal of Political Economy,* 79, 687–705.

Morgan, M., Curran, J. W., and Berkelman, R. L. (1990) The future course of AIDS in the United States. *Journal of the American Medical Association,* 263 (11), 1539–1540.

Nkowane, B. M. (1988) The impact of Human Immunodeficiency Virus infection and AIDS on a primary industry: Mining (a case study of Zambia). In A. F. Fleming, M. Carballo, D. W. FitzSimons, M. R. Bailey, and J. Mann., eds. *The global impact of AIDS.* New York: Alan R. Liss, Inc.

Osmond, D. H., and Moss, A. R. (1989) The prevalence of HIV infection in the United States: A reappraisal of the Public Health Service estimate. In P. Volberding, and M. A. Jacobson, eds. *AIDS clinical review 1989.* New York: Marcel Dekker.

Palco, J. (1989) Is the AIDS epidemic slowing? *Science,* 246, 1560.

Panem, S. (1988) *The AIDS bureaucracy.* Cambridge, MA: Harvard University Press.

Perlez, J. (1988) Africans weigh threat of AIDS to economics. *New York Times,* September 22, 1988.

Piot, P., Plummer, F. A., Mhalu, F. S., Lamboray, J. L., Chin, J., and Mann, J. M. (1988) AIDS: An international perspective. *Science,* 239, 573–579.

Quinn, T. C., Zacarias, F. R. K., and St. John, R. K. (1989) AIDS in the Americas: An emerging public health crisis. *New England Journal of Medicine,* 320 (15), 1005–1007.

Rothenberg, R., Woelfel, M., Stoneburner, R., et al. (1987) Survival with the Acquired Immunodeficiency Syndrome. *New England Journal of Medicine,* 317 (21), 1297–1302.

Rowe, M. J. and Ryan, C. C. (1988) Comparing state-only expenditures for AIDS. *American Journal of Public Health,* 78 (4), 424–429.

Salzberg, A. M., and Dolins, S. L. (1989) The relation between AIDS cases and HIV prevalence. *New England Journal of Medicine,* 320 (14), 936.

San Francisco Department of Public Health (1990) S. F. AIDS incidence and mortality by month of diagnosis or death, 1980–90. June 30, 1990.

Scitovsky, A. (1988) Estimates of the direct and indirect costs of AIDS in the United States. In A. F. Fleming, M. Carballo, D. W. FitzSimons, M. R. Bailey, and J. Mann., eds. *The global impact of AIDS.* New York: Alan R. Liss, Inc.

Shilts, R. (1987) *And the band played on.* New York: St. Martin's Press.

Statistical abstract of the United States: 1988. Washington, DC: U.S. Department of Commerce.

Transmission of HIV Infection

4

That which we call sin in others is experiment for us.

RALPH WALDO EMERSON

HIV VS. THE "AIDS VIRUS"

While most of the media coverage has focused on AIDS (the end stage of HIV infection), the major focus for education and prevention should be on reducing the rate of transmission of the Human Immunodeficiency Virus. After all, once a person has become infected with HIV, there is little in the way of prevention that can be done for that individual. Once infected, you cannot become uninfected (although there is preliminary evidence suggesting that removing the blood from an AIDS patient, heating it, and returning it to the patient may kill HIV in the blood). Too often, prevention programs emphasize the end stage of HIV infection (AIDS), and not the virus that causes the dis-

ease. Prevention programs must emphasize those behaviors that are involved in the transmission and reception of HIV, in the perspective of an infection control issue rather than an end-stage disease issue. Adolescents and young adults are oriented to the present; long-term consequences may have little meaning to someone whose activities are planned on a day-to-day basis. Consequently, emphasizing AIDS may be counterproductive as a form of health education or health promotion, since AIDS may be as remote to many young people as lung cancer or heart attacks are to smokers. These are problems about which the typical adolescent or young adult is simply not concerned.

As noted earlier, research (Bacchetti and Moss, 1989) suggests that the median incubation period for an HIV-infected person to develop AIDS is 9.8 years. These researchers analyzed data from gay men in San Francisco and found that, of those who were infected, about 45 percent came down with AIDS within nine years of being infected with the virus. Equally important, half of those who were infected will apparently take more than nine years to develop symptoms of AIDS. It is possible that some HIV infected individuals may take 15 or 20 years to develop AIDS. Of course, since AIDS has been studied for only about a decade, it is impossible to know for at least another decade how many HIV infected people will seroconvert over a 20-year period.

Moreover, it is not yet clear that an infected individual is equally infectious to other people during these years. In some cases, the person stays healthy because the immune system temporarily suppresses HIV within the blood. The infected person may be most infectious to others shortly after the initial infection occurs (at a time when there are no antibodies in the blood) and when the disease is in its final stages (when most of the antibodies have been destroyed by HIV). These lengthy time periods can be considered "silent HIV infections" (Haseltine, 1989) because they represent a time in which the person may be HIV infected, but such infection may not be identified with current ELISA and Western Blot tests, which measure only the presence of antibodies to HIV in the blood, not HIV itself.

Because of the lengthy incubation period, the term *AIDS virus* will not be used, because that terminology implies that HIV transmission and the development of AIDS are closely linked in time. Therefore, the term *HIV* will be used where appropriate. Too often, the use of the term *AIDS* where *HIV* is the more appropriate term suggests the use of fear tactics in AIDS education programs, although some psychological research suggests that messages with too much fear may lead to avoidance of the message (Jobs, 1988). As described by Janis (1984):

. . . when an authoritative warning evokes a moderate or fairly high degree of fear, any additional source of fear—whether relevant or irrelevant to the threat described in the warning—is likely to raise fear to such a high degree that it exceeds the optimal level, with the result that the authoritative recommendations are less likely to be accepted than if that additional source of fear were not present. (pp. 347–348)

The term *AIDS virus* is likely to produce more fear than the correct term, Human Immunodeficiency Virus (HIV) and suggests an unnecessarily fearful emphasis on AIDS, rather than a more appropriate emphasis on the transmission of HIV. From an educational standpoint, the question that must be answered is: "Are we trying to prevent AIDS, or are we trying to prevent infection with HIV?" The two are not necessarily the same, and how one answers that question will have a substantial impact on the content and focus of educationally based prevention programs.

ROUTES OF HIV TRANSMISSION

HIV can be transmitted from person-to-person through several major routes: sexual transmission via semen and vaginal secretions, blood transmission through needle sharing or blood transfusions, and perinatal transmission from an infected mother to child. Table 4.1 summarizes the transmission categories as described by CDC for adults, adolescents, and children.

Male-to-male sexual transmission

On a worldwide basis, the most common way of transmitting and receiving HIV is through sexual activity in which an uninfected person comes into contact with the semen or blood of an infected person. There are four possible ways of transmitting HIV: male-to-male, male-to-female, female-to-male, and female-to-female.

Table 4.1   Cumulative AIDS Cases: 1981–June 1990

Transmission Categories	Males	Females	Total
Adults/adolescents			
Homosexual/bisexual males	82,304 (66%)	0 (0%)	82,304 (60%)
Intravenous (IV) drug user	22,798 (18%)	6,689 (51%)	29,487 (21%)
Homosexual male and IV drug user	9,370 (8%)	0 (0%)	9,370 (7%)
Hemophilia/coagulation disorder	1,203 (1%)	31 (0%)	1,234 (1%)
Heterosexual cases	2,824 (2%)	4,128 (32%)	6,952 (5%)
Transfusion/blood components	2,016 (2%)	1,263 (10%)	3,279 (2%)
Undetermined cases	3,876 (3%)	899 (7%)	4,765 (3%)
Subtotal (% of all cases)	**124,385 (89%)**	**13,000 (9%)**	**137,385 (98%)**
Children			
Hemophilia/coagulation disorder			119 (0%)
Parent with or at risk of AIDS			1,966 (1%)
Transfusion/blood components			233 (0%)
Undetermined cases			62 (0%)
Subtotal (% of all cases)			**2,380 (1%)**
Total (% of all cases)	**124,385 (89%)**	**13,000 (9%)**	**137,385 (100%)**

Source: CDC (1990).

Since 1981, most male adults in the United States with AIDS (about 65%) have been homosexual or bisexual males (Curran et al., 1988). However, this percentage has been dropping as more IV drug use cases are reported (e.g., Table 1.1 in Chapter 1.), and as AZT has been increasingly used to treat gay men who are HIV infected but have not yet developed AIDS. (However, fewer AIDS cases in gay men does not necessarily mean that fewer gay men are infected with HIV).

Male-to-male transmission through anal intercourse is a very efficient way of transmitting and receiving the virus, primarily based on the anatomical structures involved. On the other hand, male-to-male mutual masturbation would not be an efficient way of transmitting the virus. Again, it is behaviors that are risky, not group affiliations.

The most risky behavior is to be the receptive partner in unprotected anal intercourse. To become infected, HIV in an infected partner must come into direct contact with the white blood cells of an uninfected partner. This can occur in several ways during anal intercourse. First, tears in the rectum may expose small veins or capillaries to HIV in the partner's semen. These tears represent a portal of entry for HIV and will allow the virus to enter the bloodstream of the uninfected partner. Second, during anal intercourse, the active partner may have minor abrasions on the penis that allow small amounts of blood to come into direct contact with his partner's rectal tissue. The blood carrying HIV can be transmitted from the active to the receptive partner, even in the absence of ejaculation.

To prevent the transmission of HIV, condoms have been widely recommended as an effective barrier method of protection. When used appropriately, latex condoms can act as a barrier to block the transmission of HIV. However, *if condoms are used, they should be used only with a water-based lubricant;* oil-based lubricants (such as petroleum jelly) cause latex condoms to deteriorate rapidly. Condoms made from sheep intestines (i.e., "skins") may offer less protection from HIV, because they are somewhat more porous than latex condoms, making it easier for HIV to pass through the condom.

Female-to-female transmission

Female-to-female transmission has been suggested as a theoretical possibility, but literature on the subject has not shown this to be a major risk factor. Sexual activity between women in which an exchange of HIV infected blood might occur is a possibility (e.g., if the couple engages in oral sex while one of the partners is menstruating, or if bleeding occurs as a result of insertive sexual practices).

Bisexual women or women who are intravenous drug users would certainly be at some risk of contracting the virus from an infected male partner or from a contaminated syringe, and could possibly pass the virus to an uninfected female partner. Most of the safer sex strategies have focused on gay male couples or heterosexual couples. Very little information has been developed for lesbian couples.

Male-to-female sexual transmissions

Male-to-female transmission is also fairly efficient. As of June 1990, there were about 13,000 AIDS cases reported in females in the United States. Approximately 3,100 (32%) contracted HIV heterosexually; contrast that with the 2,824 (2%) heterosexually transmitted cases in males. In the United States, there are about 8.5 AIDS cases in males for every AIDS case in females. In the early years of the epidemic, there were about 14 AIDS cases in males for every AIDS case in females. In other parts of the world, this ratio is closer to 2:1, or even 1:1 (Piot et al., 1988). Changes in the ratio of male-to-female AIDS cases in the United States can be seen in the following statistics (CDC, 1987, 1990):

Year	Male-to-Female Ratio
Before 1984	14.1:1
1984	13.6:1
1985	14.8:1
1986	13.8:1
1987	12.7:1
1988	8.6:1
1989	8.5:1

Early in the epidemic, AIDS was primarily a disease diagnosed in males. During the past few years, however, an increasing number of women have been diagnosed with AIDS, and the ratio of male-to-female cases will probably continue to drop during the next few years.

Anatomically, the vagina is comprised of stronger tissue than is the rectum; consequently, it appears that it is more difficult to transmit HIV via vaginal intercourse (male-to-female) than via anal intercourse (male-to-male). However, for many couples, anal intercourse is practiced as a form of birth control, and it may well be that some of the heterosexually transmitted AIDS cases occur as a result of male-to-female anal intercourse.

Female-to-male transmission

Female-to-male transmission occurs less frequently than male-to-female transmission, at least in the United States. A study of female (prostitute)-to-male transmission of HIV (Cameron et al., 1989) in Kenya found a high rate of such transmission when other sexually transmitted diseases were present, when there were genital lesions, and when the men were uncircumcised. Unprotected vaginal or anal intercourse appears to be the major route of transmission, although at least one case of transmission via oral sex by a male with a female prostitute (presumably HIV infected) has been reported in the literature (Spitzer and Weiner, 1989).

Although the above four categories briefly describe the possible modes for sexual HIV transmission, the reported AIDS cases portray a much more complex picture than these four categories allow. The CDC has identified six single modes of exposure that are responsible for about 87 percent of AIDS cases, and 24 multiple modes that are responsible for the other 13 percent of the reported cases. Space does not permit a detailed analysis of all 30 modes of exposure, but Table 4.2 provides a brief summary of the exposure modalities. Although most of the reporting on AIDS has emphasized the single modes of exposure (e.g., male homosexual, IV drug user), some individuals have had three or four different types of exposure to HIV (e.g., IV drug use, heterosexual contact, transfusion recipient)

HETEROSEXUAL TRANSMISSION: MYTH VS. REALITY

Whether HIV can be transmitted heterosexually depends, in part, on whether one wants to believe that it can be transmitted in this way. For some sexually active heterosexuals, believing that AIDS is a "gay disease" means that they won't have to change their own lifestyles. Consequently, many writers and researchers have argued about whether HIV is transmitted homosexually or heterosexually (Fumento, 1987), when the real issue is the sexual transmission of the virus. Although most AIDS cases in 1981 and 1982 were found in gay males, this does not mean that most AIDS cases in 1991 or 2001 will be found in gay males. AIDS cases in 1991 reflect patterns of HIV transmission from the prior decade. Current AIDS cases tell us only about past HIV transmission patterns, not about future transmission patterns. The Institute of Medicine (1988) has reported that

> "although the numbers are small, cases acquired through heterosexual transmission are the fastest growing group of AIDS cases in the United States."

Relative changes in the route of transmission are apparent. Since all blood has been tested since March 1985, there should be relatively few cases of HIV transmitted through blood transfusions in the future, because there is virtually no HIV-contaminated blood. Thus, transfusion-associated AIDS will become very rare. On the other hand, there is simply no way of knowing how serious HIV transmission through heterosexual behaviors will become in the next decade or so. In their review of AIDS among heterosexuals, Haverkos and Edelman (1988) note the difficulty of separating heterosexual risk factors from other risk factors, such as intravenous drug use, as well as the difficulties encountered from CDC's classification system. For example, the researchers note that

> Male intravenous drug abusers with AIDS who report homosexual activity were categorized as and presumed to be sexually transmitted cases in earlier CDC reports. In contrast, all heterosexual drug abusers with AIDS are still categorized as needle-related cases, not sexually transmitted cases. (pp. 1924–1925)

Knowing that someone with AIDS has engaged in IV drug use and homosexual behaviors does not necessarily prove which route of transmission produced the infection. Since almost all information on route of transmission is based on self-reported histories, there is no way of scientifically identifying the actual route of HIV transmission for those individuals with multiple risk factors. Heterosexual drug users may be classified as either sexually transmitted cases or as needle-related cases, but there is no way to know how the virus was actually transmitted.

Looking at all AIDS cases (in both males and females), CDC has categorized only 5 percent as the result of heterosexual contact. However, that figure is skewed by the preponderance of cases in gay and bisexual males. In males, only 2 percent of the AIDS cases are the result of heterosexual contact; in females, that figure is 32 percent—almost 16 times higher than for men.

Heterosexual transmission has been frequently documented in parts of Central Africa, and less often in the United States, although that may be due to differences in how "heterosexual contact" is defined in Central Africa and in the United States. Thus, the issue is not *whether* HIV can be transmitted heterosexually, but *how efficiently* (Padian, 1987). Absence of an animal model for HIV transmission has made laboratory research on

Table 4.2   Adult/Adolescent AIDS Cases by Single and Multiple Exposure Categories, Reported Thorough June 1990, United States

Exposure Category	AIDS Cases	
	Number	Percentage
Single mode of exposure		
Male homosexual/bisexual contact	79,013	(58)
Intravenous (IV) drug use (female and heterosexual male)	25,298	(18)
Hemophilia/coagulation disorder	742	(1)
Heterosexual contact	6,623	(5)
Receipt of transfusion of blood, blood component, or tissue	3,273	(2)
Other/undetermined	4,765	(3)
Single mode of exposure subtotal	**119,714**	**(87)**
Multiple modes of exposure		
Male homosexual/bisexual contact; IV drug use	8,452	(6)
Male homosexual/bisexual contact; hemophilia	32	(0)
Male homosexual/bisexual contact; heterosexual contact	1,641	(1)
Male homosexual/bisexual contact; receipt of transfusion	1,513	(1)
IV drug use; hemophilia	32	(0)
IV drug use; heterosexual contact	3,297	(2)
IV drug use; receipt of transfusion	652	(0)
Hemophilia; heterosexual contact	7	(0)
Hemophilia; receipt of transfusion	474	(0)
Heterosexual contact; receipt of transfusion	329	(0)
Male homosexual/bisexual contact; IV drug use; hemophilia	7	(0)
Male homosexual/bisexual contact; IV drug use; heterosexual contact	624	(0)
Male homosexual/bisexual contact; IV drug use; receipt of transfusion	247	(0)
Male homosexual/bisexual contact; hemophilia; heterosexual contact	3	(0)
Male homosexual/bisexual contact; hemophilia; receipt of transfusion	16	(0)
Male homosexual/bisexual contact; heterosexual contact; receipt of transfusion	86	(0)
IV drug use; hemophilia; heterosexual contact	3	(0)
IV drug use; hemophilia; receipt of transfusion	15	(0)
IV drug use; heterosexual contact; receipt of transfusion	187	(0)
Hemophilia; heterosexual contact; receipt of transfusion	11	(0)
Male homosexual/bisexual contact; IV drug use; hemophilia; receipt of transfusion	7	(0)
Male homosexual/bisexual contact; IV drug use; heterosexual contact; receipt of transfusion	33	(0)
IV drug use; hemophilia; heterosexual contact; receipt of transfusion	3	(0)
Multiple modes of exposure subtotal	**17,671**	**(13)**
Total	**137,385**	**(100)**

the effects of HIV difficult. However, Kestler and co-workers (1990) report the induction of AIDS in rhesus monkeys via a cloned Simian Immunodeficiency Virus. Such advances in laboratory modeling of the disease will permit significantly more control over the variables that affect progression of HIV infection to AIDS.

Nearly all the data that exist is based on self-reported data of HIV infected individuals and their partners. People do not always tell the truth about themselves. Consider how many people do not even give their real weight for their driver's license. Similar deceptions may occur when individuals are asked by government representatives to provide information about their sexual or drug-using behaviors, which may be illegal. Deception may be a form of self-protection.

TRANSMISSION VIA INFECTED BLOOD

Infected Blood

Early research on the presence of HIV in the blood suggested that most infected individuals develop antibodies within 6 to 12 weeks, although some might take considerably longer. Knowing whether one is actually infected with HIV is crucial, especially since therapy (i.e., AZT) is now available to treat those in the early stages of HIV infection. Consequently, much emphasis has been placed on the development of tests that are both highly specific and highly sensitive. Four results can occur when a blood test is taken; these are depicted in Figure 4.1 (Lilienfeld and Lilienfeld, 1980).

True positives result when a person is infected with HIV and the test accurately reports that result. False positives occur when a person is not infected with the virus but the test mistakenly classifies the person as being positive. True negatives occur when a person does not have the virus and the test shows that the person does not have the virus. False negatives occur when a person has the virus but the test report concludes that the person does not have the virus.

False positives and false negatives are not always easily determined. The concern with HIV antibody results that are false positive is that the patient will be mistakenly told that he or she has HIV. Some people have committed suicide after being given such a report. The concern with false negative results is that the patient who is infected will be told that he or she is not infected. Unless the patient adopts safer sex practices, he or she may pass the virus on to others.

The ultimate goal of HIV testing is to increase the probability that true positives and true negatives are accurately identified and to minimize the number of false positives and false negatives.

There are two measures for the accuracy of tests such as the HIV antibody test: sensitivity and specificity. The sensitivity of the HIV antibody test is the percentage of those who have HIV antibodies and are so indicated by the test. Mathematically, this is shown as

$$\text{Sensitivity (\%)} = \frac{A}{A + C} \times 100$$

In other words, sensitivity is the number of true positives divided by all of those with HIV antibodies (true positives plus false negatives.) Unfortunately, it may not be possible to know the actual number of false negatives.

Specificity is the percentage of those who do not have HIV antibodies and are so indicated by the test. Mathematically, this is shown as

$$\text{Specificity (\%)} = \frac{D}{B + D} \times 100$$

In other words, specificity is the number of true negatives divided by all of those who do not have HIV antibodies (true negatives and false positives).

Research (Horsburgh et al., 1989) suggests that at least half of the individuals who are infected with HIV will seroconvert in about two months, while 95 percent of all people infected with HIV are likely to have detectable antibodies

Test Results	HIV Antibodies	
	Present	Absent
Positive	True positive (A)	False positive (B)
Negative	False negative (C)	True negative (D)

• FIGURE 4.1   HIV test results

Box 4

How Accurate Are the HIV Antibody Tests?

The accuracy of HIV antibody tests has significant implications for preoperative screening of surgery patients (Hagen, Meyer, and Pauker, 1988), premarital screening for HIV infection (Cleary et al., 1987), physician counseling of patients (Sherer, 1988), estimating the number of Americans who are infected with HIV (Booth, 1987b), testing for life and health insurance, and other health-related issues. Although the tests are reliable if done appropriately, they cannot detect antibodies where none exist. There are other tests that involve culturing blood samples and trying to grow HIV (if it is already in the blood), but such tests are very complex, very expensive, and probably not useful for mass testing purposes at present.

Reliability vs. accuracy

Although the tests for infection with HIV are considered to be very reliable if competently done, there are some troubling statistical implications if wide-scale HIV antibody testing is considered. Assume that the tests are 99 percent reliable, and only 1 percent unreliable. If a person tests HIV positive, what is the likelihood that the person is truly infected with HIV? How accurate is that decision? Most people would answer 99 percent (or even 100%), but they would be wrong.

Following the description by Root-Bernstein (1990), assume that there are 1 million people who are infected with HIV, as estimated by the Centers for Disease Control. Of the roughly 250 million Americans, 249 million would not be infected with the virus. Assume furthermore that the HIV tests are 99 percent reliable and 1 percent unreliable, and that all 250 million

Americans are to be tested for the presence of HIV antibodies. What would be the results?

For the 1 million who are infected with the virus, the tests would correctly identify 990,000 of them (99% of 1 million) as being infected—true positives—and would incorrectly identify 10,000 (1% of 1 million) as not being infected—false negatives. For the 249 million Americans who are not infected, the tests would correctly identify 246.51 million (99% of 249 million) as not having HIV antibodies—true negatives—but would incorrectly identify 2.49 million (1% of 249 million) as having the antibodies—false positives.

In all, national testing would identify 3.48 million Americans as being HIV positive, of which only 990,000 would be true positives. In other words, there would be 3.5 false positives for every true positive. The probability that any person testing positive has been correctly identified as being infected is 990,000 divided by 3,480,000, or 28 percent! Although the tests may be highly reliable, they may still lead to inaccurate decisions. As described by Root-Bernstein, if the number of people infected with HIV is small, even a test that is highly reliable will produce more false positives than true positives if random testing is done on a large number of people.

Can accuracy be increased?

On the other hand, when a larger percentage of the population is infected (perhaps 10%) or if the test is administered only to those people who have good reason to believe that they are infected, the predictive value of the test increases drastically. For example, if there were 10 million HIV infected Americans instead of 1 million, the same testing procedure would identify 9.9 million true positives (99% of 10 million), 100,000 false negatives (1% of 10 million), 237.6 million true negatives (99% of 240 million), and 2.4 million false positives (1% of 240 million). Of the 12.4 million total positives, 80 percent would be true positives, and there would be four true positives for every false positive. The reliability of the test hasn't changed, but the accuracy of the results has improved drastically.

If HIV antibody tests were given only to those individuals who had reason to believe that they were infected (i.e., based on thorough pretest counseling), so that only the 1 million HIV-infected individuals were actually tested, the accuracy of the test would be very high indeed. The conclusions of such statistical analyses have implications for virtually every area related to AIDS, especially when random testing of large segments of the uninfected population is an issue.

within six months of infection, although some rare individuals may take longer than that (Imagawa et al., 1989).

IV drug use and needle sharing

Although not perceived as a serious problem at the beginning of the AIDS epidemic, as more and more information was gathered regarding the transmission of HIV, it became clear to researchers in major urban areas that intravenous drug users would have a major role in this disease. More and more AIDS cases are being reported in IV drug users; however, the real risk is not that one uses IV drugs, but that one shares needles, syringes, and other injection equipment with an infected user.

A study from New York City estimates that between 55 and 60 percent of IV drug users are currently infected with HIV (DesJarlais et al., 1989)—perhaps 100,000 in all. Typically, the virus is spread from one IV drug user to another during ritualistic activities in "shooting galleries," where needles and syringes ("the works") can be purchased or rented. As part of the drug subculture, the person using "the works" may draw a small amount of his or her own blood into the syringe prior to injecting a drug. After the drug is injected, a small amount of blood may remain in the syringe. The next user is likely to inject that blood

into the bloodstream when the works are passed to him or her.

For example, a person dependent on heroin may need to inject heroin 4 to 6 times per day, 28 to 42 times per week, 120 to 180 times per month, 1,500 to 2,200 times per year, so the opportunities for coming into direct contact with HIV/infected blood are considerable. The IV drug user dissolves a small amount of a drug in water and then heats the mixture in a bottlecap or spoon (a "cooker"). A small piece of cotton or a cigarette filter is added to the mixture, and the drug is drawn into the needle and syringe through the filter. The user then pierces a vein with the needle and draws back on the plunger of the syringe to ensure that a vein has indeed been penetrated. A small amount of blood is now mixed with the drug, and the entire mixture is injected. To make sure that all of the drug is out of the syringe, the plunger is pulled back again, and the contents are reinjected. The entire "works" are rinsed in water and used by the next person. At this point, the needle, the syringe, the cooker, cotton, and the water are all possibly contaminated with HIV.

Transfusions

There was considerable concern about the safety of the blood supply throughout the world when it became clear that HIV could be transmitted in blood.

HIV infected blood donors posed a particular risk for people with hemophilia and for people who required blood transfusions for surgery.

Not until March 1985 was a blood test made commercially available for testing the blood supply, although there had been some cases of HIV transmitted via infected blood before that time. Presently, all blood is screened for the presence of HIV antibodies, and all infected blood is discarded.

Because all blood donations are tested, the blood supply is considered to be extremely safe. (Other infectious diseases have been screened out as well). Nevertheless, there is that period of time (the "silent infection period") when a person newly infected with HIV has not yet developed antibodies that will be detected through routine HIV antibody screening. In such rare cases, it is possible that some HIV infected blood may still be used for transfusions.

Perinatal transmission

HIV can be transmitted from an infected pregnant woman to her child both before and after birth (CDC, 1986; Sprecher-Goldberger, 1988). A survey of newborns in New York State (Novick et al., 1989) found that the overall HIV seroprevalence rate was 0.66 percent with the highest seroprevalence rate (1.25 percent) in New York City among mothers 20 to 40 years of age who were black or Hispanic. The highest rates (over 2%) were in those areas with high rates of drug use.

MISINFORMATION ABOUT MOSQUITOES

About 27 percent of the adult American population believes that HIV can be transmitted via mosquitoes or other insects; another 21 percent doesn't know whether that is possible or not (Hardy, 1990). After all, if HIV can be transmitted from one IV drug user to another via contaminated needles or syringes, why can't it be transmitted from an infected person to an uninfected person via a contaminated mosquito? This was the argument that some people have used to explain the many cases of AIDS in Belle Glade, Florida (Booth, 1987a). After a thorough analysis of AIDS cases in Belle Glade, however, researchers concluded that the high rate of AIDS was the result of HIV transmission through sexual contact and intravenous drug use (Castro et al., 1988). Moreover, if HIV were spread by mosquitoes or other insects, there should be a wider range of HIV infection among the entire population, since mosquitoes don't bite only gay men or intravenous drug users. It would be especially high in children aged 5 to 15, since this age is frequently bitten by mosquitoes during outside play activities; however, this age group is responsible for less than 2 percent of all AIDS cases. Thus, the observation that HIV is not being seen equally throughout the population further argues against its spread via insects.

Perhaps one reason for the persistent belief in insect transmission is that it seems more acceptable to some people to contract a disease via mosquitoes than through sexual or drug-using behaviors. Some people at risk for contracting HIV may hope that mosquito transmission is a reality; then they can deny their own risky behaviors.

RISKS FROM HOUSEHOLD TRANSMISSION

Research has consistently shown that HIV is not transmitted through casual contact. Household studies have found that sexual contact is the only risk between infected and uninfected persons living in a household. A variety of studies have found that living in the same home with someone who had AIDS or AIDS/Related Complex did not put one at a higher risk for contracting HIV. Most often, spouses were infected, but children were not (Redfield et al., 1985). Despite such findings, the public continues to believe that HIV can be transmitted casually. Despite believing in transmission by working near someone with the AIDS virus

(11%), using public toilets (18%), being coughed on or sneezed on (27%), by mosquitoes or other insects (27%), and so on, 78 percent of the public believes that they have no chance of getting the virus, 18 percent rated their chances as low, 2 percent as medium, 2 percent didn't know, and 0 percent thought there was a high chance that they already had the virus (Hardy, 1990).

As far as AIDS is concerned, perceived risks are not equivalent to actual risks.

What about tears and saliva?

Very small amounts of HIV have been found in both tears and saliva (CDC, 1985; Groopman et al., 1984; Marwick, 1985). However, as pointed out by the CDC, there has been no evidence that the virus has been transmitted by either tears or saliva. To be transmitted, the virus that is in the tears or saliva of an infected person must somehow come into direct physical contact with the white blood cells of an uninfected person in sufficient quantities to produce an HIV infection. In the CDC report on isolation of the virus from tears, the CDC noted that the tears from seven AIDS patients were analyzed; one patient had the virus in her tears, three other patients showed equivocal results, and three patients were culture negative for the virus.

A possible role for circumcision?

One puzzle regarding AIDS is the different patterns of HIV transmission found in different parts of the world. For example, in the United States, homosexual behaviors seem to be the primary way HIV is spread; in Africa, heterosexual behaviors are the main way that HIV is transmitted. One possible explanation for these apparent differences in HIV transmission is the role of circumcision (Marx, 1989). Preliminary data suggest that being uncircumcised increased the likelihood of HIV transmission by a factor of 5 to 8 times, thereby increas-

ing the possibility of heterosexual transmission in those countries in which a large number of men are not circumcised. Uncircumcised men may be more likely than circumcised men to become infected with HIV from an infected female partner. However, the importance of circumcision in HIV transmission is mostly speculation at this time. Further studies will be needed to determine whether it is a significant cofactor in the transmission of HIV.

SOME METHOLOGICAL CONCERNS

What is the denominator?

Much remains to be learned about some specifics of HIV transmission. For example, it is not yet known how much of the virus is necessary for a person to become infected, or whether a person can successfully fight off a small infection with HIV. Nor is it known how many exposures are necessary for infection to occur. Single case histories often show up in the scientific literature, but a single case may or may not be significant. One question that must be asked when single case histories are reported is "What is the denominator"—in other words, one case (the numerator) out of how many possible cases (the denominator)? This disease, because of its association with sex and death, and with its high fatality rate, has an enormous potential to cause public hysteria. Educators must be particularly careful not to overemphasize the importance of anomalies in the data.

Possible contradictions

Listing all of the different behaviors associated with HIV transmission can create extreme fear, or even terror, in children and adolescents. Such fears may be counterproductive. For example, Turner, Miller, and Moses (1989) note that, although appropriate use of condoms has been recommended as an effective barrier method for HIV, some have argued that, because condoms do not provide perfect protection, they should not be recommended. As a result, some young people may believe that if condoms don't work perfectly, why use them at all? The result may be unprotected sex and a greater likelihood of contracting HIV.

What about the undetermined cases?

The fact that the route of transmission for some cases (about 3% of the total) is not identified has led some persons to speculate that the virus is being transmitted in some new ways. A closer reading of the literature shows that CDC has listed as "undetermined" those "patients on whom risk information is incomplete (due to death, refusal to be interviewed or loss to follow-up), patients still under investigation, men reported only to have had heterosexual contact with a prostitute, and interviewed patients for whom no specific risk was identified; also includes one health-care worker who seroconverted to HIV and developed AIDS after documented needlestick to blood" (*CDC Weekly Surveillance Report,* 2/20/89).

Obviously many people are reluctant to discuss their sexual or drug-using behaviors; nevertheless, further investigations have often identified the actual route of exposure. HIV is being transmitted in the same ways that it was in 1980. No new routes have been identified.

Validity and reliability

People do not always tell the truth about their sexual experiences. Thus, researchers must make every effort to obtain valid and reliable data from those individuals who are interviewed about their sexual activities. A review of much of the literature on HIV infection clearly shows that fundamental issues of validity and reliability have not been addressed in most of the published studies. Different researchers use different questions to measure the same phenomena; unfortunately, such questions may have considerable face validity (e.g., they look like they're measuring a particular phenomenon), but they lack statistical validation. Such inconsistencies among research projects make useful comparisons difficult if not impossible.

Correlation vs. cause and effect

Assumed in much of the AIDS literature is that if someone tests HIV antibody positive or is diagnosed as having AIDS and admits to a particular risk behavior (e.g., having sex with another man), the high-risk behavior actually transmitted the HIV. What may be a statistical correlation may not necessarily be a cause-and-effect relationship. Many factors might account for such spurious correlations (Hochhauser, 1979) including subject characteristics, researcher variables, and sampling biases.

1. **Subject characteristics** include expectations, attitudes, and beliefs. For example, there may be a tendency to respond in a socially acceptable fashion, reporting fewer sexual contacts or denying homosexual activities. As more and more research is done on AIDS and as findings are publicized in the media, behavioral expectations may be shaped less by personal experience and more by subtle societal pressures. For example, if researchers show a reduction in the number of sexual partners, people may *report* that they have reduced the number of sexual partners as a response to such findings, when in fact their actual behaviors may not have changed at all. It might be very difficult for a person to admit to being very sexually active when researchers are showing decreases in sexual activity.

No doubt there are differences between subjects who agree to be interviewed and those who refuse to be interviewed. Cultural and religious traditions may make it impossible for some people to tell a researcher about his or her sexual practices.

2. **Researcher variables** include the interviewer's gender, ethnic background, age, personality, experience, and attitude. The researcher may unconsciously cue the subject to respond in a particular way; thus, different researchers may get different results for the same type of project.

3. **Sampling biases** include the source of data (e.g., relying on data from a relatively small sample of gay men in San Francisco), random vs. nonrandom selection of participants, and sampling limitations based on the exclusive use of volunteers.

Many researchers have identified limitations in the interpretation of data. Barber (1976) has identified 10 major pitfalls in human research, including loose procedures, investigator fudging of data, personal attributes of the researcher, and misrecording of data. Rosenthal and Rosnow (1969) have described some unique characteristics of the volunteer subject (including higher educational level, occupational status, and need for approval, and lower authoritarianism). Diaconis (1981) has described some of the "magical" thinking found in the analysis of scientific data (e.g., seeing patterns in the data where none exist). What is known about AIDS and HIV transmission is based on the quality of the data that is collected and the quality of the researchers who interpret the data. Science may be based on objectivity, but scientists' objectivity may be colored by their own subjective characteristics. Santayana's statement, "Those who do not learn from the past are condemned to repeat it," may unfortunately sum up much of what is being done in AIDS research, education, and prevention.

SUMMARY

The Human Immunodeficiency Virus (HIV) is transmitted only in several well-known ways: sexual transmission via semen and vaginal secretions, blood transmission via needle sharing among IV drug users or blood transfusions, or perinatal transmission from an infected mother to child. Sexual transmission can occur from male-to-male, from male-to-female, from female-to-male, and possibly from female-to-female. Sharing of needles, syringes, cookers, cotton filters, and rinse water can facilitate HIV transmission among IV drug users. Once infected in this way, they can transmit the virus to their sexual partners through unsafe sex practices.

Nearly half of the American population is uncertain about whether HIV can be transmitted by mosquitoes or other insects. Transmission by this means has not been found; less than 2 percent of all AIDS cases occur in children and young adolescents, who are frequently bitten by mosquitoes during outside play activities. The fact that AIDS is not being reported equally throughout the population further suggests that HIV is not being spread by insects.

Given the sensitive, personal nature of sexual and drug-using behaviors, we must be aware of research limitations that will affect our knowledge of those behaviors that transmit HIV. Poor validity and reliability of survey questions, the tendency of subjects to respond in a socially desirable way, and the unique characteristics of people who volunteer for research studies suggest that our knowledge of the behavioral factors associated with this disease is still very incomplete.

REFERENCES

Bacchetti, D., and Moss, A. R. (1989) Incubation period of AIDS in San Francisco. *Nature,* 338 (6212), 251–253.

Barber, T. X. (1976) *Pitfalls in human research: Ten pivotal points.* New York: Pergamon Press.

Booth, W. (1987a) AIDS and insects. *Science,* 237, 355–356.

Booth, W. (1987b) A frustrating glimpse of the true AIDS epidemic. *Science,* 238, 747.

Cameron, D. W., Simonsen, J. N., D'Costa, L. J., et al. (1989) Female and male transmission of Human Immunodeficiency Virus Type 1: Risk factors for seroconversion in men. *Lancet,* August 19, 1989, pp. 403–407.

Castro, K. G., Lieb, S., Jaffe, H. W., Narkunas, J. P., et al. (1988) Transmission of HIV in Belle Glade, Florida: Lessons for other communities in the United States. *Science,* 239, 193–197.

CDC (1985) *Morbidity and Mortality Weekly Report.* Recommendations for preventing possible transmission of HTLV-III/LAV virus from tears. 34 (34), 533–534.

CDC (1986) *Morbidity and Mortality Weekly Report.* Recommendations for assisting in the prevention of perinatal transmission of HTLV-III/LAV and Acquired Immunodeficiency Syndrome. 34 (48), 721–732.

CDC (1987) *Morbidity and Mortality Weekly Report.* Update: AIDS in the United States. 36 (31), 522–526.

CDC (1990) *HIV/AIDS Surveillance Report.* May 1990: 1–22. Atlanta, GA: Centers for Disease Control.

Cleary, P. D., Barry, M. J., Mayer, K. H., et al. (1987) Compulsory premarital screening for the human immunodeficiency virus. *Journal of the American Medical Association,* 258 (13), 1757–1762.

Curran, J. W., Jaffe, W., Hardy, A. M., Morgan, W. M., Selik, R. M., and Dondero, T. J. (1988) Epidemiology of HIV infection and AIDS in the United States. *Science,* 239, 610–616.

DesJarlais, D. C., Friedman, S. R., Novick, D. M., Sotheran, J. L., Thomas, P., et al. (1989). HIV-1 infection among intravenous drug users in Manhattan, New York City, from 1977 through 1987. *Journal of the American Medical Association,* 261 (7), 1008–1012.

Diaconis, P. (1981) Magical thinking in the analysis of scientific data. In T. Sebeok, and R. Rosenthal, eds. *The Clever Hans phenomenon: Communication with horses, whales, apes and people.* New York: Annals of the New York Academy of Science, Vol. 364.

Fumento, M. (1987) AIDS: Are heterosexuals at risk? *Commentary,* November 1987, 21–27.

Groopman, J. E., Salahuddin, S. Z., Sarngadharan, M. G., et al. (1984) HTLV-III in saliva of people with AIDS-related complex and healthy homosexual men at risk for AIDS. *Science,* 226, 447–449.

Hagen, M., Meyer, K. B., and Pauker, S. G. (1988) Routine preoperative screening for HIV. *Journal of the American Medical Association,* 259 (9), 1357–1359.

Hardy, A. M. (1990) AIDS knowledge and attitudes for October–December 1989. *Advance Data from Vital and Health Statistics from the National Health Interview Survey.* No. 186. DHHS Pub. No. (PHS) 90–1250. Hyattsville, MD: National Center for Health Statistics.

Haseltine, W. (1989) Silent HIV infections. *New England Journal of Medicine,* 320 (22), 1487–1489.

Haverkos, H. W., and Edelman, R. (1988) The epidemiology of acquired immunodeficiency syndrome among heterosexuals. *Journal of the American Medical Association,* 260 (13), 1922–1929.

Hochhauser, M. (1979) Bias in drug abuse survey research. *International Journal of the Addictions,* 14 (5), 675–687.

Horsburgh, C. R., Yin Ou, C., Jason, J., et al. (1989) Duration of human immunodeficiency virus infection before detection of antibody. *Lancet,* September 16, 1989, 637–640.

Imagawa, D. T., Lee, M. H., Wolinsky, S. M., et al. *New England Journal of Medicine,* 320 (22), 1458–1462.

Institute of Medicine, 1988. *Confronting AIDS: Update 1988.* Washington, DC: National Academy Press.

Janis, I. L. (1984) The patient as decision maker. In W. D. Gentry, ed. *Handbook of behavioral medicine.* New York: Guilford Press.

Jobs, R. F. (1988) Effective and ineffective use of fear in health promotion campaigns. *American Journal of Public Health,* 78 (2), 163–167.

Kestler, H., Kodama, T., Ringler, et al. (1990) Induction of AIDS in rhesus monkeys by molecularly cloned Simian Immunodeficiency Virus. *Science,* 248, 1109–1111.

Lilienfeld, A. M., and Lilienfeld, D. E. (1980) *Foundations of epidemiology* (2nd ed.). New York: Oxford University Press.

Marwick, C. (1985) AIDS-associated virus yields data to intensifying scientific study. *Journal of the American Medical Association,* 254, 2865–2870.

Marx, J. L. (1989) Circumcision may protect against the AIDS virus. *Science,* 245, 470–471.

Novick, L. F., Berns, D., Stricof, R., Stevens, R., Pass, K., and Wethers, J. (1989) HIV seroprevalence in newborns in New York State. *Journal of the American Medical Association,* 261 (12), 1745–1750.

Padian, N. S. (1987) Heterosexual transmission of acquired immunodeficiency syndrome: International perspectives and national projections. *Reviews of Infectious Diseases,* 9 (5), 947–960.

Piot, P., Plummer, F. A., Mhalu, F. S., et al. (1988) AIDS: An international perspective. *Science,* 239, 573–579.

Redfield, R. R., Markham, P. D., Salahuddin, S. Z., et al. (1985) Frequent transmission of HTLV-III among spouses of patients with AIDS-related complex and AIDS. *Journal of the American Medical Association,* 253, 1571–1573.

Root-Bernstein, R. S. (1990) Misleading reliability. *The Sciences.* March/April, pp. 6–8.

Rosenthal, R., and Rosnow, R. L. (1969) The volunteer subject. In R. Rosenthal and R. L. Rosnow (1969) *Artifact in behavioral research.* New York: Academic Press.

Sherer, R. (1988) Physician use of the HIV antibody test. *Journal of the American Medical Association,* 259 (2), 264–265.

Spitzer, P. G., and Weiner, N. J. (1989) Transmission of HIV infection from a woman to a man by oral sex. *New England Journal of Medicine,* 320, 251.

Sprecher-Goldberger, S. (1988) Isolation of HIV virus from cell-free breast milk of seropositive mothers. In R. F. Schinazi and A. J. Nahmias, eds. *AIDS in children, adolescents & heterosexual adults: An interdisciplinary approach to prevention.* New York: Elsevier.

Turner, C. F., Miller, H. G., and Moses, L. E., Eds. (1989) *AIDS: Sexual behavior and intravenous drug use.* Washington, DC: National Academy Press.

5 Medical Aspects of AIDS

Hope springs eternal in the human breast.
ALEXANDER POPE

Much of what is known about AIDS is based on those individuals who have been diagnosed and treated for this disease, probably less than 15 percent of the total number of people infected with HIV. Given that AIDS is a newly identified disease, it should not be too surprising that methods for diagnosing and treating AIDS have been constantly evolving.

Human Immunodeficiency Virus—a retrovirus

When a person becomes infected with HIV, the virus attaches itself to a protein called an antigen (the T4) on the surface of a cell. Many cells, including T-helper lymphocyte cells (an important part of the immune system), carry this T4 antigen. After attaching to its target cell, the virus enters the cell and sheds its protein coat, exposing the viral RNA inside. The enzyme reverse transcriptase then converts viral RNA to viral DNA, which becomes part of the target cell's DNA. Viral DNA then instructs the cell to make new virus particles, which leave to infect other cells. Thus, HIV has been identified as a "retrovirus," a type of virus that contains the genetic materials RNA plus the ability to copy this RNA into an infected cell. As HIV replicates within the T-helper cells, for example, the infected cells are slowly destroyed. If enough of the T-helper cells are destroyed, the immune system itself becomes weaker and weaker, and the HIV infected individual becomes more and more susceptible to opportunistic infections that are normally fought off. In a similar fashion, HIV may penetrate cells in the central nervous system (brain and spinal cord), and by inserting genetic material into the cells within that system, slowly destroy it, leading to brain damage and dementia. Figure 5.1 depicts how the immune system works, and how drugs can fight off the Human Immunodeficiency Virus.

Diagnostic criteria

Diagnostic criteria for AIDS have changed; there were the "old" criteria (before the HIV antibody test was developed) for AIDS, the "recent" criteria (after the HIV antibody test was available), and the "new" criteria (CDC, 1987b). The diagnostic criteria were changed because researchers believed that many people with AIDS were not being accurately diagnosed under the old criteria. For example, one new diagnostic criterion for AIDS is the HIV wasting syndrome—the loss of substantial amounts of weight in a relatively short time. The symptom was seen quite frequently in some Central African AIDS patients (where it was called "slim disease"), but did not become part of the U.S. diagnostic criteria until the late 1980s. Another new diagnostic criterion is HIV encephalopathy (or AIDS dementia); this refers to the psychological problems (such as memory loss) that occur in some AIDS patients.

Although such changes are necessary because of our continually increasing understanding of AIDS, they do present some significant statistical problems. Before 1987, many people may have actually died of AIDS but had not been counted as an AIDS case or death because their symptoms did not meet the earlier criteria. Thus, the actual number of AIDS cases in the United States is no doubt considerably higher than the official reports based on the old or new diagnostic criteria. Changing the diagnostic criteria in the middle of an epidemic makes it very difficult to accurately observe the course of the epidemic over time. As our understanding increases, it would not be surprising to see the diagnostic criteria modified yet again.

Media reports have not often shown the wide range of illnesses that can be found in people with AIDS; despite the presence of *Pneumocystic carinii pneumonia* (PCP) and Kaposi's sarcoma in many AIDS patients, a rather wide variety of diseases can be used to diagnose AIDS. For example, Table 5.1 shows AIDS cases by initial diagnosis in San Francisco from 1981 through June 1990. Although PCP and Kaposi's sarcoma account for about 71 percent of the old case definition for AIDS, about 13 other diseases have been used to diagnose AIDS.

Table 5.2 shows the AIDS cases by initial diagnosis in San Francisco using the new case definition; in addition to the 15 old criteria for AIDS, 16 new criteria are listed. We are all exposed to some of these diseases on a daily basis if we have pets such as parrots or cats. But we do not become ill, because our immune system is not suppressed. A person who is HIV infected often becomes ill when exposed to these same diseases, because his or her immune system has been compromised and is simply unable to fight off these infections.

About 13 percent of the AIDS cases in San Francisco were diagnosed using the new case definition, suggesting that the old case definition may have underdiagnosed and underreported AIDS cases within the city. Had the new diagnostic criteria not been in place, it is possible that the 1,100 AIDS cases reported under the new criteria would not have been reported under the old criteria. If such figures can be projected nationally (which may or may not be appropriate), the national number of reported AIDS cases from 1981 through 1987 may have been underestimated by about 10 percent. In those geographic areas with relatively few AIDS cases, some physicians may not have the diagnostic expertise to identify AIDS, thus reducing the reported number of cases even more.

HOW DRUGS FIGHT AIDS

How the immune system works

1. A virus invades the body.

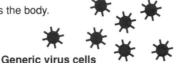

Generic virus cells

Macrophage cell

2. An early line of defense is a macrophage, a white blood cell that engulfs a virus and displays a portion of it for contact with a T4 cell. T4 cells activate the immune system's defenses.

Virus cells

3. Macrophages also stimulate the T4 cells to reproduce themselves into thousands of cells to fight the virus.

Macrophage cell

T4 cell

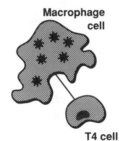

T4 cell

4. When T4 cells encounter the virus, they send out chemical signals to other types of white blood cells, known as B cells and "killer" T8 cells.

"Killer" T8 cell

5. Killer T8 cells destroy infected cells with the help of some T4 cells.

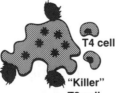

T4 cell

"Killer" T8 cell

6. T4 cells send chemical signals to B cells causing them to reproduce and divide into two groups: plasma B cells and memory B cells. Plasma cells produce antibodies that disable invaders. Memory cells speed up immune response if virus is encountered again.

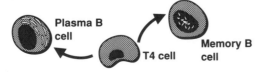

Plasma B cell   **T4 cell**   **Memory B cell**

How drugs fight HIV

1. HIV invades body.

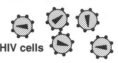

HIV cells

2. Macrophage engulfs virus. An HIV cell attaches to a T4 cell. Other HIV cells remain in the macrophage. *Treatment: A drug called Soluble CD4 can block the infection of T4 cells.*

Macrophages remain chronically infected and do not die. *Possible treatment: A new drug called GLQ223 may kill HIV-infected macrophages.*

Macrophage cell

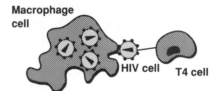

HIV cell   **T4 cell**

RNA

T4 cell

3. After the HIV cell attaches to the T4 cell, the HIV cell sheds its coating and its genetic material (RNA) enters the T4 cell.

4. The viral RNA is changed into DNA with direction from an enzyme called reverse transcriptase. *Treatment: AZT slows reverse transcriptase.*

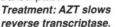

T4 cell

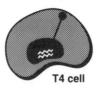

5. Viral DNA is incorporated permanently into the cell's genes. The virus is duplicated by the cell's own protein factories, or ribosomes.

T4 cell

6. New HIV cells bud from the surface of infected cells. T4 cells eventually die. *Possible treatment: GLQ223 blocks replication in Infected T4 cells.*

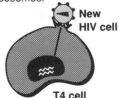

New HIV cell

T4 cell

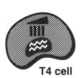

• FIGURE 5.1   How drugs fight AIDS. Reprinted with permission from *The San Francisco Examiner* © 1990 *San Francisco Examiner.*

TABLE 5.1   Acquired Immunodeficiency Syndrome (AIDS) Monthly Surveillance Report Summary of Cases Meeting the Old CDC Surveillance Definition in San Francisco Cases Reported Through June 30, 1990

Initial Diagnosis (old definition)[a]	Number	Percent
Pneumocystis carinii pneumonia; definitive	4,205	48.0
Kaposi's sarcoma, <60 yrs.; definitive	2,007	22.9
Non-Hodgkins lymphoma, HIV+; definitive	307	3.5
Cryptococcosis, extrapulmonary; definitive	272	3.1
Mycobacterium avium complex or M. Kansasii disease, disseminated; definitive	198	2.3
Candidiasis of the esophagus, trachea, bronchi, or lungs; definitive	193	2.2
Cryptosporidiosis, chronic intestinal; definitive	130	1.5
Cytomegalovirus disease; definitive	130	1.5
Herpes simplex virus infection; definitive	57	0.7
Toxoplasmosis of the brain; definitive	56	0.6
Progressive multifocal leukoencephalopathy; definitive	40	0.5
Primary lymphoma of the brain, <60 yrs.; definitive	23	0.3
Isosporiasis, chronic intestinal, HIV+; definitive	15	0.2
Histoplasmosis; disseminated; HIV+; definitive	14	0.2
Lymphoid interstitial pneumonia/pulmonary lymphoid hyperplasia, <13 yrs.; definitive	4	0.0
Subtotal (old definition)	**7,651**	**87.4**

Source: *S. F. AIDS incidence and mortality by month of diagnosis or death, 1980–1990.* San Francisco Department of Public Health, July 1990.
[a] AIDS Cases by initial diagnosis, San Francisco, 1981–1990.

TABLE 5.2   Acquired Immunodeficiency Syndrome (AIDS) Monthly Surveillance Report Summary of Cases Meeting the New CDC Surveillance Definition in San Francisco Cases Reported Through June 30, 1990

Initial Diagnosis (new definition)[a]	Number	Percent
HIV wasting syndrome; definitive	268	3.1
Pneumocystis carinii pneumonia; presumptive	225	2.6
HIV encephalopathy ("AIDS dementia"); definitive	218	2.5
Toxoplasmosis of the brain; presumptive	118	1.3
M. tuberculosis, extrapulmonary; definitive	68	0.8
Kaposi's sarcoma; presumptive	66	0.8
Cytomegalovirus retinitis with loss of vision; presumptive	58	0.7
Candidiasis of the esophagus; presumptive	46	0.5
Mycobacterial disease (not *M. Tuberculosis*), disseminated; definitive	11	0.1
Mycobacterial disease (unspecified species), disseminated; presumptive	6	0.1
Pneumocystis carinii pneumonia, HIV–	6	0.1
Salmonella septicemia, recurrent; definitive	5	0.1
Coccidioidomycosis, disseminated; definitive	4	0.0
Lymphoid interstitial pneumonia/pulmonary lymphoid hyperplasia, <13 yrs.; presumptive	2	0.0
Bacterial infections, recurrent, <13 yrs.; definitive	1	0.0
Primary lymphoma of the brain, any age; definitive	1	0.0
Subtotal (new definition)	**1,103**	**12.6**
Total	**8,754**	**100.0**

Source: *S. F. AIDS incidence and mortality by month of diagnosis of death, 1980–1991.* San Francisco Department of Public Health, July 1990.
[a] AIDS Cases by initial diagnosis, San Francisco, 1981–1990.

e CDC change in the case definition of AIDS has had a substantial impact on the number of AIDS cases diagnosed and reported. Selik and co-workers (1990) reviewed nearly 30,000 AIDS cases from the time of the case definition change through 1988. They found that about 28 percent of those cases met the new criteria only; moreover, the characteristics of some AIDS cases have changed. The risk category "heterosexual IV drug abuser" accounted for 18 percent of the cases under the old criteria, but 35 percent of the cases under the new criteria. Changing the definition of AIDS is changing our view of this disease.

Presumptive diagnosis

A diagnosis of AIDS can be made on the basis of certain clinical signs, such as PCP or Kaposi's sarcoma. Surprisingly, a person need not necessarily test positive for HIV antibodies to be diagnosed as having AIDS; the presence of certain opportunistic infections may be sufficient for an AIDS diagnosis to be made. Although some people believe that there is an "AIDS test," it is possible to be diagnosed with AIDS even though one is HIV antibody negative. A person can pass the HIV antibody test and still have AIDS. San Francisco reported AIDS cases of two patients—based on presumptive criteria—who were HIV negative but who had PCP. Figure 5.2 is a flow diagram for the revised CDC case definition of AIDS (1987), illustrating that a positive diagnosis for AIDS can be made if laboratory results are positive, negative, or unknown/inconclusive.

DEVELOPING TREATMENTS

Although many drugs are being developed to treat people with AIDS, no drug has yet been developed that can cure AIDS. AZT (also known as Zidovudine or Retrovir) is currently the most widely used drug for treating AIDS patients; it appears to be able to extend the lifespan of people who use

it by several years. However, AZT does have serious side effects and it is expensive ($2,000–$6,000 per year without the necessary blood tests that accompany it). Although Burroughs-Welcome, the manufacturer of AZT, lowered the cost of the drug in the fall of 1989, it may still be prohibitively expensive for many AIDS patients. Although originally developed for patients with AIDS, AZT is being used prophylactically for those people who have tested HIV positive but who have not developed any opportunistic infections. By administering AZT as soon as possible after a person becomes infected, physicians hope that the drug will help keep the immune system strong and slow the rate at which it deteriorates.

People with AIDS die not only from the disease, but from suicide as well. A study of suicides in New York (Marzuk et al., 1988) found that the relative risk for suicide in men with AIDS aged 20 to 59 was about 36 times the rate of similarly aged men without AIDS, and 66 times that of the general population. However, these data are from 1985, when virtually no treatments were available. Whether such trends will continue with the development of treatments such as AZT remains to be determined. Effective treatments for AIDS will likely have an impact not only on deaths directly related to AIDS itself, but also on suicide-related deaths as well.

Cost issues are not irrelevant in the development of a safe and effective treatment for AIDS. The drug manufacturer hopes to offer a treatment that will be safe, effective, and profitable. The patients hope to use a drug that will be safe, effective, and inexpensive, especially if the drug has to be taken for the rest of one's life. Developing an effective treatment for AIDS is only one problem; the distribution of an effective treatment to hundreds of thousands of people (perhaps millions) is quite another.

The Food and Drug Administration has developed protocols for testing of new drugs for safety and efficacy. These protocols are based on fundamental scientific principles and tend to be rather time consuming. It may take a decade or

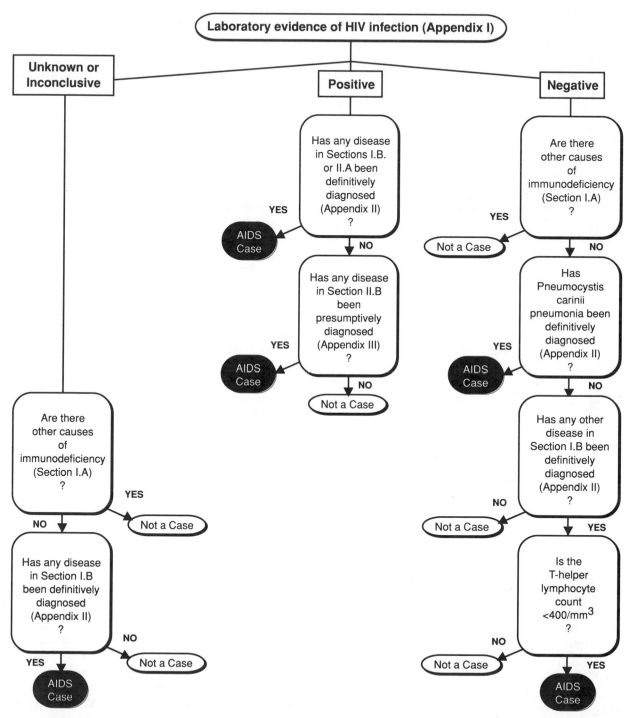

• FIGURE 5.2   Revised case definition of AIDS: September, 1987.

more for a drug manufacturer to get final approval for a new drug. Because AIDS is such a fatal disease, many AIDS organizations have been protesting the slowness of the federal bureaucracy in its testing and approval of new drugs. Because of pressures from groups such as AIDS Coalition to Unleash Power (ACT-UP), the Food and Drug Administration has developed a two-track system for testing new drugs. One track is to continue standard research testing protocols as has been done for decades. The other track is to make the drug available to patients as soon as possible.

AIDS has focused attention on some of the inherent conflicts between regulatory agencies and patients who must live with a fatal disease. On the one hand, the FDA does not want to make available to the public dangerous drugs (such as Thalidomide) that might be neither safe nor effective. In an effort to document safety and efficacy, massive amounts of data are required that may take years (or decades) to collect. The advantage of this system to the public is that drugs made available for public consumption have been appropriately tested and reviewed. The disadvantage is that it takes so long, and many people who might have benefited from the drug are no longer alive to receive those benefits.

People with AIDS have been arguing for almost a decade that because the disease is ultimately fatal, why should they die waiting a decade for a drug to make it through the federal bureaucracy? What does an AIDS patient have to lose, if he or she is going to die anyway? Some federal officials believe that the government is now moving too quickly in making AIDS drugs available to AIDS patients; some AIDS patients believe the government is still moving too slowly. The conflict between scientific data collection and matters of life and death is not likely to be completely resolved any time soon. The desired end is the same for both groups: a safe and effective treatment for AIDS.

Treatment for AIDS involves more than just drug therapy, however. Most, if not all, AIDS patients will require some hospital care to treat the infections that develop throughout the course of the disease. Inpatient hospital care is expensive. Early estimates of the lifetime costs of treating a patient with AIDS ranged from $25,000 to $147,000 (Sisk, 1987). More recent estimates—$75,000 for lifetime health–care costs (Hellinger, 1990)—suggest that the costs will not be quite so high, especially if outpatient programs are more frequently used and coordinated with community services.

San Francisco, in particular, has developed a coordinated system of providing care to AIDS patients that includes inpatient hospitalization, outpatient medical care, housing, meals, and social support. Despite the large number of AIDS cases in San Francisco, the cost of providing treatment and services to people with AIDS has been reduced in comparison to those cities whose primary treatment consists of inpatient hospitalization. Given the large number of AIDS cases in San Francisco, however, recent reports suggest that this system is simply becoming overwhelmed. In 1983, 250 AIDS cases were reported to the San Francisco Department of Health, about 21 per month; by the summer of 1990, that number had increased to 180 per month. In about seven years, the number of AIDS cases had increased by about 900 percent. Such rapid increases in a fatal disease make planning, organizing, staffing, and funding of organizations incredibly difficult, because no one really knows six years in advance how many AIDS cases will be diagnosed.

Despite such communitywide effort, treatment costs are likely to escalate. As drugs such as AZT prolong life, people with AIDS will live longer and they will require more medical care. Cities with large numbers of AIDS patients will not have enough hospital beds to treat all of those patients who need inpatient treatment, whether AIDS related or not. New York City, which had contemplated closing some hospitals in the late 1970s and early 1980s, may have to build new hospitals to provide medical services for the thousands of New Yorkers (up to 200,000) who are estimated to be HIV infected. A 600-bed hospital cannot be planned, built, and staffed in a short period of time; that process takes years. In the meantime, what will, or can, be done if there is a sudden rapid increase in the number of people who develop AIDS? Despite almost a decade of AIDS treatment, about 22 percent of all AIDS cases since 1981 (1 of 5) were reported in the first ten months of 1990.

As treatments become more sophisticated, AIDS may well become a chronic, treatable disease rather than an acute, fatal disease. Costs of providing such long-term care may be substantial, because many AIDS patients will not have their own health insurance and will have to rely on publicly funded health-care facilities for their lifetime care.

PROBLEMS IN VACCINE DEVELOPMENT

Many people are hoping for a vaccine for HIV. As with the problems identified in developing treatments for AIDS, however, numerous problems exist in the development of an HIV vaccine. Fauci and Fischinger (1988) have identified a number of general difficulties in developing an AIDS vaccine, including the ability of HIV to mutate, the ability of the virus to lie dormant in cells, and the lack of a good animal model for AIDS, although recent works suggest that an effective animal model may not be too far off.

The changing face of HIV

The molecular structure of HIV is capable of change. A vaccine that was effective against one form of HIV might not protect a person against another form of the virus. Although the media generally call the virus the ''AIDS virus,'' researchers have identified at least two AIDS-related viruses; the first is HIV-1, the virus that is responsible for AIDS as we know it today. The second is HIV-2, a virus of fairly recent identification (mid-1980s) in parts of Western Africa and Central America. Researchers do not yet know

whether HIV-2 is as serious as HIV-1 in terms of its ability to destroy the immune system. If it is, then two vaccines might be necessary. If more Human Immunodeficiency Viruses are detected, then more vaccines will be required. Given the molecular differences in each virus, the development of a vaccine for protection from all HIVs may take a very long time indeed.

Difficulty with animal models

Many vaccines and drug treatments have been developed and tested in animals before being used on human beings. Unfortunately, the only animal that can be infected with HIV is the chimpanzee, which is relatively expensive and in fairly short supply. However, research by Kestler and co-workers (1990) has shown that AIDS can be induced in rhesus monkeys through the use of a Simian Immunodeficiency Virus (SIV). To the extent that these findings can be replicated, it may be possible to study both the development of AIDS and potential treatments (and vaccines) in a controlled experimental setting.

Mice and rats do not develop AIDS and so are unsuitable for vaccine development purposes. Moreover, many animal-rights advocates are trying to eliminate all animal-based laboratory research. Even if animal models for HIV infection can be developed, they may not be implemented, given the climate surrounding the issue of animal rights (e.g., picketing and protesting of laboratories, caged animals being let loose by protestors). Since drugs must be certified as safe and effective by the Food and Drug Administration before general distribution, the inability to first test the safety and efficacy of an AIDS vaccine on animals presents significant medical and ethical problems.

Uniqueness of HIV

Unfortunately, methods that have been successful in developing vaccines for other diseases (polio, measles, mumps, rubella, etc.) are not likely to be successful in developing an AIDS vaccine (Matthews and Bolognesi, 1989). HIV is a retrovirus, a class of viruses that has been studied for less than a decade. Since HIV inserts its own genes into the cells it infects, it establishes a permanent home and may remain dormant for years, or perhaps even decades. A vaccine might be able to stimulate the immune system when the virus began to multiply, but there is not yet a way of getting the HIV genetic material out of the cells it has infected.

Fear of the vaccine

One way that vaccines are developed is to inject a person with a small quantity of a dead or weakened viral agent, so that the body's immune system will develop a response to that agent. The polio vaccine consists of a component of dead or weakened polio virus injected into the body; the body's immune system develops a response not only to the virus, but to any live virus that subsequently infects the immunized person. In a very few cases, some children given the polio virus did develop polio as a result of the vaccination, perhaps because not all of the polio cells had been killed before the vaccination was given.

Similar problems will occur with an HIV vaccine. Would the general public be willing to be immunized if the vaccine contained dead components of HIV? How would the media describe the vaccine—as being injected with inactivated AIDS? Unless a significant portion of the public underwent vaccination, the impact of the vaccine on future AIDS cases might be minimal.

AIDS is a disease surrounded by denial. As noted earlier, national surveys by the National Center for Health Statistics have found that 78 percent of the public believes that they have no chance of getting the AIDS virus, 17 percent a low chance, 2 percent a medium chance, and 0 percent a high chance. If the perceived risk is so low, why

bother with vaccination, especially if there is a chance that one could "get" AIDS from the vaccination itself?

Equally important are the risks that the vaccine manufacturer would take in terms of financial liability if someone who developed AIDS as a result of the vaccine sued the manufacturer. One such lawsuit would probably eliminate the likelihood that the general public would continue to be vaccinated. One report of a person becoming HIV positive three months after being vaccinated would probably set off a public panic regarding the safety of the vaccine, even if 50 million people were safely vaccinated. Again, what is the denominator, and how much influence should be given to a relatively rare occurrence?

Such concerns have apparently caused many drug manufacturers not to seek a vaccine for AIDS unless there can be some federal guarantees that they will not be sued in cases in which the disease developed after the vaccine was administered. No manufacturer will take on the financial and public relations risks of an HIV vaccine alone; many have already abandoned birth control drugs and products for the same reason.

Some people—perhaps many people—would not want to be vaccinated, not because they are concerned about the safety or efficacy of the vaccine, but because of what it means psychologically to them to be vaccinated against AIDS. Would being vaccinated against AIDS be seen as an admission that one needed to be vaccinated because one engaged in risky behaviors? Would such a vaccination be an admission that one was gay or an IV drug user? How would being vaccinated (which implies a certain amount of perceived personal vulnerability) fit in with the denial of not being at risk that is expressed by so many people?

Some would see the vaccine as giving implicit approval for what might be considered to be immoral or illegal acts. If the fear of AIDS keeps people from engaging in risky behaviors, then a vaccine would reduce people's fears of such behaviors and might lead to increases in such behaviors. No doubt some would argue that an AIDS vaccine would promote homosexuality. Similar arguments were used when treatments became available for syphillis; fear of syphillis was thought to keep many young people sexually inactive. Eliminate the fear, increase the activity. No doubt many religious and political leaders would advocate against being vaccinated against HIV.

Obviously, the effectiveness of an AIDS vaccine will depend not only on the biological aspects of the vaccine itself, but on the social, psychological, cultural, political, and religious acceptance of such a vaccine.

HIV ANTIBODY TEST

In the absence of a vaccine for AIDS, HIV antibody testing takes on an important role. Although a person infected with HIV may not be able to do very much to forestall the inevitable development of AIDS, that person can reduce the likelihood of spreading the virus to uninfected people.

Testing for infection with HIV was not available until the spring of 1985. At that time, many people who engaged in high-risk behaviors did seek out antibody testing in the hope that they would find out whether or not they were infected with HIV. However, it soon became apparent that the results of one's HIV antibody test could have a profound impact on one's health and life insurance, job, and housing.

What the test does

The testing process is really a sequence of tests— as many as three. The blood sample is first analyzed by the Enzyme Linked Immunosorbent Assay (ELISA). If the result is negative, that result is communicated to the patient. However, if the result of the test is positive (suggesting that the person has HIV antibodies in his or her blood), a second ELISA test is run. If that test is positive, then a third test, the Western Blot, is used to analyze the blood. Only if the two ELISA tests are positive along with the Western Blot is the patient considered to be HIV positive. Three positive test results are necessary to confirm HIV seropositivity.

Who does the test

Not all labs that provide ELISA and Western Blot tests are equally competent. Using the same blood samples, not all labs arrive at the same conclusion (Gross, 1989). Recommendations for mass screening must take into account the accuracy of the lab doing the HIV antibody test (Barnes, 1987), given the serious consequences of false positive and false negative results.

People at risk

Many of those who sought testing in 1985 and 1986 were gay men who believed that they were at risk for having contracted the virus. However, once it became clear that the results of the HIV antibody test could be used to fire employees, cancel their life or health insurance, or evict them from their homes, the socially negative consequences of being HIV positive began to outweigh the medical consequences of finding out one's HIV status. Equally important was the fact that there was no treatment for people who tested positive—nothing could be done medically to treat HIV positive patients, and relatively little could be done to treat those who had developed full-blown AIDS.

The requests for HIV antibody testing began to decrease among high-risk individuals, in part because of the lack of any sort of effective medical treatment, and in part because many gay men decided that they simply didn't need to know their HIV status. Since they had changed their behaviors to incorporate safer sex activities into their lives, what would be the personal benefit of knowing that one was infected with HIV? Indeed, the fear

Box 5

The Importance of Counseling

Much emphasis has been placed on the importance of one's HIV status (e.g., knowing the results of one's "AIDS test"). Unfortunately, the counseling component of the counseling and testing protocol has not received adequate public attention or discussion. Counseling is important because it helps the individual cope with his or her seropositivity status and promotes responsible behavior, regardless of whether one's test results are positive or negative. Test results alone will not, and cannot change behaviors. Given the importance of behavioral change, counseling takes on an even more important role than test results. Although HIV testing facilities were originally called "anonymous testing sites" in many communities, the terminology has changed to "alternative counseling and testing sites," as the anonymity component of the program was eliminated and the counseling component became more prominent.

Detailed strategies for counseling and testing have been disseminated (CDC, 1987a). Basic issues that should be addressed prior to testing include the following:

- Finding out why the person wants to be tested,

- Asking the person about his or her risky behaviors,

- Explaining the purpose of the antibody test and the possible results,

- Describing safer sex and other prevention activities,

- Assessing the anticipated impact of the test results; what would a positive test mean; what would a negative test mean; what is the willingness to refer drug-using or sex partners,

- Describing confidentiality of test results and how the results are to be obtained (i.e., in person, not by phone or letter).

Posttest counseling—*if negative*—should include the following:

- Giving the results and dealing with possible responses of guilt, anger, relief, and so on,

- Identifying plans for remaining negative and reviewing overall risk reduction strategies.

Posttest counseling—*if positive*—should include the following:

- Giving the results and dealing with the emotional reaction, such as anxiety, fear of death, guilt, depression, and anger,

- Explaining the results of the test; what it means, what it doesn't mean,

- Referring the patient for professional assistance, if needed,

- Discussing motivations for protection of self and others,

- Seeking a drug-using or sex partner referral for follow-up contact tracing,

- Planning for a medical evaluation.

Everyone who seeks out HIV antibody testing should receive both pre- and posttest counseling by a trained counselor. Testing without counseling trivializes the issue and misses an opportunity to help change behaviors during a "teachable moment," especially with adolescents and young adults who have probably not addressed these issues in such detail.

Informed consent

Although informed consent from the patient is routinely recommended before testing, a review of HIV antibody testing at one midwestern hospital from April 1985 through August 1986 found that only 10 percent of the HIV antibody test results provided documentation of informed consent (Henry, Maki, and Crossley, 1988). Equally important, these researchers found several misuses of the test:

- In 6 cases, a positive ELISA and a negative Western Blot were interpreted as a positive test,

- In 5 cases, patients who were HIV positive were recorded as having AIDS,

- In 11 cases, no details were recorded in the chart about who ordered the HIV antibody test or why it was ordered.

In the absence of such informed consent protocols, it falls to the person who is being tested to be knowledgeable about issues of informed consent, anonymity, and confidentiality and to raise these issues if the health-care provider does not.

Knowledge and behavior change

Knowing one's seropositivity status may or may not be beneficial. In a study of gay men in Chicago (Ostrow et al., 1989), learning that one was seronegative had a positive effect on mental health status, while discovering that one was seropositive had a significant adverse impact on most measures of mental health (depression, anxiety, obsessive-compulsive behavior, and total distress). Equally important, knowing one's seropositivity status did not result in changes in HIV-transmitting sexual behavior. (Of course, knowing that one is intoxicated does not always lead to a reduction in driving behavior either.) Ostrow and others suggest that behavioral change as a result of educational interventions may not increase if HIV status is known, and that implementation of widespread HIV antibody testing programs should be considered carefully.

Other studies (Coates et al., 1988) have found beneficial results of knowing one's antibody status on risk-taking behaviors, although studies are limited in terms of study population (gay and bisexual men, IV drug users) and geographic area (major cities such as San Francisco, New York, Chicago, and Baltimore). How such knowledge might affect the behavior of other individuals at risk (e.g., heterosexual females in rural parts of America) is not yet known. If the goal is behavior change, testing (and the knowledge of one's test results) may be less important than competent counseling and skill-building for the development of "safer" behaviors.

Such behavioral change is crucial for those individuals who are currently seronegative—and want to stay that way. We must remember that it "takes two" to transmit HIV: one to transmit it and one to receive it. Emphasis on the person who is HIV infected and exclusion of the person who is HIV negative will not reduce the spread of the virus.

and anxiety of knowing that one was HIV positive might produce severe psychological distress. Many believed that it was better not to know but to take precautions sexually and to live a healthier lifestyle.

People not at risk

As the mass media continued to report about the AIDS epidemic, thousands of "worried well" individuals sought out HIV antibody testing. The worried well were primarily middle-class heterosexuals who thought that they might have contracted HIV from a past sexual encounter. Perhaps a few did, but most did not. Unfortunately, although many gay men changed their sexual behaviors as a result of AIDS, many heterosexuals probably did not. For some, a negative test result only served to reassure them that AIDS was a gay disease, not one that heterosexuals needed to be concerned about.

Obviously, some heterosexuals have tested positive, and many of those have developed AIDS. But that number is so small, in comparison to gay and bisexual men, that many heterosexuals simply do not perceive themselves to be at risk. It will probably take an increase in the number of reported heterosexual cases for the vast majority of heterosexuals to believe that they are at risk and to take appropriate precautions. Many gay men changed their behaviors because they saw their lovers and friends dying of AIDS; until heterosexuals begin to see their lovers and friends dying of AIDS, individual motivation to change will probably be minimal.

Mass screening

Periodic suggestions have been made that all citizens of the United States should be tested for HIV antibodies, or that, at the very least, all couples applying for marriage licenses should be tested. References to the historical mass screenings for other communicable diseases, such as syphillis, have been used to justify such recommendations. However, it must be remembered that mandatory reporting and contact tracing for syphillis was not completely successful. While public health physicians often reported the names of infected patients, private physicians were less likely to do so (Ostrow, Eller, and Joseph, 1988).

Following these suggestions, Illinois did institute premarital HIV testing in 1988 for all couples who planned to be married, but the following year the requirement was abandoned. It was abandoned because (1) very few people were identified as being HIV positive, (2) many couples

went to a neighboring state to be married, thus avoiding the cost and consequences of the antibody test, and (3) some couples apparently decided to live together without marrying. Those couples who could not afford the cost of the testing and counseling from a private physician (as much as $200–$300), would probably have to use the public health system; the cost to the state would be substantial. Estimates by Cleary and coauthors (1987) suggested that compulsory premarital screening in the United States would

• Detect fewer than 1/10 of 1 percent of HIV infected individuals,
• Cost more than $100 million,
• Identify more than 350 false positives,
• Not identify about 100 false negatives.

Despite the apparent limitations of compulsory screening efforts, arguments have been put forth for widespread voluntary HIV antibody testing (Rhame and Maki, 1989; Maki, 1989). They have suggested that HIV antibody testing be routinely administered to all adults under the age of 60 who newly enter the health-care system (e.g., all hospital admissions), and recommended that HIV testing become as common as blood pressure monitoring, cholesterol testing, and mammography.

Any recommendations for a national policy on HIV testing will continue to generate debate (Falco and Cikins, 1989). Moreover, inconsistencies in laws from state to state (Gostin, 1989) are likely to impede the development of a national consensus on many AIDS-related issues. Gostin found that

• 19 states require written, informed consent for HIV antibody testing,
• 7 states permit mature minors to give informed consent without parental agreement,
• about half the states protect the confidentiality of HIV-related information by state statute.

Given such inconsistencies, the state of residence may play a key role in one's decision not only to be counseled and tested, but in the quality of the counseling and testing provided.

Impact of a negative test

While being told that one's HIV antibody test is positive can be devastating, being told that one's test is negative can produce a variety of emotions and responses. A negative test simply means that the test was not positive at the time that the blood sample was taken—perhaps more time was needed for the person to seroconvert. Although most people seroconvert within 8 to 12 weeks after exposure to HIV, some take longer. Thus, a negative result should not be taken to mean that one is positively not infected with the virus (unless the person has not engaged in any risky behaviors at all).

Some businesses have tried to take advantage of the AIDS hysteria. Typically they provide (for a fee) certification, such as an ID card, that one was "AIDS free." Of course, that statement would be only accurate until the person's next sexual or IV drug-using encounter. Indeed, if the person were tested only shortly after being infected, the test results might be negative, even though the person was HIV infected. What these testing services were really promising was permission to continue to engage in sexual practices without a change in one's behavior. After all, if you had sex only with other people who had HIV-negative ID cards, why bother to use safer sex practices?

Some people who have tested negative mistakenly believed that being negative somehow confers "immunity" to them, especially if they have been repeatedly negative. Unfortunately, there are some people who have tested negative once, twice, or three times, only to become positive on the fourth test. Too often, being negative can produce a false sense of security (Goldblum and Marks, 1988), not only that one might have beaten the odds of contracting the virus from a single potential exposure but also that perhaps one cannot contract the virus.

Negative test results can occur when people have consistently engaged in safer sex practices, have avoided other routes of exposure, or simply have had good luck. Continued safer sex practices reduces the likelihood of becoming infected; continued risky sex practices increases the likelihood. Unfortunately, seropositivity can't be undone; you can go from being uninfected to infected, but you can't become uninfected.

Anonymity vs. confidentiality

In the early days of testing, every effort was made to get as many people tested as possible, in the hope that the spread of the virus could be reduced if HIV positive people knew their HIV status and practiced safer sex so as to limit subsequent infections. To encourage people to be tested, many states set up "anonymous" testing programs, in which the individual's identity was not recorded; only code numbers would be used when the person returned for his or her test results.

Many gay men believed that if their names were made available by the testing center to state or federal agencies, opportunities for discrimination against them would increase. On the other hand, traditional public health methods for dealing with transmittable diseases—(such as sexually transmitted diseases)—have emphasized case finding and contact tracing as a way of slowing down the spread of the disease. Conflicts between public health and medical confidentiality are not easily resolved. Serious discrimination does exist (Sherer, 1988):

> "In 1985, I was the primary physician for a young man whose life was ruined by the inappropriate disclosure of a positive human immunodeficiency virus (HIV)—antibody test. A physician ordered the test without consent and notified the local health department of the positive result. The health department notified the individual's employer and he was promptly fired. These events became common

knowledge at his workplace and in his rural Midwestern town and he was shunned. His landlord asked him to move. Ten days after testing, the life he had known for the past ten years was permanently ruined and he left town. With the loss of his job came loss of health insurance and insurability; he has been unable to obtain health or life insurance since then.'' (p. 264)

Such discrimination is likely to discourage people at high risk from taking the HIV antibody test unless they can be tested with complete assurance of anonymity. Researchers (Fehrs et al., 1988) have found that anonymous testing increased the overall demand for such testing by about 50

percent over confidential testing, especially for gay men (125% increase in demand).

In a confidentially based public health program, the testing agency requests the name of the infected individual and the names of those people with whom he or she had sexual contact (or needle-sharing contact) within the last 5 to 10 years. It may be difficult, if not impossible, for people to remember all the names and addresses of sexual partners from that long ago. The health department would contact and inform the partner that he or she might be infected with the virus and should probably seek HIV antibody testing. It is important to note that at no time is the name of the person who may have transmitted the virus ever divulged to the partner.

SUMMARY

HIV damages the immune system by attaching itself to cells, inserting genetic material into the cells, and causing those immune system cells to generate defective new cells. As new information has been collected regarding how HIV functions to destroy both the immune system and cells within the central nervous system, the Centers for Disease Control have changed the diagnostic criteria for AIDS. Such changes will provide a somewhat different picture of the AIDS epidemic.

Effective treatment for AIDS is limited; AZT is the only anti-viral drug that has been approved by the Food and Drug Administration for AIDS patients, although many more are being investigated. Conflicts between federal agencies and people with AIDS have led to changes in the speed with which new drugs will be tested and made available.

Although a vaccine for AIDS remains a possibility, the lack of a good animal model, the uniqueness of HIV, and the possible psychological fear that many would have of being injected with

an AIDS vaccine may reduce the likelihood of success for such a vaccine.

HIV antibody counseling and testing efforts will continue to play a major role in dealing with AIDS. The importance of true positive results, false positives, true negatives, false negatives, anonymity, and confidentiality must be understood before someone volunteers for the antibody test.

REFERENCES

Barnes, D. M. (1987) New questions about AIDS test accuracy. *Science,* 238, 884–885.
CDC (1987a) *Recommended additional guidelines for HIV antibody counseling and testing in the prevention of HIV infection and AIDS.* Atlanta, GA: Centers for Disease Control.
CDC (1987b) *Morbidity and Mortality Weekly Report. Revision of the CDC surveillance case definition for Acquired Immunodeficiency Syndrome.* Atlanta, GA: Centers for Disease Control.
Cleary, P. D., Barry, M. J., Mayer, K. H., et al. (1987) Compulsory premarital screening for the Human Immunodeficiency Virus. *Journal of the American Medical Association,* 258 (13), 1757–1762.

Coates, T. J., Stall, R. D., Kegeles, S. M., et al. (1988) AIDS antibody testing: Will it stop the AIDS epidemic? Will it help people infected with HIV? *American Psychologist,* 43 (11), 859–864.

Falco, M., and Cikins, W. I. eds. (1989) *Toward a national policy on drug and AIDS testing.* Washington, DC: Brookings Institution.

Fauci, A. S., and Fischinger, P. J. (1988) The development of an AIDS vaccine: Progress and promise. *Public Health Reports,* 103 (3), 230–235.

Fehrs, L. H., Fleming, D., Foster, L. R., et al. (1988) Trial of anonymous versus confidential human immunodeficiency virus testing. *The Lancet,* August 13, 1988, 379–382.

Goldblum, P., and Marks, R. (1988) The HIV testing debate. *Focus: A guide to AIDS research.* 3 (12), 1–3.

Gostin, L. O. (1989) Public health strategies for confronting AIDS: Legislative and regulatory policy in the United States. *Journal of the American Medical Association,* 261 (11), 1621–1630.

Gross, M. (1989) HIV antibody testing: Performance and counseling issues. In: P. O'Malley, ed. *The AIDS epidemic.* Boston, MA: Beacon Press.

Hellinger, F. J. (1990) Updated forecasts of the costs of medical care for persons with AIDS, 1989–1993. *Public Health Reports,* 105 (1), 1–12.

Henry, K., Maki, M., and Crossley, K. (1988) Analysis of the use of the HIV antibody testing in a Minnesota Hospital. *Journal of the American Medical Association,* 259 (2), 229–232.

Kestler, H., Kodama, T., Ringler, D., et al. (1990) Induction of AIDS in rhesus monkeys by molecularly cloned Simian Immunodeficiency Virus. *Science,* 248, 1109–1112.

Maki, D. G. (1989) AIDS: Serologic testing for the Human Immunodeficiency Virus—to screen or not to screen. *Infection Control and Hospital Epidemiology,* 10 (6), 243–247.

Marzuk, P. M., Tierney, H., Tardiff, K., et al. (1988) Increased risk of suicide in persons with AIDS. *Journal of the American Medical Association,* 259 (9), 1333–1337.

Matthews, T. H., and Bolognesi, D. P. (1989) AIDS vaccines. In: *The science of AIDS: readings from Scientific American.* New York: W. H. Freeman and Company.

Ostrow, D. G., Eller, M., and Joseph, J. G. (1988) Epidemic control measures for AIDS: A psychosocial and historical discussion of policy alternatives. In: I. B. Corless and M. Pittman-Lindeman, eds. *AIDS: Principles, practices, and politics.* Washington, DC: Hemisphere Publishing Corp.

Ostrow, D. G., Joseph, J. G., Kessler, R., et al. (1989) Disclosure of HIV antibody status: behavioral and mental health correlates. *AIDS Education and Prevention,* 1 (1), 1–11.

Rhame, F. S., and Maki, D. G. (1989) The case for wider use of testing for HIV infection. *New England Journal of Medicine,* 320, 1248–1254.

Sherer, R. (1988) Physician use of the HIV antibody test. *Journal of the American Medical Association,* 259 (2), 264–265.

Selik, R. M., Buehler, J. W., Karon, J. M., et al. (1990) Impact of the case definition of Acquired Immunodeficiency Syndrome in the United States. *Journal of Acquired Immune Deficiency Syndromes,* 3 (1), 73–82.

Sisk, J. E. (1987) The costs of AIDS: A review of the estimate. *Health Affairs,* Summer 1987, 5–21.

6 Populations Affected by AIDS

The only thing necessary for the triumph of evil is for good men to do nothing.

EDMUND BURKE

Our understanding of the U.S. populations affected by AIDS is based primarily on data provided by the Centers for Disease Control, which maintains the national data base describing the statistical part of the AIDS epidemic. Diagnosed AIDS cases are reported by the state health departments to CDC on a regular basis; however, incomplete or inaccurate data may provide a blurred picture of the AIDS epidemic. For example, a report by Laumann and colleagues (1989) suggested that CDC data might have substantially underestimated the prevalence of AIDS in higher socioeconomic status whites and in the Midwest, while overstating the relative prevalence of AIDS in minorities and in the East. Moreover, lag time in the reporting of

AIDS cases may skew the data somewhat. The Centers for Disease Control (1990) have noted that, although half of all AIDS cases are reported within three months of diagnosis, 15 percent are not reported until a year or more after the diagnosis has been made.

Worldwide, the situation is somewhat more complicated. The World Health Organization (WHO) provides AIDS statistics on a worldwide basis, as well as prevention and treatment programs to many countries. As of the summer of 1990, WHO estimated that 8 to 10 million people worldwide had already been infected with HIV, and that up to 3 million women and children would die of AIDS in the 1990s—six times as many deaths as in the 1980s (Altman, 1990). Although most of the AIDS cases in the United States have been reported in gay and bisexual men, WHO reported that on a worldwide basis, about 60 percent of the AIDS cases have been attributed to heterosexual intercourse, a figure that may rise to 80 percent of all cases by the beginning of the twenty-first century.

One can argue the strengths and weaknesses of the different methodologies for estimating HIV infection and future AIDS cases, but the point of such discussion is that there is simply not a national consensus regarding the best method. Such limitations will probably always be with us, because different researchers use different methods to attempt to reach the same goal. More time and more data will be necessary to resolve such conflicts; consequently, current data should not be taken as representing the complete picture of AIDS.

HIGH-RISK "GROUPS"

Early in the AIDS epidemic, the Centers for Disease Control identified "high-risk" groups of people thought to be at risk for contracting HIV. After all, the first AIDS cases were all diagnosed in gay men. The use of such categories can be helpful in some cases, for example, in targeting health education messages to those individuals at most risk (such as by making information available in gay bars) or in providing a framework for health-care providers who must provide health-care services and sexuality or drug abuse counseling (e.g., at STD clinics). However, an overreliance on "risk groups" alone may blur the risks for those individuals who engage in risky behavior, but who do not identify with a particular "high-risk" group. Moreover, placing people with AIDS into a transmission category is based exclusively upon self-reports; people have been known to be less than accurate (or honest) regarding their sexuality and drug-using behaviors. Cultural differences in

homosexuality and bisexuality (de la Vega, 1989) may not always be reflected in the CDC data.

Because of the complexity of these risk issues, only brief descriptions of the affected populations will be provided. Such brevity should not be construed to minimize the impact of this disease. Table 6.1 is a statistical summary of adult and adolescent AIDS cases by gender, exposure category, and race or ethnicity for males and females through June 1990.

ADULT AND ADOLESCENT CATEGORIES

Homosexual and bisexual males have comprised 66 percent of all AIDS cases since 1981. Most of the reported AIDS cases have been diagnosed in this transmission category, thus leading to the early perception of AIDS as a "gay plague." However, because HIV can be transmitted via specific homosexual activities does not mean that AIDS is a "gay disease." Many gay men who have been in monogomous relationships for lengthy periods of time or who have been practicing safer sex are at no risk for contracting HIV.

Urban areas with large numbers of gay men, such as San Francisco and New York have been hard hit by AIDS. This disease has affected not only those gay men who are HIV positive, who have been diagnosed with AIDS, or who have died of AIDS, but also their lovers, their families, their friends, physicians, co-workers, neighbors, and others.

Because of the concentrations of gay men in major urban areas, support systems and educational programs developed early in the epidemic. Gay organizations provided safer sex information years before federal and state government agencies responded to the health crisis. In particular, the San Francisco AIDS Project and the Gay Men's Health Crisis in New York City took leadership positions on providing accurate and timely information about AIDS to the gay community. The fact that a gay "community" existed meant that it was possible to disseminate information to gay

TABLE 6.1   Adult and adolescent AIDS Cases in the United States by Sex, Exposure Category, and Race or Ethnicity, Reported Through June 1990

Male Exposure Category	White, not Hispanic Number (%)	Black, not Hispanic Number (%)	Hispanic Number (%)	Asian/Pacific Islander Number (%)	American Indian/ Alaskan Native Number (%)	Total[a] Number (%)
Male homosexual/bisexual contact	59,000 (80)	13,717 (44)	8,673 (46)	633 (81)	101 (62)	82,304 (66)
Intravenous (IV) drug use (heterosexual)	4,551 (6)	10,889 (35)	7,250 (39)	23 (3)	18 (11)	22,798 (18)
Male homosexual/bisexual contact and IV drug use	5,494 (7)	2,475 (8)	1,347 (7)	16 (2)	24 (15)	9,370 (8)
Hemophilia/coagulation disorder	1,008 (1)	76 (0)	92 (0)	15 (2)	8 (5)	1,203 (1)
Heterosexual contact	459 (1)	2,117 (7)	237 (1)	6 (1)	1 (1)	2,824 (2)
Sex with IV drug user	*292*	*589*	*155*	*2*	*1*	*1,039*
Sex with person with hemophilia	*4*	*1*	*—*	*—*	*—*	*5*
Born in Pattern-II country	*3*	*1,342*	*8*	*3*	*—*	*1,359*
Sex with person born in Pattern-II country	*29*	*25*	*4*	*—*	*—*	*58*
Sex with transfusion recipient with HIV infection	*21*	*9*	*1*	*—*	*—*	*32*
Sex with HIV-infected person, risk not specified	*110*	*151*	*69*	*1*	*—*	*331*
Receipt of blood transfusion, blood components, or tissue[b]	1,504 (2)	295 (1)	163 (1)	42 (5)	1 (1)	2,010 (2)
Other/undetermined[c]	1,573 (2)	1,325 (4)	890 (5)	43 (6)	9 (6)	3,876 (3)
Male subtotal	73,589 (100)	30,894 (100)	18,652 (100)	778 (100)	162 (100)	124,385 (100)
Female **Exposure Category**						
IV drug use	1,413 (40)	3,888 (57)	1,348 (52)	12 (17)	15 (56)	6,689 (51)
Hemophilia/coagulation disorder	24 (1)	6 (0)	1 (0)	—	—	31 (0)
Heterosexual contact	986 (28)	2,156 (32)	940 (36)	25 (36)	7 (26)	4,128 (32)
Sex with IV drug user	*510*	*1,268*	*786*	*11*	*4*	*2,588*
Sex with bisexual male	*225*	*132*	*50*	*6*	*1*	*415*
Sex with person with hemophilia	*53*	*6*	*1*	*1*	*—*	*61*
Born in Pattern-II country	*2*	*494*	*3*	*1*	*—*	*502*
Sex with person born in Pattern-II country	*4*	*37*	*1*	*—*	*—*	*43*
Sex with transfusion recipient with HIV infection	*55*	*9*	*11*	*1*	*—*	*77*
Sex with HIV-infected person, risk not specified	*137*	*210*	*88*	*5*	*2*	*442*
Receipt of blood transfusion, blood components, or tissue	831 (24)	254 (4)	151 (6)	24 (34)	2 (7)	1,263 (10)
Other/undetermined	242 (7)	484 (7)	145 (6)	9 (13)	3 (11)	889 (7)
Female subtotal	3,496 (100)	6,788 (100)	2,585 (100)	70 (100)	27 (100)	13,000 (100)
Total	77,085	37,682	21,237	848	189	137,385

[a]Includes 310 males and 34 females whose race or ethnicity is unknown.
[b]Includes 12 transfusion recipients who received blood screened for HIV antibody, and 1 tissue recipient.
[c]"Other" refers to three health-care workers who seroconverted to HIV and developed AIDS after occupational exposure to HIV-infected blood. "Undetermined" refers to patients whose mode of exposure to HIV is unknown. This includes patients under investigation; patients who died, were lost to follow-up, or refused interview; and patients whose mode of exposure to HIV remains undetermined after investigation.

men who were part of that community. In areas where such communities do not exist, reaching gay men with potentially life-saving health information was considerably more difficult.

Data have clearly shown changes in risky behavior among many gay men (Stall et al., 1988), although the cause(s) of such behavioral change have not yet been specifically identified. Most educational programs have not had a strong evaluation component (Sisk, 1988), so it is not known whether the behavioral changes that have been reported are a result of health education messages, the impact of having friends die of AIDS, personal fear of contracting the virus, or some combination of those factors.

Men who identify themselves as gay men are likely to have been exposed to considerable amounts of safer sex information during the past few years. However, those men who have not "come out of the closet" are less likely to have been affected by safer sex messages. For those individuals who are leading double lives—such as some bisexual men—the difficulties in developing and providing appropriate counseling and prevention programs may be enormous (Paul, 1989).

Although AIDS has been viewed as a uniformly fatal disease, the survival rate has been increasing during the past few years. Again, most of the data is based on studies from San Francisco or New York and may not be generalizable to other parts of the country. In a study of nearly 6,000 AIDS patients who were diagnosed before 1986, Rothenberg and associates (1987) found that the group with the most favorable survival rate was white homosexual men 30 to 34 years of age who had Kaposi's sarcoma; some survived as long as nine years after diagnosis. They concluded: "It is perhaps too soon to know whether AIDS is universally fatal. Previous case reports and general clinical experience suggest that there is a spectrum of severity and that long-term survival is possible" (p. 1301). Since it may have taken some of those men as long as nine years to go from being infected with HIV to developing AIDS, and they

may have survived as long as nine years after being diagnosed with AIDS, a few may have lived as long as 18 years after becoming infected. That's an important point when trying to educate young people about AIDS; it may be fatal, but death may be a relatively long way away, at least for some. If nothing else, such statistics should provide a degree of hope for those who have recently been told that they are HIV positive.

Intravenous drug users (IVDUs) account for approximately 18 percent of the reported AIDS cases since 1981. Among women, IVDUs comprise about 52 percent of reported AIDS cases. A review of 92 studies of HIV infection among IVDUs (Hahn et al., 1989) found seroprevalence rates of 0 to 60 percent among IVDUs in drug treatment programs, with estimates that 5 to 33 percent of the total IVDUs in the United States were HIV infected—between 61,000 and 398,000 people. The vast majority of AIDS cases in these HIV infected individuals will come from New York City. Des Jarlais, Friedman, Novick, and their fellow researchers (1989) have estimated that the number of AIDS cases as a result of IV drug use in New York City is comparable to the total number of all cases in San Francisco, and half the cases in Europe!

In their analysis of stored blood samples from intravenous drug users, Des Jarlais and other researchers (1989) concluded that the introduction of HIV-1 into the IVDU community probably occurred in 1975 or 1976, or perhaps even earlier. Since recognition of AIDS cases did not occur until 1981 (in gay men), the virus had six or more years to spread without any sort of public health or medical intervention.

Perhaps 100,000 IVDUs are infected with HIV in New York City; each one may develop AIDS. These IVDUs (as well as bisexual males) may represent the "bridge" that permits the transmission of HIV into the general population, contrary to the original belief that AIDS would be almost exclusively a disease of gay men with little impact beyond that group. The major issues associated with IVDU transmission are threefold: (1)

HIV transmission via needle sharing; (2) efforts to distribute "clean" syringes and needles to IVDUs; and (3) pharmacological treatments for drug addiction.

- HIV transmission via needle sharing. In many states, the purchase of needles and syringes without a prescription is illegal. Thus, most IVDUs do not have a source of sterile needles and syringes (their "works") and must resort to sharing them. Such sharing has become a ritualistic part of the IV drug using subculture and represents an opportunity for sharing HIV as well. Narcotic addicts must inject heroin several times a day, usually every four to six hours. Since sterile "works" cannot be purchased legally, those "works" that are available are often rented and shared among many users. Blood (and hepatitis B, HIV and other diseases) can easily be shared along with the works.

  Cocaine use represents a significant new opportunity for HIV transmission. A survey in San Francisco (Chaisson et al., 1989) found that intravenous use of cocaine significantly increased the risk of HIV infection, especially among blacks. Because the duration of the cocaine high is relatively short compared to that of heroin and the degree of dependency to cocaine is relatively powerful, cocaine users may inject 10 or more times per day, perhaps twice as often as heroin users. If the "works" are being shared, the cocaine IVDU may be sharing two or three times as often as the heroin IVDU.

  Efforts to reduce the potential spread of HIV among IVDUs are based on three major approaches. First, increasing the number of treatment slots (especially for methadone maintenance) is crucial for getting more of the IVDUs completely off illicit narcotics and shared "works." Unfortunately, there are not an extra 200,000 treatment slots available in New York City, and even if the funds were available for such programs, there would probably still be a shortage of trained drug abuse counselors. Charles Schuster (1988), Director of the National Institute on Drug Abuse, has estimated that, on a national basis, 59,000 additional staff members may be necessary to meet the increasing demand for treating intravenous drug users. Professional training programs, however, are not likely to be sources of such staff; Campos, Brasfield, and Kelly (1989) found that 75 percent of the graduate programs in clinical and counseling psychology that they surveyed did not cover AIDS at any point in their curricula and that fewer than half of the programs trained students in human sexuality. The demand for trained counselors will clearly exceed the supply. Consequently, some programs have had waiting lists of six months or more and those who want help in getting off heroin or cocaine are being turned away. Nevertheless, both federal and state governments are increasing funds for such treatment programs, although staff for such programs may be inadequately trained.

- Efforts to distribute "clean" (i.e., sterile) syringes and needles to IVDUs. From a public health standpoint, the argument has been made that supplying IVDUs with sterile "works" will reduce the spread of HIV. However, such efforts are often viewed as encouragement to become an IVDU by the law enforcement community.

- Pharmacological treatments for drug addiction. Methadone (a legal narcotic) has been used effectively to get heroin addicts off heroin. They are given oral methadone on a daily basis in an effort to eliminate (or at least reduce) their need to inject heroin. Thus, methadone functions as a chemical diversion for heroin addicts. Although not everyone agrees philosophically or practically about the merits of methadone treatment, AIDS issues may make it a more appealing alternative than it has been in the past. Unfortunately, there is no chemical diversion for cocaine that is comparable to methadone. Given the highly addictive nature of cocaine and the absence of a chemical substitute, the successes in reducing HIV transmission in heroin users may be offset by increases in HIV transmission in cocaine users.

IV drug users represent a risk not only to other IV drug users, but to their sexual partners and offspring as well. HIV infected male IVDUs can pass the virus on to their female partners. If the partner becomes pregnant, there is some chance (perhaps 50%) that the baby will be HIV infected and will later develop AIDS. Cases have been reported of the father, mother, and baby all being HIV infected; in some families the mother and father have died, leaving an HIV infected baby. Some of these babies cannot be placed in foster homes, some have no other family members, others spend the rest of their lives living in an acute care hospital at enormous financial cost.

HIV is most efficiently transmitted through sexual and drug-using behaviors in which an uninfected person comes into contact with the blood or semen of an infected person. When both behaviors are present in the same individual, the risk of transmitting the virus greatly increases.

On a percentage basis, three times as many women as men have IV drug use as their primary risk factor for AIDS. Because a dependency is expensive to maintain, some drug-using women turn to prostitution as a way of financially supporting their drug habits. Thus, the chain of HIV infection can be rather extensive: An HIV infected male drug user can transmit the virus to his uninfected female partner; she can in turn transmit the virus to male sexual partners through prostitution; or on to her fetus if she becomes pregnant. Theoretically, one infected person becomes three (or more) infected people. Research into the effects of HIV on mother and child mortality has found that HIV may become one of the five leading causes of death in women of reproductive age by 1991, with an increasing impact on infant mortality as well (Chu et al., 1990).

The risk of contracting HIV is not from being an IVDU per se, but from engaging in risky behaviors that expose one to the virus. Chemical dependency is not unknown in the medical profes-

sion; both physicians and nurses have been known to inject narcotics. If disposable needles and syringes are used and needle sharing does not occur, there is no risk of contracting HIV. By emphasizing IV drug use as a risk factor, however, risks may not be perceived by those individuals who use IV drugs but do not identify themselves as "addicts."

Adolescents and young adults may experiment with narcotics or cocaine once or twice with their friends. They may share the "works," but they are not likely to see themselves as drug dependent—or at risk for contracting HIV. Some athletes (and nonathletes) inject steroids and share needles and syringes with their friends. They probably don't view themselves as "addicts" either. Indeed, one case has been reported of HIV transmission in a body builder who had been injecting anabolic steroids and sharing a hypodermic needle with a fellow body builder (Scott and Scott, 1989). Although the risk of contracting HIV this way may be relatively low at present, there will undoubtedly be some cases of AIDS in high school and college athletes that originated this way. A study of anabolic steroid use by male high school seniors (Buckley et al., 1988) found that 6.6 percent of twelfth-grade male students use or have used anabolic steroids, and that more than two-thirds began using steroids when they were 16 or younger. As states begin to categorize steroids as a controlled substance, they are likely to become available only on the black market. If needles and syringes are also illegal, some steroid users may find themselves in the same situation with respect to HIV as heroin users.

While many believe that IVDUs care little about their own health and would be very resistant to behavioral change, researchers have found risk-reduction behaviors being used among Manhattan IV drug users (Des Jarlais et al., 1985; Selwyn et al., 1987). Nevertheless, reaching IVDUs is not always easy, since they are not organized into social and political groups as are many gay men. With much of their daily life focused on ways of getting money to pay for the next dose of heroin or cocaine, many IVDUs tend not to be in touch with the media. The latest information about AIDS in the *New York Times* or on the "Six O'Clock News" will probably not reach the IVDUs in New York City. Informational strategies that worked for gay men (such as distributing safer sex brochures in gay bars and publicizing AIDS information in gay newspapers) would not work for IVDUs.

Homosexual and bisexual males who use IV drugs comprise about 8 percent of the reported AIDS cases, although it cannot be determined which behavior actually resulted in contraction of the virus. This group may have served as the "bridge" between the HIV infected homosexual groups to the as yet uninfected IVDU groups in the early 1970s (Des Jarlais et al., 1989).

Research is not yet clear about how many times one must be exposed to HIV or how much of the virus is necessary for infection to take place. Some people have apparently become infected with HIV after only one exposure; others have not become infected even after many exposures. Differences in the virulence of the virus itself, or individual differences in the immune system may account for much of this variation in infectivity. Being a homosexual male (who engages in unsafe sex) and an IVDU (who shares needles or syringes) puts one at risk for potentially many more exposures to the virus, since the virus can be contracted through both sexual and drug-using activities.

Heterosexual cases have accounted for about 5 percent of all AIDS cases since 1981. Although only 2 percent of all male AIDS cases were the result of heterosexual transmission, 31 percent of the female cases were the result of heterosexual transmission. In fact, the heterosexual transmission category is the only one in which the absolute number of female cases (4,128) is higher than the number of male cases (2,824) as of April 1990 (Centers for Disease Control, 1990). The data suggest that male-to-female transmission of HIV is more efficient than female-to-male transmission.

Women seem to be more likely to receive the virus than to transmit it, but this might be a function of sexual practices, such as engaging in unprotected anal intercourse.

Much has been written about the potential for heterosexual spread of HIV. Recall that Masters and fellow researchers (1988) estimated that 3 million Americans were HIV infected (in contrast to the 950,000 to 1.5 million estimate of the CDC at that time) and concluded that, "The AIDS virus is now running rampant in the heterosexual community" (p. 7). At about the same time, Fumento (1987) argued that AIDS was not putting heterosexuals at risk, and that "it will not explode into the heterosexual population" (p. 24). Such diverse perspectives are unlikely to be completely resolved until more is known about how the disease moves through the population.

In a survey of sexual partners, the Centers for Disease Control (1986) reported that "a sizeable percentage of young, never-married men report more than 10 partners in the past 12 months: 4.6% of those aged 18–29 years and 2.9% of those aged 30–44 years. When these percentages are applied to the total number of such men in the United States . . . over 700,000 single men 18–29 years and over 100,000 single men 30–44 years may have 10 or more partners per year and hence appear to be at considerable risk of sexual exposure to HIV-1 and other STDs" (p. 567).

Unfortunately, the survey did not attempt to measure the number of lifetime sexual partners. The survey covered only February through April of 1987 to February through April of 1988; respondents who reported 0 or 1 partner during that year may have had more partners 5 or 10 years ago, when they were 5 or 10 years younger.

A survey of high-risk behavior among Canadian college students (MacDonald et al., 1990) found that about 70 percent of the students were sexually active. Of those sexually active students, 14 percent of the men and 19 percent of the

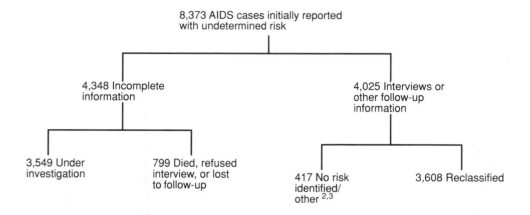

8,373 AIDS cases initially reported
with undetermined risk

4,348 Incomplete
information

4,025 Interviews or
other follow-up
information

3,549 Under
investigation

799 Died, refused
interview, or lost
to follow-up

417 No risk
identified/
other [2,3]

3,608 Reclassified

[1] Excludes 62 children under 13 years of age who have an undetermined risk: 55 children are under investigation and 7 have died, refused interview, or were lost to follow-up. An additional 96 children who were initially reported with an undetermined risk have been reclassified after investigation.

[2] **Health-care workers.** 3 of the 417 adults/adolescents are classified as "other" and are health-care workers who seroconverted to HIV and developed AIDS after occupational exposure to HIV-infected blood. For the remaining 414, the mode of exposure to HIV remains undetermined after investigation. 65 of these are health-care workers, 58 of whom responded to a standardized questionnaire. 34 (59%) reported needlesticks and/or mucous membrane exposures to blood and other body fluids of patients. None of the source patients was known to be infected with HIV at the time of the exposure and none of the health-care workers was evaluated at the time of the exposure to document seroconversion to HIV antibody. See MMWR, "Update: Acquired Immunodeficiency Syndrome and Human Immunodeficiency Virus Infection Among Health-Care Workers," (April 22, 1988) 37:229-234, 239.

[3] **Heterosexual transmission.** 350 of the 414 patients who had no risk identified after follow-up responded to a standardized questionnaire; 114 (36%) of 214 persons responding to questions related to sexually transmitted disease gave a history of such disease and 74 (35%) of 214 interviewed men reported sexual contact with a prostitute. Some of these persons may represent unreported or unrecognized heterosexual transmission of HIV. See *MMWR* "Update: Heterosexual Transmission of AIDS and HIV Infection — U.S.," (June 23, 1989) 38:423-424, 429-434.

• FIGURE 6.1   Description of "undetermined" AIDS cases. HIV/AIDS Surveillance Record, July 1990, p. 16

women had engaged in anal intercourse, but only 25 percent of the men and 16 percent of the women reported always using a condom. Among those students who had 10 or more partners, 27 percent of the men and 35 percent of the women practiced anal intercourse. Such data are fairly consistent with those of Reinisch and co-workers (1988), who estimated that 18 percent (probably an underestimate) of heterosexual males had engaged in anal intercourse, and 39 percent of women have had at least one experience with anal intercourse.

Defining a heterosexual case of AIDS is not always easy. CDC, in its definition of heterosexually transmitted cases "includes . . . per-sons who have had heterosexual contact with a person with AIDS or at risk for AIDS and . . . per-sons without other identified risks who were born in countries in which heterosexual transmission is believed to play a major role although precise means of transmission have not yet been fully defined." Thus, heterosexual transmission is *presumed* to be the route of HIV infection in those U.S. cases in which the patient was born in certain other countries.

Despite the desire for absolute information regarding such issues as heterosexual transmission, the general public may simply have to learn to wait for more data before conclusions can be reached with any degree of accuracy.

Undetermined cases represent about 3 percent of the total AIDS cases since 1981. This category is the one that concerns many people, because the implication is that there might be some new route of transmission, if the cause of AIDS is "undetermined."

A thorough investigation of more than 2,000 AIDS patients who had no previously identified risk factors (Castro et al., 1988) found the following:

- 596 of these cases were currently still under investigation,

- in 325 cases, further information was unavailable because of the patient's death, refusal to be interviewed, or failure to follow up,

- 860 cases were reclassified into the other transmission categories,

- 281 cases remained in the no-identified-risk category, although some potentially risky activities were identified, such as sexually transmitted diseases, sexual contact with prostitutes, receipt of products from human plasma, tattoos, acupuncture, and human bites. No data were available on the HIV status of the possible source, however.

Given the stigma that is associated with AIDS, it shouldn't be too surprising that people are not always willing to admit their risky behaviors to an interviewer. Furthermore, given the dementia that is found in some AIDS patients, the memory for past events may deteriorate to the point that the patients honestly cannot remember past events that might have put him or her at risk for HIV infection.

Transfusion and blood components represent 2 percent of all AIDS cases since 1981, but 11 percent of AIDS cases in women, probably because women visit physicians more than do men and are more likely to undergo surgical procedures. Because the tests for HIV antibodies were not available until March 1985, people who received blood transfusions since about 1977 to March 1985 were at some risk of contracting HIV from infected blood donations. Some blood banks have been sued, since there were recommendations that they screen for hepatitis (a surrogate marker for HIV) as a way of screening the blood supply. The blood banking industry did not believe at that time in the early 1980s that such an approach was feasible. Some blood banks have been found liable, and some have not.

All donated blood is currently screened for HIV antibodies; blood that is found to be infected is destroyed. The blood banks claim that the blood supply is safer than it has ever been, not only in terms of HIV, but in terms of other diseases as well. Nevertheless, many people who plan elective surgery are banking their own blood (autologous banking) rather than relying on donated blood that might be contaminated. Interestingly, in late 1987, about 22 percent of the public thought it likely that a person could get the AIDS virus from donating or giving blood (Dawson and Thornberry, 1988), apparently not understanding the difference between IVDUs who share needles and the use of needles in a blood bank setting, where disposable needles and syringes are used for each donor.

By the late fall of 1989, 27 percent of the public believed that the present blood supply was not safe for transfusions, and 24 percent didn't know (Hardy, 1990). Despite testing of all blood donations, despite the destruction of all infected donations, despite the recommendations that some people not donate blood, and despite the very low rate of HIV infected blood in the blood supply, more than 50 percent of the public is uncertain as to the safety of the blood supply. Miller and fellow researchers (1990) have noted that estimates of the number of HIV infected units of blood that are not detected range from 1 in 40,000–50,000 to 1 in 153,000 units. They suggest a number of strategies that might be used to reduce even further the likelihood of transfusion-related HIV infection: recruiting "safe" donors, decreasing the unnecessary use of blood products, increasing autologous donations, decreasing patient need for blood products, and others.

Hemophilia/coagulation disorders comprise about 1 percent of the total AIDS cases since 1981 and 1 percent of the cases in 1989. Of the 20,000 hemophiliacs in the United States, about half are HIV infected, and AIDS has become the chief cause of death for this group (Ragni, 1989). Since 1985, blood and plasma products for hemophiliacs in the United States have been heat treated to kill HIV and other viruses (CDC, 1987).

Children accounted for about 1.7 percent of reported AIDS cases. According to CDC, childhood cases "includes all patients under 13 years of age at time of diagnosis." Nearly 80 percent of the cases in children were the result of having a parent with AIDS or at risk of AIDS; the virus was presumably transmitted from an infected mother to her fetus or infant during the perinatal period. Other cases are the result of transfusions and blood components, or a result of hemophilia or coagulation disorders. Although the number of diagnosed cases is not high, HIV infection in children will have an impact on issues such as day care, foster care, school attendance and immunizations (Rogers et al., 1987).

The geographic dispersion of AIDS cases in children as well as adults means that some areas will have heavier case loads of HIV infected children or children with AIDS. New York City has been hit particularly hard by AIDS, with about 26,000 reported AIDS cases since 1981. A survey of newborns (Novick et al., 1989) found HIV infection in 1 of every 77 childbearing women. In some New York City hospitals, between 3 and 4 percent of the newborns were HIV infected.

RISKS IN CHILDHOOD AND ADOLESCENCE

Although CDC has developed broad categories for the classification of AIDS cases, there are a variety of circumstances in which HIV can be transmitted that would not be identified in that classification system. For example, although not likely to be a problem of immense proportions, the risk of HIV transmission to a child through sexual abuse is a real one (Bruner, 1988). As more and more people become infected with HIV, the probability increases that a child who is sexually assaulted will be infected with the virus.

Adolescent runaways are potentially vulnerable to HIV. Many young people who run away from home support themselves on the street by turning to prostitution. Media reports have suggested that some men have been seeking out younger and younger prostitutes because they assume that the younger prostitutes have had fewer partners and are less likely to be HIV infected. Some runaways get involved with drugs and may resort to prostitution to support their drug habits; in such cases, the opportunity for HIV infection increases because of participation in two risky behaviors. Fullilove and fellow researchers (1990) found that 41 percent of the black, teenaged crack cocaine users they surveyed had reported a history of sexually transmitted diseases. For girls, risky behaviors were associated with a history of selling crack and the number of drugs used on a daily basis. For boys, risky behaviors were associated with a description of "I don't know ahead of time if I'm going to have sex—it just happens" and the number of drugs they used on a daily basis. Intravenous drug use is the only drug use that puts one at risk for HIV infection.

Young people are sexually active and are susceptible to sexually transmitted diseases. In 1987, 12 percent of all reported primary and secondary cases of syphillis and 24 percent of all gonorrhea cases occurred in 15-to-19-year-olds (CDC, 1988a).

THE ROLE OF ALCOHOL

In the emphasis to view IV drug use as a major factor in HIV transmission, the role of alcohol has often either been overlooked completely or relegated to the role of a minor cofactor in AIDS.

Box 6

People of Color

AIDS has had a disproportionate impact upon people of color. Originally viewed by many as a disease of gay white males, the disease has increasingly affected minority populations. Although blacks (12%) and Hispanics (6%) comprise 18 percent of the U.S. population, they account for 40 percent of the AIDS cases. Blacks and Hispanics have been particularly hard hit, accounting for 70 percent of the cases in heterosexual men, 70 percent of those in women, and 75 percent of those in children (CDC, 1988b). There is no doubt that HIV is being heterosexually transmitted among blacks and Hispanics; there is also no doubt that racism (like homophobia) will play an important role in AIDS. Even with the minority communities, leaders have often been slow to address AIDS issues, in part because the disease had been viewed primarily as a disease of gay white males, and in part because of the difficulty of discussing sex, drug use, and death.

Issues Among Minority Populations

Des Jarlais and Friedman (1989) have noted that in all of the U.S. studies that found significant differences in HIV infection among ethnic groups, "minority IV drug users had higher rates of exposure to HIV than did white IV drug users" (p. 25), although they have no satisfactory explanation for such observations. There is no question that minority populations will continue to be significantly affected by AIDS. However, educators must recognize the unique characteristics of the different ethnic populations and not lump all minorities together. For example, although the Centers for Disease Control identify "Hispanics" as an ethnic category, there are differences between Puerto Rican IV drug

users and non-Puerto Rican Hispanics (Mexican-Americans, Cuban-Americans, and others of Central and South American origin).

Regarding Puerto Rican IV drug users, Serrano (1990) emphasized the importance of the family as a way of coping with AIDS. She notes that some "shooting galleries" may contain photos, religious items, or other family-related objects as a way of reminding the addict of his or her family life. Marin (1990), in her review of non-Puerto Rican Hispanics, notes the importance of "simpatia"—the maintanence of smooth social relations based on politeness, respect, and the avoidance of assertiveness or criticism. One result of simpatia is that taboo subjects (e.g., AIDS, condom use, IV drug use) are to be avoided in conversation. The strategy of getting people to talk with their partners about sex and drug-use histories may be appropriate for some (e.g., white gay males) but completely inappropriate for others (e.g., non-Puerto Rican Hispanic heterosexual couples).

In the black community (Bean, 1989), there is often a perception that homosexuality is a white phenomenon, often as way of denying one's own homosexuality. Reaching gay black males, for example, becomes incredibly difficult, given the relative absence of black gay bars and the tendency to deny one's homosexual orientation. Bean suggests targeting the black family as an effective way of reaching these men.

In the Asian and Pacific Islander population (Chinese, Filipino, Japanese, Vietnamese, Pacific Islander), relatively few AIDS cases have been reported, and the Asian community tends to be somewhat isolated. On the one hand, such isolation may make it more difficult to reach Asians and Pacific Islanders at risk. On the other hand, such relative isolation may have limited the introduction of HIV into Asian communities (Iguchi et al., 1989).

AIDS and the "General Population"

Too often, asking whether HIV will spread into the "general" population really means whether HIV will spread into the "white middle-class heterosexual" population. Such a question means that as long as AIDS is viewed as a disease of gay men, IV drug users, blacks, Hispanics, Asian Americans, and others who are not seen as belonging to the "general population," individual and organizational change will not be necessary. In this view, AIDS is a disease of "them" rather than of "us."

Some have argued that AIDS is a form of genocide being applied by the federal government to minorities in a concerted effort at extermination. Military research in which people were unknowingly exposed to "harmless" bacteria, and the Tuskeegee experiment, in which black men diagnosed with syphillis were allowed to go untreated in order to observe the ultimately fatal course of the disease (Jones, 1981), have been cited as precedent for such actions. Clearly, the minority perspective on AIDS is very different from the white, middle-class perspective and must be taken into account in epidemiology, education, prevention, and treatment.

Although HIV is not transmitted via alcohol, a person under the influence of alcohol or other intoxicants may take behavioral chances that put him (or her) at risk of contracting the virus. In a review of the relationship between alcoholism and AIDS, Molgaard, Nakamura, Hovell, and Elder (1988) identified three areas in which alcohol and AIDS may be interrelated: alcohol and the immune system, alcoholism and sexuality, and alcohol and sexual practices.

Alcohol and the immune system

Heavy users of alcohol are susceptible to infection and a weakened immune system. HIV infected individuals (or people with AIDS) who continue to drink heavily may be further reducing the ability of their immune system to fight off opportunistic infections. Uninfected individuals who drink too much may reduce the ability of their immune system to fight off the HIV when exposed to the virus.

Alcoholism and homosexuality

Drinking seems to play a role in helping some homosexuals to cope with the isolation, stigmatiza-

tion, and homophobia that characterize the homosexual experience. Gay bars may represent a supportive environment for a sexual orientation that may be viewed as unacceptable by parents, siblings, peers, and co-workers.

Alcohol and sexual practices

Alcohol, through its disinhibitory effects, may result in behavior that is out of control. Risky behaviors that would not be acceptable in a sober state become acceptable in an intoxicated state.

DYING OF AIDS OR LIVING WITH AIDS?

AIDS has often been portrayed in the media as a uniformly fatal disease, and such fatality has been used as a fear tactic to presumably motivate young people not to use drugs, or not to engage in homosexual activities. Despite years of research which clearly show that frightening young people will have little, if any, impact upon their risk-taking behaviors, AIDS is still being portrayed as a disease that kills everyone who is diagnosed with it.

Because AIDS originally was detected in gay men, and because some people, including religious leaders, stated that AIDS was a punishment from God, dying of AIDS was perceived by many as divine punishment for one's immoral acts.

Since 1981, medicine has become more sophisticated in treating AIDS; AZT has been an effective anti-viral therapy for many AIDS patients, and aerosolized pentamadine has been helpful in preventing the development of pneumocystis in some HIV infected individuals. Emphasis on the end stage of AIDS (death) tends to obscure the rather lengthy process that one may take to eventually die of AIDS. The spectrum of HIV infection shows a rather different picture:

Date of infection to HIV antibodies found: 6 weeks to 6 months

HIV antibodies to diagnosis of AIDS: 1 to 10 years or more

Survival with AIDS: 1 to 10 years or more

The overall picture shows a disease that may take from 1 to 20 years or more from date of initial infection until death. Since the disease was only identified in 1981, *it is not yet possible to estimate the outer limits of survival with only ten years of historical data.* Nevertheless, with increasing medical advances, many HIV infected individuals may live 20 or 30 or 40 years before dying of AIDS-related illnesses.

SUMMARY

Although emphasis was originally placed on "high-risk groups," it is clear that the real risk for contracting HIV is based on behaviors, not on group affiliations. In the mid-1980s, about 70 percent of AIDS cases were reported in gay or bisexual men; by 1990, that had dropped to about 57 percent. In contrast, cases in intravenous drug users have increased from about 15 percent of the cases in the mid-1980s to almost 25 percent of the cases in 1989. Ethnic differences show that blacks and Hispanics have been hit very hard by AIDS. Although they comprise 18 percent of the population, they make up 40 percent of the AIDS cases.

AIDS cases among heterosexuals make up about 5 percent of the total cases; however, among women, heterosexual contact now accounts for nearly one-third of the reported AIDS cases. Not only are sexual and drug-using behaviors an important part of the AIDS epidemic, but as more information becomes available, issues of age, gender, and race or ethnicity will become increasingly relevant.

Children and adolescents may find themselves at increasing risk for HIV infection from such factors as child sexual abuse and running away from home (and supporting themselves through prostitution). In addition, young people are sexually active, with 15-to-19-year-olds accounting for nearly a quarter of all gonorrhea cases. Adding to these issues, alcohol and other drugs (especially crack cocaine) may contribute to HIV infection, insofar as these substances may weaken a person's immune system or contribute to the loss of behavioral control that makes otherwise risky behaviors seem more acceptable.

Despite the tendency to view AIDS as a uniformly fatal disease that quickly results in death, the overall picture of AIDS shows a disease that may take from 1 to 20 years or more from date of initial infection until death. Even without a vaccine, AZT or other treatments may enable HIV infected individuals to live 20 or 30 or 40 years before dying of AIDS-related illnesses.

REFERENCES

Altman, L. (1990) AIDS rise seen for women and young. *New York Times,* July 28, 1990, Y 11.

Bean, C. (1989) The minority A.I.D.S. Project: Dealing with AIDS in a Black community in Los Angeles. In *AIDS and intravenous drug abuse among minorities.* Rockville, MD: National Institute on Drug Abuse.

Bruner, B. (1988) Sexual abuse in children and adolescents. In R. F. Schinazi and A. J. Nahmias, eds. *AIDS in children, adolescents and heterosexual adults.* New York: Elsevier.

Buckley, W. E., Yesalis, C. E., Friedl, K. E., et al. (1988) Estimated prevalence of anabolic steroid use among male high school seniors. *Journal of the American Medical Association,* 260 (23), 3441–3445.

Campos, P. E., Brasfield, T. L., and Kelly, J. A. (1989) Psychology training related to AIDS: Survey of doctoral graduate programs and predoctoral internship programs. *Professional Psychology: Research and Practice.* 20 (4), 214–220.

Castro, K. G., Lifson, A. R., White, C. R., et al. (1988) Investigations of AIDS patients with no previously identified risk factors. *Journal of the American Medical Association,* 259 (9), 1338–1342.

Centers for Disease Control (1987) *Morbidity and Mortality Weekly Report. Human Immunodeficiency Virus infection in the United States: A review of current knowledge.* 36 (Suppl. no. S–6), 1–48.

Centers for Disease Control (1988a) *Sexually transmitted disease statistics: 1987.* Atlanta, GA: U.S. Department of Health and Human Services.

Centers for Disease Control (1988b) *Morbidity and Mortality Weekly Report. Number of sex partners and potential risk of sexual exposure to Human Immunodeficiency Virus.* 37 (37), 565–568.

Centers for Disease Control (1990) *HIV/AIDS Surveillance Report.* May 1990, 1–18.

Chaisson, R. E., Bacchetti, P., Osmond, D., et al. (1989) Cocaine use and HIV infection in intravenous drug users in San Francisco. *Journal of the American Medical Association,* 261 (4), 561–565.

Chu, S. Y., Buehler, J. W., and Berkelman, R. L. (1990) Impact of the Human Immunodeficiency Virus epidemic on mortality in women of reproductive age, United States. *Journal of the American Medical Association,* 264 (2), 225–229.

Dawson, D., and Thornberry, O. T. (1988) AIDS knowledge and attitudes for December 1987. Provisional data from the National Health Interview Survey. *Advance Data from Vital and Health Statistics.* No. 153. Hyattsville, MD: U.S. Public Health Service.

de la Vega, E. (1989) Homosexuality and bisexuality among Latino men. *Focus: A guide to AIDS research and counseling.* 4 (7), 3–4.

Des Jarlais, D. C., Friedman, S. R., and Hopkins, W. (1985) Risk reduction for the acquired immunodeficiency syndrome among intravenous drug users. *Annals of Internal Medicine,* 103, 755–759.

Des Jarlais, D. C., and Friedman, S. R. (1989) Ethnic differences in HIV seroprevalence rates among intravenous drug users. (In *AIDS and intravenous drug abuse among minorities.* Rockville, MD: National Institute on Drug Abuse.)

Des Jarlais, D. C., Friedman, S. R., Novick, D. M., et al. (1989) HIV-1 infection among intravenous drug users in Manhattan, New York City, from 1977 through 1987. *Journal of the American Medical Association,* 261 (7), 1008–1012.

Fullilove, R. E., Fullilove, M. T., Bowser, B. P., et al. (1990) Risk of sexually transmitted disease among black adolescent crack users in Oakland and San Francisco, Calif. *Journal of the American Medical Association,* 263 (6), 851–855.

Fumento, M. A. (1987) AIDS: Are heterosexuals at risk? *Commentary,* 11, 21–27.

Hahn, R. A., Onorato, I. M., Jones, T. S., and Dougherty, J. (1989) Prevalence of HIV infection among intravenous drug users in the United States. *Journal of the American Medical Association,* 261 (18), 2677–2684.

Hardy, A. M. (1990) AIDS knowledge and attitudes for October–December 1989. Provisional data from the National Health Interview Survey. *Advance Data from Vital and Health Statistics.* No. 186. DHHS Publication No. (PHS) 90–1250. Hyattsville, MD: U.S. Public Health Service.

Iguchi, M. Y., Aoki, B. K., Ngin, P., and Ja, D. Y. (1989) AIDS prevalence in U.S. Asian and Pacific Islander populations. In *AIDS and intravenous drug abuse among minorities.* Rockville, MD: National Institute on Drug Abuse.

Isay, R. A. (1989) *Being homosexual: Gay men and their development.* New York: Farrar, Straus, Giroux.

Jones, J. H. (1981) *Bad blood: The Tuskeegee syphilis experiment.* New York: The Free Press.

Laumann, E. O., Gagnon, J. H., Michaels, S., et al. (1989) Monitoring the AIDS epidemic in the United States: A network approach. *Science,* 244, 1186–1189.

Marin, B. V. (1990) AIDS prevention for non-Puerto Rican Hispanics. In C. G. Leukefeld, R. J. Battjes, and

Amsel, Z., eds. *AIDS and intravenous drug use: Future directions for community-based prevention research. NIDA Research Monograph* 93. Rockville, MD: National Institute on Drug Abuse.

Masters, W. H., Johnson, V. E., Kolodny, R. C. (1988) *Crisis: Heterosexual behavior in the age of AIDS.* New York: Grove Press.

MacDonald, N. E., Wells, G. A., Fisher, W. A., et al. (1990) High-risk STD/HIV behavior among college students. *Journal of the American Medical Association,* 263 (23), 3155–3159.

Miller, H. G., Turner, C. F., and Moses, L. E., eds. (1990) *AIDS. The second decade.* Washington, DC: National Academy Press.

Molgaard, C. A., Nakamura, C., Hovell, M., and Elder, J. P. (1988) Assessing alcoholism as a risk factor for Acquired Immunodeficiency Syndrome (AIDS). *Social Science Medicine,* 27 (11), 1147–1152.

Novick, L. F., Berns, D., Stricof, R., et al. (1989) HIV seroprevalence in newborns in New York State. *Journal of the American Medical Association,* 261 (12), 1745–1750.

Paul, J. P. (1989) AIDS counseling and prevention among bisexual men. *Focus: A guide to AIDS research and counseling.* 4 (7), 1–2.

Ragni, M. W. (1989) Medical aspects of hemophilia and AIDS. *Focus: A guide to AIDS research.* 4 (6), 1–2.

Reinisch, J. M., Sanders, S. A., and Ziemba-Davis, M. (1988) The study of sexual behavior in relation to the transmission of Human Immunodeficiency Virus: Caveats and recommendations. *American Psychologist,* 43 (11), 921–927.

Rogers, M. F., Thomas, P. A., Starcher, E. T., et al. (1987) Acquired immunodeficiency syndrome in children: Report of the Centers for Disease Control national surveillance, 1982–1985. *Pediatrics,* 79 (6), 1008–1014.

Rothenberg, R., Woelfel, M., Stoneburner, R., et al. (1987) Survival with the acquired immunodeficiency syndrome. *New England Journal of Medicine,* 317 (21), 1297–1302.

Schuster, C. R. (1988) A federal agency perspective on AIDS. *American Psychologist,* 43 (11), 846–848.

Scott, M. J., and Scott, M. J. (1989) HIV infection associated with injections of anabolic steroids (letter). *Journal of the American Medical Association,* 292 (2), 207–208.

Selwyn, P. A., Feiner, C., Cox, C. P., et al. (1987) Knowledge about AIDS and high-risk behavior among intravenous drug abusers in New York City. *AIDS,* 1, 247–254.

Serrano, Y. (1990) The Puerto Rican intravenous drug user. In C. G. Leukefeld, R. J. Battjes, and Z. Amsel, eds. *AIDS and intravenous drug use: Future directions for community-based prevention research. NIDA Research Monograph* 93. Rockville, MD: National Institute on Drug Abuse.

Sisk, J. (1988) *How effective is AIDS education?* Washington, DC: Office of Technology Assessment, Congress of the United States.

Stall, R. D., Coates, T. J., and Hoff, C. (1988) Behavioral risk reduction for HIV infection among gay and bisexual men. *American Psychologist,* 43 (11), 878–885.

Prevention Strategies: Education Is Cognitive, AIDS Is Behavioral

7

> *Nothing is so firmly believed as that which is least known.*
>
> EDMUND BURKE

In the absence of a cure for AIDS, and the likelihood of a safe and effective vaccine being perhaps decades away, education has been recommended as the major, if not the only strategy for preventing future cases of HIV infection (Institute of Medicine, 1988). Towards that goal, a variety of strategies have begun on both the federal (Mason et al., 1988) and the professional level (Sy et al., 1989). While education may be effective in changing knowledge and attitudes, it is much less likely to have a long-term impact on 33behavior change. Some expectations are unreasonably optimistic:

> "Education works to prevent the spread of AIDS by altering the behavior through which the virus is transmitted. . . . The Centers for Disease Control (CDC) argues that behavior can be changed if people are told which of their activities increase the probability of

93

"catching AIDS," and are told of "safe" alternatives" (Aiken, 1987, p. 90).

Far too often, those advocating prevention through education have simply not been familiar with the successes and failures of previous education-based prevention programs. Educating people to avoid unhealthy behaviors is not a new recommendation; information about the health risks of smoking cigarettes, using alcohol and other drugs, driving without wearing a seat belt, and so on has been made available for decades. One can be either optimistic or pessimistic about the impact of such educational activities. Some changes in behavior have occurred (e.g., the percentage of Americans smoking has decreased from about 50% in 1964 to about 26% in 1988), but there are many factors in addition to education that may have contributed to that decline. These include the passage of laws prohibiting smoking in public places, the designation of smoking and non-smoking areas, increased costs of smoking by increased taxation, recommendations and interventions by medical providers, more research data on the health hazards of smoking, data on the impact of secondhand smoke, and the elimination of TV advertising for cigarettes.

It is difficult to sort out the effects of education from the other variables in the environment. Broad-based prevention efforts are essential; although education is important, it is not the only method for preventing the spread of HIV. As suggested by Cates and Bowen (1989), expanding methadone maintenance treatment programs, improving control of sexually transmitted diseases, providing family planning outreach for HIV positive women, and extending social support systems will be necessary adjuncts to the strictly "educational" programs.

MEDIA CAMPAIGNS

Early educational efforts were primarily the result of gay organizations in San Francisco (e.g., San Francisco AIDS Project) and New York (e.g., Gay Men's Health Crisis). At the beginning of the epidemic, when it seemed as though AIDS was largely a gay disease, gay organizations were responsible for developing educational materials and programs in an attempt to protect the health of gay men. It was not until seven years into the AIDS epidemic that federally supported media campaigns were put into place. Between May 26 and June 30, 1988, the federal government mailed 107 million copies of a brochure, "Understanding AIDS," to virtually every household in the United States (CDC, 1988c). That was the first time in American history that the federal government tried to contact every resident by mail regarding a major public health problem. However, it was nearly five years earlier that Secretary of Health and Human Services Margaret Heckler stated at a conference in Denver (June 14, 1983): "Nothing I will say is more important than this: that the Department of Health and Human Services considers AIDS its number-one health priority" (Shilts, 1987, p. 324).

The media is a powerful force in the United States. By the time they have graduated from high school, typical students have spent more hours watching television than in class. From the standpoint of audience penetration, the mass media—especially television—represents a way of presenting important health information to literally millions of Americans in a cost-effective manner. Unfortunately, research also shows that many viewers do not remember what they have seen on television even after only a few hours; consequently, messages must be repeated with some degree of frequency.

Media campaigns, although reaching many people, may be severely limited in the content of the message. As noted by Check (1987), much of the coverage on AIDS has been flawed. In particular, the need of the media to appeal to a large mainstream audience (without alienating them), the reliance on single authorities, and a tendency to emphasize sensationalism over factual stories tends to provide a limited, and occasionally inaccurate,

Drug Abuse Prevention: A Model for AIDS Prevention?

AIDS prevention programs do not have to be developed in a vacuum; there is a relatively extensive history regarding the development, implementation, and evaluation of alcohol and drug abuse curricula in the schools. While the relationship between drug abuse and AIDS may not be exactly the same, there are some warnings from drug abuse programs that should be heeded when developing AIDS prevention programs.

Do drug abuse prevention programs work?

Comprehensive assessments of alcohol and drug education prevention programs have simply failed to demonstrate significant changes in behavior as a result of the typical school-based drug intervention education program. Typical programmatic changes were found with knowledge and attitudes, but not behaviors (Bangert-Drowns, 1988). A review (Hopkins et al., 1988) of a comprehensive alcohol education program ("Here's Looking at You") found that the curriculum had no systematic impact on subsequent drinking behaviors, despite the fact that the program was developed on a sound theoretical base.

A survey of junior and senior high school students (Mauss et al., 1988) found that, although contemporary alcohol education programs do focus on variables (e.g., self-esteem, decision-making skills, coping) that seem to be related to drinking, they have very little impact on drinking behavior. Although some smoking prevention programs appear to be successful in delaying the onset of cigarette smoking in adolescents, drug and alcohol prevention programs have not been similarly successful. An evaluation of 30 school-based alcohol and drug abuse prevention programs (Rogers et al., 1989) found that while a few programs did report reductions in drug use, many of the programs did not. In their review of five high school curricula, they reported the following:

Program 1: Significant but uneven changes in behavioral intentions to use drugs

Program 2: Strong positive effects on drug-using behaviors, but only in one of the two sites where it was tested

Program 3: No effects on the reduction of substance use

Program 4: Reduction of drug use reported, but no statistics provided to support that conclusion

Program 5: No evidence available regarding the program's impact on substance use.

Another 51 curricula were identified but not reviewed, for a variety of reasons. Of the 51 programs, 20 (40%) could not be reviewed, because no evaluation of the program was available.

Why recommend education?

Given the rather poor track record of educational programs in preventing substance use and abuse in young people, one must ask: "Why has education received such a prominent role in AIDS prevention"? There are several reasons why education has been promoted:

1. Education is not too controversial. No matter what the problem, one can always be safe by recommending more education as the solution. This is not to imply that AIDS education is not controversial—certainly

the concept of AIDS education and the content of such education has raised considerable controversy in many school districts. But it is a recommendation that can be and has been made with little fear of contradiction, although the philosophy and content of particular programs may generate considerable discussion.

2. Education can be delegated. In many ways, the AIDS crisis has highlighted the lack of leadership from key politicians on the state and federal level. Despite former Surgeon General Koop's leadership role on AIDS, former President Reagan had almost nothing to say on the topic until late in his presidency. Relatively few political leaders have been willing to take a stand on the importance of AIDS as a public health issue. The reluctance to approach AIDS issues "from the top down" means that leadership has been slow in coming. A double message may be the result. On the one hand, key public health leaders have described AIDS as the "nation's number one health priority". On the other hand, influential political leaders remained silent. Is AIDS important, or isn't it?

3. The United States was unprepared for a health crisis of this magnitude. The "system" was simply not capable of responding to this crisis. Lack of leadership, administrative red tape, absence of a comprehensive health-care "system," homophobia, fear of sexual frankness, ignorance about IV drug use all came together through AIDS. It is easier to recommend educational changes that will "change the individual" than it is to "change the system," despite the fact that sexuality and drug use do not occur in a vacuum.

portrayal of AIDS. Basic distinctions between "HIV infection" and "AIDS" are often not made in the media, despite the recommendation by the Presidential Commission on the Human Immunodeficiency Virus Epidemic that the term "HIV infection" be used instead of the ubiquitous "AIDS." The language that we use to communicate about this disease (Gayle, 1989; Hochhauser, 1988) will shape our perceptions, our goals, and our strategies.

Thus far, media efforts have not had a great effect on behavior, although effects on knowledge and attitude have been found. An analysis (Sherr, 1987) of a British health education campaign on AIDS (consisting of whole-page newspaper ads) found increases in knowledge, but little effect on attitude or behavior. While about half of the higher risk group reported reading the ads, only about 30 percent of the lower risk group read the materials.

From a somewhat different perspective D'Augelli and Kennedy, 1989), a brochure that was more sexually explicit produced some discomfort in senior undergraduates. The researchers note that it is possible to overestimate how accepting an audience may be for sexually explicit materials, especially if same-sex activities are described. Discomfort, embarrassment, and guilt may be overwhelming enough to cause avoidance of the message.

Even if the material is presented in a format that is readable, even if it is presented in a way that does not embarrass the reader, the content may still not be understood. In a different context, Jacoby and Hoyer (1987) studied the extent to which magazine readers understood (or misunderstood) the meaning of what they read. They found that 63 percent correctly understood what they had read, 21 percent incorrectly understood what they had read, and 16 percent didn't know.

In addition to these limitations of material and audience, the choice of media remains an important consideration. As noted by the General Accounting Office (GAO, 1989), media selection should be determined by two factors: which media provide the best access to the target audience, and which media permit the best use of available (limited) resources? If the wrong medium is chosen, the message will not be conveyed. These observations suggest that effective use of the media for prevention messages will be a difficult task at best. Moreover, different media approaches are necessary to reach whites, African-Americans, Hispanics, Native Americans, and other ethnic groups.

Disease prevention or infection control

From a prevention standpoint, the language that is used helps set the objectives. For someone who is diagnosed with AIDS, prevention will not work. For someone who is uninfected, the goal of prevention must be to prevent infection. Using AIDS as a scare tactic will likely be as effective as using the fear of alcoholism to prevent alcohol use or using lung cancer as a reason to not begin smoking. From this perspective, the goal is infection control, not disease prevention.

SAFER SEX STRATEGIES

When it became known that HIV could be transmitted sexually, recommendations came from many AIDS organizations regarding what were called "safe sex" techniques. That term still can be found in much of the AIDS literature. However, the term "safe sex" implies a degree of safety that simply may not exist in the real world, when decisions made in the heat of passion (or under the influence of alcohol or drugs) may not always be "safe." Moreover, even if used appropriately, condoms can and do fail. As a result of these limitations, the term *safe sex* was replaced with *safer sex,* suggesting that sexual behaviors could be made safer, but not always completely safe.

A content analysis of "risk reduction/safe-sex" brochures (Siegel et al., 1986), found some important limitations and omissions. First, none of the brochures reviewed contained an action plan suggesting strategies that could be used to deal with the threat of AIDS, although some of the

brochures did offer concrete suggestions that could be one part of such a plan. It is one thing to simply describe behavioral changes, but it's quite another to incorporate new behaviors into one's life. Finally, about half of the brochures were ambiguous regarding key objectives, such as reducing or limiting one's sexual partners or the frequency of engaging in specific risky behaviors. Such limitations may well produce counterproductive outcomes in people who understand the brochures at a cognitive level, but who do not know how to develop such new behaviors.

Few brochures provided any information at all about "self-efficacy"—reassurances to the reader that behavior changes could be accomplished as part of a constructive, positive lifestyle. As noted by Stall, Coates, and Hoff (1988), a belief in personal efficacy has been found in a number of studies to be a powerful variable in the adoption of low-risk sexual behaviors. McKusick and fellow researchers (1990) found personal efficacy to be an important variable in reducing unprotected anal intercourse among San Francisco gay men. They also identified several additional program characteristics for the reduction of high-risk behaviors, including the challenging of peer norms, the promotion of HIV antibody testing, and the eroticizing of safer sexual activities.

Abstinence

From the standpoint of sexual transmission of HIV, abstinence is the only definite method of not contracting the virus (although one could be sexually abstinent and contract the virus through needle sharing). Unfortunately, as with much of the language surrounding AIDS, the meaning of "abstinence" is not always clear. For many people, abstinence means not engaging in vaginal sexual intercourse. Does abstinence also include the avoidance of mutual masturbation, or deep kissing, or petting, or even oral sex? It is possible that a person could be abstinent (not having vaginal intercourse) and still be engaging in risky behaviors (e.g., anal intercourse, oral sex) that could result in transmission of HIV.

By the time they have graduated from high school, about 70 percent of young people have already been sexually active. Surveys of 13-to-18-year-old high school students (CDC, 1990) found that over half (56%) reported having had sexual intercourse at least once, with about 21 percent having had four or more sexual partners. Among those who have dropped out of high school, the percentage is probably higher. As a method for preventing HIV transmission, abstinence may reinforce those students who have been abstinent and choose to continue to be abstinent. For those young people, the message of abstinence may be very effective.

For those students who have already been sexually active, recommendations of abstinence may not be so effective. Some young people may choose to follow that message and return to being abstinent; others may choose to continue to be sexually active. Adolescence is a time of risk taking, of trying to establish one's identity, or rebelling against authority figures. For some adolescents, being told to be abstinent by an adult authority figure is likely to be counterproductive. Miller, Turner, and Moses (1990), note that the CDC (1988a) "Guidelines for Effective School Health Education to Prevent the Spread of AIDS" recommend that school programs encourage sexually active students to "stop engaging in intercourse until they are ready to establish a mutually monogamous relationship within the context of marriage" (p. 4). However, these researchers also note that such guidelines do not reflect the diversity of values or behaviors in the United States, but seem to impose a particular set of values on all adolescents. One result of this prevention effort, should it be successful, would be that many young people might get married in order to have sex (as they did in earlier decades). However, marriages based on the need to legitimize sexual activity might not be the best basis for a successful long-term relationship.

Mutually monogamous partners

After abstinence, having a relationship with only one person has been suggested as a method of avoiding HIV. As with abstinence, the term *mutual monogamy* means different things to different people. For married couples, mutual monogamy should be the norm, yet data on the percentages of married people who have extramarital affairs is not encouraging. In their review of sexual behavior, Reinisch, Sanders, and Ziemba-Davis (1988) estimated that 37 percent of husbands and 29 percent of wives have had at least one extramarital relationship. Young people, who are just beginning to date, may find the concept of a "mutually monogamous" relationship difficult.

Adolescence and young adulthood is a time of psychological and sexual exploration and growth. In contrast to the 1950s or 1960s, when dating several people simultaneously was an accepted practice, many young people in the 1980s and 1990s engage in "serial monogamy," in which the person dates only one person at a time. In this context, the adolescent may perceive himself or herself to be faithful to his or her partner for the duration of the relationship. Perhaps the relationship will lead to marriage, in which case it may serve as a mutually monogamous relationship. On the other hand, if the relationship ends, after one year or so, the adolescent or young adult may move into another relationship. The young people involved in this dating sequence consider themselves to be faithful to their partner for as long as the relationship lasts. If it does not last until marriage and they move into another relationship, they do not necessarily perceive themselves as being promiscuous, but only being faithful to another person. Referring to such behaviors as "promiscuity" may do little to enhance communication between young people (who believe they are being faithful to their current partner) and adults.

Condoms

Condoms, especially those made of latex with a spermicide, have been recommended (CDC, 1988b) as an effective barrier method for protecting one from sexually transmitted diseases, as well as HIV. However, condoms are not foolproof. Condoms can fail for a variety of reasons:

- *Defective manufacturing.* Condoms are tested by being filled with water or air until they burst. If 4 or more per 1,000 fail, the entire lot fails. For those lots that have passed, the average failure rate is 2.3 per 1000 (CDC, 1988b).
- *Improper use.* Using a condom seems fairly straightforward; however, there are ways that it can be used improperly, resulting in pregnancy or transmission of sexually transmitted diseases. Some people open the package with their teeth (perhaps tearing the condom inside the package); some people use an oil-based lubricant (which will cause latex to disintegrate); some people put the condom on too late (after some semen has been discharged); some people take off the condom improperly (causing seminal leakage).
- *Misunderstandings.* Although condoms come with instructions, often in the heat of passion (or in the dark) one cannot read the instructions or

does not take time to follow the step-by-step procedures. Moreover, condom instructions may be hard to understand by those who have limited reading skills or who may be functionally illiterate. A readability analysis of 14 sets of condom instructions (Richwald et al., 1988) found that 8 of the 14 required a reading level of at least a high school graduate; none required less than a 10th-grade level. Simply telling people to use condoms, without showing them how to use them and how not to misuse them may reduce their risk of HIV infection by only a small amount. Moreover, if condoms are used regularly but improperly, they may convey a false sense of security to both partners, and other aspects of safer sex may be ignored. Table 7.1 describes the CDC (1988b) recommendations for the proper use of condoms to reduce the transmission of sexually transmitted diseases.

- *Condom promotion.* Discussions about condoms, or even recommendations that they be used, may not be translated into safer sex behaviors. In a study of condom promotion, Solomon and DeJong (1989) found that not only was education (i.e., a soap opera–style videotape on STDs) important in influencing attitudes about condom use, but making condoms more accessible by redeeming condom coupons at a clinic increased

TABLE 7.1   Recommendations for Condom Use[1]

1. Latex condoms should be used because they offer greater protection against viral STD than natural-membrane condoms.
2. Condoms should be stored in a cool, dry place out of direct sunlight.
3. Condoms in damaged packages or those that show obvious signs of age (e.g., those that are brittle, sticky, or discolored) should not be used. They cannot be relied upon to prevent infection.
4. Condoms should be handled with care to prevent puncture.
5. The condom should be put on before any genital contact occurs, to prevent exposure to fluids that may contain infectious agents. Hold the tip of the condom and unroll in onto the erect penis, leaving space at the tip to collect semen, yet assuring that no air is trapped in the tip of the condom.
6. Adequate lubrication should be used. If exogenous lubrication is needed, only water-based lubricants should be used. Petroleum- or oil-based lubricants (such as petroleum jelly, cooking oils, shortening, and lotions) should not be used, because they weaken the latex.
7. Use of condoms containing spermicides may provide some additional protection against STD. However, vaginal use of spermicides along with condoms is likely to provide greater protection.
8. If a condom breaks, it should be replaced immediately. If ejaculation occurs after condom breakage, the immediate use of spermicide has been suggested. However, the protective value of postejaculation application of spermicide in reducing the risk of STD transmission is unknown.
9. After ejaculation, care should be taken so that the condom does not slip off the penis before withdrawal; the base of the condom should be held while it is withdrawn. The penis should be withdrawn while it is still erect.
10. Condoms should never be reused.

[1] CDC, 1988b.

the request for condoms, especially among those patients with fewer years of formal education.

Solomon and DeJong (1989) targeted individual patients in their project. In designing interventions for intravenous drug users, Stone and other researchers (1989) recommended that interventions for IV drug users should target the couple, rather than just the individual. Strategies that target couples will have to be very different from those that target individuals, which suggests that a variety of condom promotional techniques must be developed. A generic recommendation for condoms will probably be ineffective.

TALKING AND LISTENING

Many health educators have recommended that partners talk with each other about their past sexual experiences. This may be difficult, if not impossible, because many young people have grown up either ignorant about sex or unable to discuss human sexuality. It's not easy to tell another person about your sexual history; neither is it easy to listen to another person tell you about his or her sexual experiences. Nevertheless, from the standpoint of risk-reduction behaviors, such conversations can do much to help identify the risks that have been taken in the past and to suggest what risk-reduction activities should be used with each other. Such communication skills must be taught, not just recommended.

Despite a person's or a couple's best efforts, behavior change is not always consistent. As with people who quit smoking, drinking, or using drugs, some relapses must be expected. During the past few years, substantial declines in gonorrhea in homosexual and bisexual men have been reported. However, a report on gonorrhea in homosexually active men in King County, Washington (CDC, 1989) suggests that gonorrhea will triple in 1989 from 1988. Behavioral change successes are not always permanent.

IV DRUG USE

Being an IV drug user per se does not put one at risk for contracting HIV; the sharing of needles and syringes (the "works") is the risky behavior. Telling a heroin addict to simply "Just say no" is not likely to reduce needle-sharing behaviors, especially since such sharing may be a major part of the IV drug-using culture. HIV transmission via needle sharing is a major problem for several reasons. Although IV drug use is generally viewed as a problem of inner city addicts, a survey of high school students aged 13 to 18 (CDC, 1990) found that an average of 3 percent (2–5%) had injected cocaine, heroin, or other drugs, while 0.9 percent (.2–3%) reported that they shared needles. Nationally, there are about 13 million high school students; if these statistics are generalizable (and they may not be), then between 260,000 and 650,000 may have injected drugs at least once, while 26,000 to 390,000 may have shared needles. Although many of these students may not become dependent on drugs, their experimental use may still put them at risk for contracting HIV.

IV drug use issues

Uninfected drug users can contract the virus from infected drug users by using the same "works." Since many states require a physician's prescription to purchase syringes and needles, IV drug users must recycle their "works" because the supply is limited. To complicate the issue even more, DesJarlais and Friedman (1989) have noted that some IV drug users do not consider themselves to be "sharing" their "works" if those works are being used by sexual partners or very close friends. The analogy that Des Jarlais and Friedman use is that a couple who eats a meal together would not describe that meal as "sharing their food," since the food is possessed by both of them.

Because of the dependency-producing nature of heroin, cocaine, crack, and other street drugs, some drug users have turned to prostitution as a way of obtaining money for their drug habit. Those who become infected by their "works" may transmit the virus to their customers, or vice versa. Moreover, while heroin users may get "high" every four to six hours and may have to inject four to six times per day, intravenous users of cocaine may have to inject a dozen times per day because the "high" lasts for a much shorter period of time (Booth, 1988). More injections require more syringes; more injections probably mean more sharing of "works"; more sharing probably means more spread of HIV infection.

Needles and syringes have taken on a completely new importance during the past few years. Similar risks exist in a health-care setting, where a needlestick injury from an HIV infected patient can lead to HIV infection in the health-care worker who was stuck. In IV drug use and in the health-care setting, the needle and syringe serve as the vehicle of viral transmission.

Nonstick technology

One response from the health-care industry has been to develop a "nonstick" technology for needles and other invasive devices, such as catheters. Syringes are available that can be used only once and must then be disposed of in a puncture-proof container. During the next few years, reusable syringes may become harder and harder to obtain, as nonstick technology comes to predominate. However, the cost of these "safer" syringes is significantly higher than the reusable syringes, and the health-care industry may be relatively slow to adopt such an expensive alternative. Nevertheless, at some point in the future, the "works" that become available to drug users may not be able to be shared, although it is possible that some of the single-use syringes might be able to be modified for multiple uses. Given the subcultural value of needle sharing for IVDUs, a black market in reusable needles and syringes may well develop as a way of meeting that particular need.

Needle exchanges

One way of trying to slow the transmission of HIV via needles and syringes is to provide IV drug users with clean needles and syringes upon demand. However, state and federal laws may make such exchange programs legally difficult to accomplish. For example, in some states, it is illegal to sell or possess a syringe and needle without a physician's prescription (Pascal, 1988). Fearing arrest, users are unlikely to carry their needles with them. By sharing needles, the user can inject drugs without taking the risk of carrying his or her own injection equipment, although social factors such as trust also play a role in needle sharing (Battjes and Pickens, 1988).

Although needle-exchange programs have been suggested, only a few have been tried. One program (Buning et al., 1988) in Amsterdam, the Netherlands, made the following discoveries:

- IV drug addicts who participated in the exchange reported less sharing than those who did not participate,
- needle sharing still continued, although many addicts reported changing their sharing behavior,
- providing clean needles did not encourage addicts to inject more, as had been feared by some.

Bleach

Another method for helping to slow down the rate of HIV transmission due to IV drug use is to teach IV drug users how to clean their "works," typically by twice flushing the needle and syringe in household bleach (Newmeyer, 1988). Bleach was selected as the disinfectant of choice because it is

1. quick, taking less than 60 seconds,
2. inexpensive,
3. conveniently available,
4. safe to the user and to his or her equipment,
5. effective at neutralizing viruses.

This, too, is a politically sensitive issue, with some arguing that providing bleach simply encourages users to keep using drugs and may help recruit new drug users, because the perception may be that syringes are now safer than they were in the past.

U.S. differences

All patterns of IV drug use are not the same. Seroprevalence rates for IV drug users vary considerably by region (Hahn et al., 1989). Nationally, 5 to 33 percent of the IV drug-using population is thought to be infected—between 61,000 and 398,000 people. Highest rates of infection were in New York City (as high as 65% in Brooklyn) and Puerto Rico (45–59%), while lower rates were found in San Francisco (7–13%) and Tampa, New Orleans, and Tacoma (less than 2%). Such differences may be due to patterns of mobility with considerable mobility in the Northeast (between northern New Jersey and New York City, for example), or the use of shooting galleries (which may be more of a Northeastern phenomenon), or simply the number of HIV infected individuals in the community.

RISK ASSESSMENT AND PREVENTION

How do people assess their own risks with respect to AIDS? Unfortunately, much of the commentary on AIDS has relied more on the author's conception of risk than of the scientific community's definition. Much of what is known about AIDS is based upon epidemiological research; nevertheless, despite massive amounts of data, many fundamental scientific standards may be omitted or even violated in the subsequent interpretation of these data (Feinstein, 1988). One crucial point made by Feinstein is that if the epidemiological research is flawed, researchers may make erroneous associations that lead the public to believe that a risk exists when, in fact, the risk does not exist. Much of

the hysteria and fear surrounding AIDS may be due to the categorization of "risk groups" with the disease—fear of people substituted for fear of behaviors.

As a result, many Americans believe it is likely or very likely that a person will get AIDS or the AIDS virus infection from casual contact (living, working, or simply being near someone who is infected). Detels and coauthors (1989) concluded that:

> "This paper underscores the fact that transmission of HIV-1 is associated with specific sexual activities, not with sexual orientation. Anal-genital intercourse is not an exclusively homosexual practice. . . . Thus, it seems reasonable that AIDS cases reported by the state and federal governments might better be classified by most-likely activity, which may be associated with transmission, rather than by sexual orientation, e.g., anal-genital intercourse, vaginal intercourse, IV drug use, and transfusion. This method of reporting would underscore to the community the specific activities that should be avoided. Currently, there is considerable concern by the public that casual contact with individuals who have specific sexual preferences could result in infection. Reporting by specific activity likely to be associated with transmission could do much to reduce this fear." (p. 83)

After all, a close reading of the CDC "exposure categories" (male homosexual or bisexual contact, intravenous drug use, heterosexual contact, etc.) does not really describe exactly *how* the virus is transmitted. What does "homosexual contact" or "heterosexual contact" mean? How many ways can those terms be interpreted—and misinterpreted?

Some researchers have concluded that the public's perception of health risk is not always based on fact, but on the public's understanding of technical information, how the "facts" are presented to the public, the public attitudes and understanding of science, and a national preoccupation with health and selected political factors (Burger, 1988).

In a review of personal risks, Weinstein (1989) notes that although people often overestimate the general harm caused by some problems, they tend to consistently *underestimate* their own personal risks. A few of Weinstein's conclusions are very relevant to AIDS education and prevention.

1) Optimism is greater for those hazards with which people have had little personal experience, with a low probability of occurring, and with a possibility of personal control. Someone who has never seen a person with AIDS (or HIV infection), who believes that the likelihood of becoming infected is low (most Americans say they have little or no chance of contracting the HIV), and who believes that he or she can avoid HIV by avoiding casual contact with infected people, may have an overly optimistic perspective of health. Such optimism may prevent the development of safer sex and drug-using behaviors if the person believes that the likelihood of becoming HIV infected is essentially zero.

2) Most people desire to be better than others. We may enhance our own self-esteem by attributing AIDS to risky behavior by "others." To the extent that the disease occurs to someone else who behaves in ways that we do not behave (or at least say that we do not), we can protect our feeling of competence and justify not having to change our behaviors.

3) Errors in thinking may produce overly optimistic expectations about risks. If an education or prevention program creates a stereotype of an AIDS patient, some may translate this stereotype into a standard. In comparison with this standard, some people conclude incorrectly that since they are not the same as the standard, they are not at risk. (The logic would be "Gay men get AIDS. I am not a gay man. Therefore, I cannot get AIDS.")

The way that risks are presented by educators may not be the way that risks are perceived by students. Unless a more complete understanding of the social and psychological aspects of risk (Freudenberg, 1988) becomes incorporated into prevention programs, the outcome of AIDS prevention programs will demonstrate very few successes.

SUMMARY

Education is a cognitive process; AIDS is behavioral. Despite the emphasis on education as an effective prevention strategy, education is likely to be effective in changing knowledge and perhaps attitudes and is likely to be ineffective in changing behaviors. Even if mass media are used, information may be presented in ways that cannot be understood by the audience, in ways that may offend the audience, or in ways that frighten the audience so much that they avoid the message.

Being HIV infected and being diagnosed with AIDS are not the same. A crucial objective for any educational program is to decide whether the focus of the program is on AIDS prevention (which may be 10 years in the future for many young people) or on HIV infection control (which is a more immediate concern). Terminology such as "abstinence," "safer sex," and "mutual monogamy" may mean different things to different people, depending on their gender, age, ethnic background, and sexual orientation. Clearly defined terms are essential.

Research on risk assessment shows that many people are overly optimistic about their own personal risks. Because of ambiguities in the description of "exposure categories," many people may believe that they are avoiding HIV infection by avoiding those people who have the disease, rather than their own behaviors which may place them at risk. Rationalizations based on a lack of personal experience with people with AIDS, a stereotypical image of a person with AIDS, or a need to maintain self-esteem by viewing AIDS as a disease of "other people" all contribute to the overly optimistic perception that one is not at risk and does not have to change.

REFERENCES

Aiken, J. H. (1987) Education as prevention. In H. L. Dalton, S. Burris, and the Yale AIDS Law Project, eds. *AIDS and the law.* New Haven: Yale University Press.

Bangert-Drowns, R. L. (1988) The effects of school-based substance abuse education—A meta-analysis. *Journal of Drug Education,* 18 (3), 243–264.

Battjes, R. H., and Pickens, R. W. (1988) Needle sharing among intravenous drug abusers: Future directions. In R. J. Battjes and R. W. Pickens, eds. *Needle sharing among intravenous drug abusers: National and international perspectives. NIDA Research Monograph 80.* Rockville, MD: National Institute on Drug Abuse.

Booth, W. (1988) AIDS and drug abuse: No quick fix. *Science,* 239, 717–719.

Buning, E. C., H. A. van Brussel, G., and van Santen, G. (1988) Amsterdam's drug policy and its implications for controlling needle sharing. In R. H. Battjes and R. W. Pickens, eds. *Needle sharing among intravenous drug abusers: National and international perspectives. NIDA Research Monograph 80.* Rockville, MD: National Institute on Drug Abuse.

Burger, E. J. (1988) How citizens think about risks to health. *Risk Analysis,* 8 (3), 309–313.

Cates, W., and Bowen, G. S. (1989) Education for AIDS prevention; not our only voluntary weapon. *American Journal of Public Health,* 79 (7), 871–873.

CDC (1988a) *Morbidity and Mortality Weekly Report.* Guidelines for effective school health education to prevent the spread of AIDS. 37 (S–2), 1–14.

CDC (1988b) *Morbidity and Mortality Weekly Report.* Condoms for prevention of sexually transmitted diseases. 37 (9), 133–137.

CDC (1988c) *Morbidity and Mortality Weekly Report.* Understanding AIDS: An information brochure being mailed to all U.S. households. 37 (17), 261–269.

CDC (1989) *Morbidity and Mortality Weekly Report.* Trends in gonorrhea in homosexually active men—King County, Washington, 1989. 38 (44), 762–764.

CDC (1990) *Morbidity and Mortality Weekly Report.* HIV-related knowledge and behaviors among high school students—Selected U.S. sites, 1989. 39 (23), 385–389; 395–397.

Check, W. A. (1987) Beyond the political model of reporting: Nonspecific symptoms in media communication about AIDS. *Reviews of Infectious Diseases,* 9 (5), 987–1000.

D'Augelli, A. R., and Kennedy, S. P. (1989) An evaluation of AIDS prevention brochures for university men and women. *AIDS Education and Prevention,* 1 (2), 134–140.

DesJarlais, D. C., and Friedman, S. R. (1989) Ethnic differences in HIV seroprevalence rates among intravenous drug users. In *AIDS and intravenous drug abuse among minorities.* Rockville, MD: National Institute on Drug Abuse.

Detels, R., English, P., Visscher, et al. (1989) Seroconversion, sexual activity, and condom use among 2915 HIV seronegative men followed up to 2 years. *Journal of Acquired Immune Deficiency Syndrome,* 2 (1), 77–83.

Feinstein, A. R. (1988) Scientific standards in epidemiologic studies of the menace of daily life. *Science,* 242, 1257–1263.

Freudenberg, W. R. (1988) Perceived risk, real risk: Social science and the art of probabilistic risk assessment. *Science,* 242, 44–48.

GAO (1989) *AIDS education. Reaching populations at higher risk.* Washington, DC: U.S. General Accounting Office.

Gayle, J. A. (1989) The effect of terminology on public consciousness related to the HIV epidemic. *AIDS Education and Prevention,* 1 (3), 247–250.

Hahn, R. A., Onorato, I. M., Jones, T. S., and Dougherty, J. (1989) Prevalence of HIV infection among intravenous drug users in the United States. *Journal of the American Medical Association,* 261 (18), 2677–2684.

Hochhauser, M. (1988) Communicating about AIDS. *Focus: A guide to AIDS research.* 3 (11), 1–3.

Hopkins, R. H., Mauss, A. L., Kearney, K. A., and Weisheit, R. A. (1988) Comprehensive evaluation of a model alcohol education curriculum. *Journal of Studies on Alcohol,* 49 (1), 38–50.

Institute of Medicine (1988) *Confronting AIDS. Update 1988.* Washington, DC: National Academy Press.

Jacoby, J., and Hoyer, W. D. (1987) *The comprehension and miscomprehension of print communications: An investigation of mass media magazines.* Hillsdale, NJ: Lawrence Erlbaum Associates.

Ledbetter, C. A., and Johnson, D. (1989) AIDS: Reading level analysis of public information. *AIDS & Public Policy Journal,* 4 (3), 11–14.

Mason, J. O., Noble, G. R., Lindsey, B. K., et al. (1988) Current CDC efforts to prevent and control human immunodeficiency virus infection and AIDS in the United States through information and education. *Public Health Reports,* 103 (3), 255–260.

Mauss, A. L., Hopkins, R. H., Weisheit, R. A., and Kearney, K. A. (1988) The problematic prospects for prevention in the classroom: Should alcohol education programs be expected to reduce drinking by youth? *Journal of Studies on Alcohol,* 49 (1), 51–61.

McKusick, L., Coates, T. J., Morin, S. T., et al. (1990) Longitudinal predictors of reductions in unprotected anal intercourse among gay men in San Francisco: The AIDS Behavioral Research Project. *American Journal of Public Health,* 80 (8), 978–983.

Miller, H. G., Turner, C. F., and Moses, L. E. (1990) *AIDS. The second decade.* Washington, DC: National Academy Press.

Newmeyer, H. A. (1988) Why bleach? Development of a strategy to combat HIV contagion among San Francisco IV drug users. In R. H. Battjes and R. W. Pickens, eds. *Needle sharing among intravenous drug abusers: National and international perspectives. NIDA Research Monograph 80.* Rockville, MD: National Institute on Drug Abuse.

Pascal, C. B. (1988) Intravenous drug abuse and AIDS transmission: Federal and state laws regulating needle availability. In R. H. Battjes and R. W. Pickens, eds. *Needle sharing among intravenous drug abusers: National and international perspectives. NIDA Research Monograph 80.* Rockville, MD: National Institute on Drug Abuse.

Reinisch, J. M., Sanders, S. A., and Ziemba-Davis, M. (1988) The study of sexual behavior in relation to the transmission of Human Immunodeficiency Virus. *American Psychologist,* 43 (11), 921–927.

Richwald, G. A., Wamsley, M. A., Coulson, A. H., and Morisky, D. E. (1988) Are condom instructions readable? Results of a readability study. *Public Health Reports,* 103 (4), 355–359.

Rogers, T., Howard-Pitney, B., Bruce, B. L. (1989) *What works? A guide to school-based alcohol and drug abuse prevention curricula.* Palo Alto, CA: Health Promotion Resource Center, Stanford Center for Research in Disease Prevention.

Sherr, L. (1987) An evaluation of the UK government health education campaign on AIDS. *Psychology and health: An international journal,* 1 (1), 61–72.

Shilts, R. (1987) *And the band played on.* New York: St. Martin's Press.

Siegel, K., Grodsky, P. B., and Herman, A. (1986) AIDS risk-reduction guidelines: A review and analysis. *Journal of Community Health,* 11 (4), 233–243.

Solomon, M. Z., and DeJong, W. (1989) Preventing AIDS and other STDs through condom promotion: A patient education intervention. *American Journal of Public Health,* 79 (4), 453–458.

Stall, R. D., Coates, T. J., and Hoff, C. (1988) Behavioral risk reduction for HIV infection among gay and bisexual men. *American Psychologist,* 43 (11), 878–885.

Stone, A. J., Morisky, D., Detels, R., and Braxton, H. (1989) Designing interventions to prevent HIV-1 infection by promoting use of condoms and spermicides among intravenous drug abusers and their sexual partners. *AIDS Education and Prevention,* 1 (3), 171–183.

Sy, F. S., Richter, D. L., and Copello, A. G. (1989) Innovative educational strategies and recommendations for AIDS prevention and control. *AIDS Education and Prevention,* 1 (1), 53–56.

Weinstein, M. C., Graham, J. D., Siegel, J. E., and Fineberg, H. V. (1989) Cost-effectiveness analysis of AIDS prevention programs: Concepts, complications and illustrations. In C. F. Turner, H. G. Miller, and L. E. Moses, eds. *AIDS: Sexual behavior and intravenous drug use.* Washington, DC: National Academy Press.

Weinstein, N. D. (1989) Optimistic biases about personal risks. *Science,* 246, 1232–1233.

8 Education vs. Information

> *Beware of false knowledge; it is more*
> *dangerous than ignorance.*
>   GEORGE BERNARD SHAW

EDUCATION VS. INFORMATION

Different professionals define prevention in different ways (Leventhal et al., 1985). For example, physicians are likely to support a biomedical perspective emphasizing the use of medical interventions (such as AIDS vaccines) to prevent the development of AIDS. Public health professionals promote an environmental method for blocking the spread of disease (e.g., HIV antibody testing, reporting of names and contact tracing). Behavioral scientists focus on methods of altering an individual's risk behavior (e.g., teaching safer sex practices, and cleaning needles and syringes). Although the ultimate objective—the reduction or elimination of HIV infection—may be the same for all three professions, the methods of achieving that objective may be quite different. To some extent, each profession has recognized its particular limitations in dealing with AIDS, and all have identified education and information as a method of prevention.

Education and information are not the same, but many AIDS educators seem to believe that merely providing AIDS information to young people is the same as educating them about AIDS. Education is

> "The process of educating, teaching, or training; a part of or a stage in this training. . . . the process of imparting or acquiring skills for a particular trade or profession,"

while information is

> "News or intelligence communicated by word or in writing; facts or data; knowledge derived from reading or instruction. . . ." (*Living Webster Encyclopedic Dictionary of the English Language,* 1975).

There is no shortage of information about AIDS. Books, journal articles, brochures, magazine articles, television specials, and documentaries have provided the American public with a considerable amount of information concerning AIDS. However, information alone is not likely to result in significant behavior change. Indeed, information-based prevention programs may help to change the knowledge base of the person receiving the information, but they will probably have little effect on behavior change.

Information is essentially atheoretical; there is no system for motivating or reinforcing the person who has received such information. Consequently, although information alone may be interesting for the audience, it does not provide a system for initiating and maintaining behavior change. Because AIDS information often occurs randomly, without placement in a relevant context, knowing the basic "facts about AIDS" does not imply that a person will necessarily know how to protect himself or herself from the virus nor how to maintain such behavioral changes over the course of a lifetime.

Winett (1986), in an intriguing chapter titled "Information and Health Behavior: Futile Attempts or Small-Wins," suggests that health problems must be viewed within a contextual system (e.g., organization of cities and towns) before new information can be used to positively affect health behaviors. Ultimately, Winett asks, "Will these information-based, small-win strategies make any difference in health outcomes?" (e.g., the Stanford Five City Project to improve cardiovascular health). He concluded that only time will provide the answer to that question. Given the limitations that have been experienced when trying to change health behaviors, we may have to scale down our expectations for our definition of "success" regarding AIDS prevention programs.

Level of education

Education does have more of a theoretical base than does information. However, educational programs tend to focus more on cognitive changes rather than on attitudes and behaviors. Even recommendations for further education about AIDS tend not to have a theoretical basis. For instance, one way that AIDS education could be developed throughout the school curriculum would be to incorporate Bloom's (1986) taxonomy of educational objectives. Surgeon General Koop received considerable criticism when he recommended that AIDS education take place as early as elementary school, as some thought that this meant educating very young children about such issues as condoms and safe sex. Bloom's taxonomy offers one method for incorporating AIDS education throughout the curriculum, based not so much on the content of the prevention program, but on the cognitive abilities of students and the changes in those abilities from kindergarten through the twelfth grade. Briefly summarized, AIDS education programs might have the following components:

1. Knowledge; of specifics, of terminology, of categories
   - Defining AIDS terminology; knowledge of the history of AIDS; knowing the difference between AIDS and HIV
2. Comprehension; interpretation and extrapolation
   - Understanding health education materials; interpreting different types of AIDS research data; predicting the future of AIDS
3. Application
   - Applying educational principles to medical or psychological phenomena
4. Analysis; of elements, of relationships, of organizational principles

- Recognizing unstated assumptions (e.g., political, religious), checking the consistency of health-related hypotheses with given information
5. Synthesis; producing a communication; deriving abstract relations
   - Telling a personal experience about AIDS; planning a teaching unit for AIDS; formulating new hypotheses about AIDS
6. Evaluation; judging internal and external criteria
   - Judging the accuracy of information about AIDS; finding logical fallacies in AIDS-related arguments; comparing major theories.

If such a comprehensive plan were put into place, students would no doubt have a better knowledge base and conceptual understanding of AIDS-related issues. However, such academic accomplishments do not necessarily mean that students will modify their risky behavior in appropriate ways.

AIDS is a political as well as a social and medical issue. The cost of developing, implementing, and evaluating comprehensive AIDS education programs is likely to be rather high. As noted by Booth (1987), some politicians have been offended by explicit AIDS educational materials and have threatened to withhold federal funds for programs they find offensive. Even if effective prevention programs are developed, funding may be insufficient for their wide-scale implementation. Education may be acceptable, but ineffective; behavioral change may be effective, but unacceptable. Thus, recommending more and more education to deal with a problem is a relatively safe strategy, since education tends to focus on abstract principles rather than on concrete behaviors. However, sexual behaviors and IV drug-using behaviors are *behaviors* and may require behavioral rather than educational intervention. This means that some people would have to be trained in how to use a condom, how to clean one's ''works,'' and so forth. This would require hands-on training, per-

haps through classroom educational activities. We would not expect airline pilots to improve their flying skills by just reading a manual and taking a multiple-choice test; we would expect them to do some actual flying (either in a simulator or in the air). Similar activities may be necessary for significant behavioral changes to occur in sex and drug use.

PRINCIPLES OF BEHAVIOR CHANGE

Most AIDS prevention programs have not had any sort of theoretical basis to guide the program. The standard strategy has simply been to distribute as much information as possible through brochures, pamphlets, student programs and assemblies, and other means without any forethought as to what approach is likely to be effective in changing behavior. Simply telling people to change is not enough.

On the one hand, it has been suggested (Baum and Nesselhoff, 1988) that one component of AIDS education is to reduce people's irrational fear of the disease so that more effective interventions can take place. On the other hand, many of the AIDS prevention programs have tried to increase fear through the use of scare tactics, in the hope that such fear would result in behavior changes. However, Becker and Joseph (1988) note that ''Nonetheless, there is little actual evidence that an individual's knowledge and attitudes toward AIDS significantly shape his or her behavior.'' (p. 408)

Attitudes and behavior

Research on the relationship between attitudes and behavior is complex. Although one might expect that our attitudes will determine how we behave, sometimes it is just the opposite: What we do determines what we believe. If so, practicing safer sex would lead to positive attitudes about safer sex, while having a positive attitude about safer sex might not lead to abstinence or safer sex practices. Is the goal for people to know about abstinence, to have a positive attitude about abstinence, or to practice abstinence? The answer to that question will help determine what kind of education intervention should be developed.

Siegel and Gibson (1988) have identified some of the barriers to changes in sexual behavior among heterosexuals. Some of the barriers are attitudinal and perceptual, and these authors believe that such health education programs must focus on changing these attitudes and perceptions. Key barriers to change include

- a perception of low vulnerability,
- an unwillingness to use condoms,
- confusion regarding the actual threat to heterosexuals,
- the stigma of AIDS.

Although health educators often assume that attitude change is necessary before behavior change can take place, there is considerable literature in psychology suggesting that in some cases, attitudes change after behavior changes.

Scare tactics

Historically, the standard method for getting young people to change their behaviors with regard to alcohol, drugs, and sex has been to scare them by describing the long-term consequences of such behaviors (e.g., alcoholism, drug dependency, and death from AIDS). Unfortunately, although scare tactics may be helpful for some individuals who have not yet engaged in the particular at-risk behavior (by reinforcing their choice not to take that specific risk), such tactics will probably not work for the vast majority of young people. Scare tactics will not work for the following reasons:

1. The fearful consequences are in the distant future. To try to convince a teenager that he or she shouldn't smoke cigarettes because of the risk of getting lung cancer in 30 or 40 years is an exercise in futility. First, adoles-

cents have a difficult time projecting themselves that far into the future; indeed, it is difficult for adults to project their own health (or unhealthy) behaviors 1 year or 5 years or 10 years into the future. Sixteen-year-olds cannot imagine what it's like to be 46 years old.

2. Medical cures and treatments will be found. Because of all the medical advances that have occurred during the past few decades, many young people believe that cures will be developed for whatever health problems they may develop in the future. Some adolescents may believe that they can participate in risky behaviors now, because medicine will have a cure for what ails them in the next year or in just a few short years.

3. Adolescents rebel against authority. Telling adolescents not to do something is often good motivation for them to do it—adolescent rebellion can be a powerful motivator. As well intentioned as health warnings from adults can be, for many adolescents such warnings may be taken as simply another way for adults to control the adolescent's life.

4. Scare tactics may contradict experience. Young people's decisions are often based on the here and now; the pleasure principle is a primary motivator. Personal experiences with alcohol, drugs, or sex may differ from the message that is delivered by adults. If one's personal experience with alcohol, marijuana, or sex has been essentially positive, negative warnings from adults will probably not be taken too seriously. Experiences are concrete, while warnings are abstract.

5. Lack of a "scare tactics" model. Too often, scare tactics are simply presented as scare tactics, without much analysis of the role of fear and how fear can serve as a motivator to change behavior. For example, from the psychological literature, much is known about approach-avoidance conflicts. For a young

person, sexuality and the fear of AIDS would combine into a classic approach-avoidance conflict. On the one hand, the young person wants to approach the sexual experience; on the other hand, she or he may be afraid of contracting HIV as a result of that sexual experience.

6. Fear may actually produce misperceptions of risk. Even among some gay men who were at risk for contracting HIV, some tended to show an unrealistic optimism in assessing their perceived risk (Bauman and Siegel, 1987). These researchers identified several reasons for such unrealistic optimism which apparently produced high-risk activities:

- Risk-reduction guidelines may increase the likelihood of perceiving oneself at low risk (since one may engage in only one or two risky behaviors).
- Inaccurate health beliefs (engaging in high-risk practices with fewer partners was "safe").
- Some ineffectual precautions produced a false sense of security.
- Misperceptions may lower anxiety, which may reduce the motivation for engaging in safer sex.

Behavior change on a large scale is difficult because of the strength of the motivation for sex and drugs. First, people must believe that they are at risk and have a strategy for coping with the risk. Second, they must believe in their own power to change and control their own behaviors. Third, the new behaviors must become the community norm (Booth, 1988).

Self-efficacy

Self-efficacy is the belief that one is a competent person with some degree of mastery over the environment (Bandura, 1986). This is particularly important with respect to HIV infection, because if people do not believe that they have any personal control over becoming infected, they are likely to take risks that may lead to infection. The development of self-efficacy can be a major objective of AIDS education programs.

More specifically, considerable research has been done on the concept of locus of control (whether a woman believes that she is internally controlled—in control of one's own destiny—or externally controlled—being controlled by change or outside factors). A woman who believes that she is in control of her sexuality can purchase condoms and try to persuade her partner to use them. A woman who believes that she is not in control of her sexuality can wait for her partner to decide whether they will engage in safer sex.

In those cases in which external events cannot be predicted or controlled by the individual, learned helplessness may result (Seligman, 1975). When repeatedly experiencing events they can neither predict nor control, many people tend to feel helpless; such helplessness may produce severe depression. In contrast, people who repeatedly experience events they can predict and control tend to be able to cope more effectively. When feeling helpless, one may do nothing; when feeling in control, one will do something.

Adolescent sexuality often tends to be spontaneous, because many adolescents and their parents believe that it is inappropriate to plan for sex—that makes it wrong. If it just happens, well, that's another story. The problem with sex "just happening," however, is that after a few experiences, an adolescent may believe that he or she is helpless to really do anything about it. Pregnancy, sexually transmitted diseases, and AIDS may be justified by saying "It just happened," or "We didn't plan for this to happen." A sense of self-efficacy is vital for the development and maintenance of safer sex behaviors.

Indeed, the issue of self-efficacy has broader implications beyond basic AIDS education. Since AIDS has been portrayed as a disease that is uniformly fatal to those who contract it, people with AIDS often develop severe depression. One attitudinal change that bears on the self-efficacy issue is the transition from ''dying of AIDS'' to ''living with AIDS.'' In the former, a person with AIDS would be resigned to his or her fate, recognizing that death is inevitable and probably forthcoming very shortly. Nothing can be done, so why try? In the latter case, people with AIDS have realized that they may have a short time left or a long time, but some time nevertheless. The emphasis shifts to living a healthier life (e.g., better nutrition, more exercise, stress reduction activities, maintaining a social life) for as long as possible. A sense of mastery may make a real difference, not only in AIDS prevention, but in AIDS treatment as well.

Knowing someone with AIDS

One factor that may influence people's behavior is knowing someone who has AIDS. Many of the sexual behavior changes that have been found in gay men in major cities may, in part, result from them knowing a friend or lover with AIDS. To see firsthand what a person with AIDS is going through can serve as a powerful motivator to some people, although others may avoid changing their behaviors simply because they know someone with AIDS. In particular, if the person with AIDS has changed his or her behavior, friends may change their behaviors via the ''modeling'' process (Bandura, 1986).

In some cities that have reported a large number of AIDS cases, it is not uncommon for some people to know a dozen, or two dozen, or three dozen people with AIDS. To know that many people who have the disease can be a devastating experience, as one attends funeral after funeral. The impact of seeing friends test HIV positive, be diagnosed with AIDS, develop *Pneumocystis carinii pneumonia* or Kaposi's sarcoma, and lose half their body weight is a painful experience.

As of October–December 1989, about 14 percent of the American population reported personally knowing someone having AIDS or the AIDS virus (Hardy, 1990); that figure has more than doubled from 6 percent in late 1987 (Dawson and Thornberry, 1988). Personal behavior may change as a result of seeing what has happened to one's friends, the same way that behavior may change if a family member is killed in an automobile accident or develops lung cancer from smoking. Given the secrecy that still surrounds this disease, many more Americans may have a friend or family member with the disease, but they are simply not aware of it.

Cultural sensitivity

For some time after AIDS was first identified, it was characterized as a disease of gay white males; many minority leaders simply did not believe that AIDS was a threat to their community or to their race. However, since the number of diagnosed AIDS cases in minority populations has been growing steadily, the need for culturally sensitive AIDS education programs has become apparent. Early on in the epidemic, virtually all of the educational programs were developed by gay men for other gay men; many of those messages were seen as irrelevant or inappropriate in minority communities.

Numerous recommendations have been made for the development of culturally sensitive and educationally effective programs for people at risk whose cultural and ethnic background is not white, middle class. For example, information must contain the appropriate vocabulary and be appropriate for the level of sophistication of the audience. Cultural values and attitudes of the target group should be reflected in the program. The program should not be just a translation of the materials that were targeted at gay white males and white male IV drug users (Peterson and Marin, 1988).

Messages for black and Hispanic/Latina women (Mays and Cochran, 1988) must occur in a context in which conservative religious beliefs and church affiliations are recognized, where models of sexual relationships may be different, and where

Developmental Issues

We all experience stages of physical, psychological, and social development, and a variety of theories have been developed to explain such changes (Miller, 1989): Piaget's Cognitive-Stage Theory, Freud and Erikson's Psychoanalytic Theory, Social Learning Theory, Information Processing Theory, Ethological Theory and Perceptual Development Theory. Since HIV infection has occurred in newborns, children, adolescents, young adults, middle-aged adults, and the elderly, a life-span developmental perspective can be useful for developing and understanding prevention programs. Indeed, each theory probably has some relevance for understanding some part of the AIDS crisis. However, just a few examples will be presented to highlight the value of a developmental viewpoint, with emphasis on adolescence and young adulthood.

Erikson's Psychosocial Development Theory

Adolescence is a time for identity formation or role confusion. It is during this time that the sense of self develops, and new roles are experienced via peer groups, religion, political associations, and sexual experimentation. Adolescents will put on and cast off these roles until they find a comfortable one. Experimentation is critical and natural, but it must be encouraged in a healthy context. The immediacy of a developing personality takes precedence over the distance of future health problems.

Young adulthood is a time of intimacy or isolation. Interestingly, one part of early adulthood is an "us versus them" perception, perhaps contributing to the attitudes of homophobia that are often seen in young people. Those who are only beginning to form one identity (e.g., heterosexual) may feel threatened by those who are forming a different identify (e.g., homosexual).

Kohlberg and Gilligan:
Stages of Moral Development

Depending upon levels of moral development, adolescents and young adults are likely to judge based on standards of convention or postconventional morality. For those at the stage of conventional morality, law and social convention determine moral reasoning strategies. One obeys the law because it is the law; for these individuals, AIDS educational messages that emphasize federal and state laws (or religious laws) might be effective. As with other AIDS educational efforts, however, moral reasoning does not always lead to moral actions.

Unfortunately, the relationship between reasoning ability and sexual behaviors has not yet been studied, despite the fact that it is well known (Brooks-Gunn et al., 1988) that younger adolescents tend to be more concrete (rather than abstract) in their thinking, self-centered (rather than other-centered), and focused on the present (rather than on the future). Older adolescents (and young adults), should be more abstract in their thinking, more other-centered, and oriented to the future; such developmental differences between younger and older adolescents are highly relevant to the development of effective prevention programs.

Developmental differences between males and females may be key factors for the development of effective prevention programs during adolescence and early adulthood. As suggested by Gilligan (1982), women's emphasis on the maintenance of relationships may be a crucial factor in understanding why couples may or may not incorporate safer sex recommendations into their relationship.

Prevention across the life span

Although a life-span developmental perspective is necessary for AIDS prevention programs, very little is known about preventive health behavior across the life span. Leventhal and fellow researchers (1985) summarized the field and identified 11 points for a life-span developmental perspective on prevention. The major points included the following:

- Little is known about developmental influences on the outcome of intervention programs.

- Reductions in risk behaviors are seen in 50 to 70 percent of persons who complete a prevention program.
- Less intense communications strategies change knowledge and attitudes but have less impact on behavior.
- Most programs have had difficulty maintaining behavioral change over long periods of time; relapses seem to be inevitable.
- Self-directed motivation for change may be more important than simply providing an intervention program; if one is not motivated to change, one won't.
- More emphasis has been placed on teaching health promotion than on preparing and motivating people to decide to begin to adopt healthier lifestyles.

social responsibility may be more of a motivation than individual safety (e.g., men practicing safer sex to survive as a father or support for parents, women practicing safer sex to stay alive to care for their parents or children). The development and implementation of effective AIDS prevention programs in different cultures will depend less on what is known about AIDS and more on what is known about the characteristics of the community and its culture. Although it is often assumed that characteristics of minority communities put them at more risk for HIV, an understanding of minority strengths is essential for the development of effective programs. Hahn and Castro (1989) note several characteristics of the Latino community that may help in an effective response to AIDS, including traditional support systems by family members, the importance of family and childbearing, and the role of Latino organizations. School-based educational programs should be aware of these issues when developing AIDS prevention programs, so that the programs are consistent with the cultural characteristics of the students.

Increasing rate of STDs

The rate of sexually transmitted diseases has been fluctuating during the past 15 years, depending on the particular disease. The incidence of gonorrhea began to rise in 1966, peaked in 1975, and has been declining since then. However, gonorrhea rates for young people are relatively high. In 1987 there were 780,000 reported gonorrhea cases: 24 percent in 15-to-19-year-olds, and 36 percent in 20-to-24-year-olds. Combined, the 15-to-24-year-olds comprised 62 percent of all gonorrhea cases. Such a high rate of gonorrhea in young people suggests that many engage in unprotected sex and may be putting themselves at risk for HIV.

Although the vast majority of AIDS cases have been diagnosed in adults, the long incubation period for the disease suggests that many adults may have become infected with HIV during adolescence. A survey of 19 college campuses found that an average of two students in every thousand were infected with HIV (Biemiller, 1989). The infection rate was as low as zero on some of the campuses. The highest was 9 per 1,000 at one campus. No doubt, some of these

TABLE 8.1   Gonorrhea: Rates per 100,000 Population by Age Group and Sex (1980–1987)

Age	Calendar Year	Male Cases	Female Cases	Total Cases	Male Rates	Female Rates	Total Rates
10–14	1980	2,199	6,674	8,874	23.6	74.8	48.7
	1981	2,341	6,330	8,871	25.1	70.9	47.5
	1982	2,125	6,232	8,357	23.0	70.7	46.3
	1983	1,945	5,892	7,837	21.4	67.8	44.1
	1984	2,024	5,815	7,839	22.5	67.8	44.6
	1985	2,087	6,078	8,164	23.8	72.9	47.7
	1986	2,013	6,075	8,088	23.7	75.2	48.8
	1987	1,775	5,267	7,041	21.0	65.6	42.7
15–19	1980	99,994	147,245	247,239	953.4	1424.6	1187.3
	1981	97,055	137,807	234,862	954.3	1379.7	1165.1
	1982	97,015	138,071	235,086	979.2	1423.3	1198.9
	1983	88,787	131,598	220,385	926.0	1401.8	1161.4
	1984	83,935	126,585	210,520	895.8	1375.9	1133.7
	1985	86,510	132,311	218,821	930.5	1455.1	1189.9
	1986	83,462	132,245	215,707	893.3	1451.2	1168.8
	1987	73,570	114,663	188,233	793.2	1269.2	1028.1
20–24	1980	224,091	155,365	379,000	204.1	1460.7	1824.0
	1981	217,326	154,076	371,402	101.2	1428.1	1757.5
	1982	217,488	145,687	363,135	102.6	1353.6	1720.6
	1983	199,005	141,373	340,378	923.7	1320.0	1616.6
	1984	187,946	141,530	329,476	860.7	1340.4	1594.8
	1985	193,714	147,932	341,645	947.7	1420.6	1678.1
	1986	186,889	147,858	334,747	931.1	1461.0	1690.8
	1987	164,739	128,199	292,938	758.5	1306.3	1527.2

Note: Adopted from Centers for Disease Control, 1988.

TABLE 8.2   AIDS Cases in Adolescents and Adults Under Age 25 by Exposure Category (through June 1990)

Exposure Category	13–19-Year-Olds		20–24-Year-Olds	
	Number	Percent	Number	Percent
Male homosexual/bisexual	152	28	3,393	57
IV drug use (female and heterosexual male)	61	11	957	16
Male homosexual/bisexual and IV drug use	24	4	560	9
Hemophilia/coagulation disorder	167	31	151	3
Heterosexual contact	65	12	539	9
Sex with IV drug user	38		297	
Sex with bisexual male	3		44	
Sex with person with hemophilia	1		14	
Born in Pattern II country	13		104	
Sex with person born in Pattern II country	—		6	
Sex with transfusion recipient with HIV infection	—		6	
Sex with HIV-infected person, risk not specified	10		68	
Receipt of blood transfusion/blood components or tissue	42	8	88	1
Undetermined	30	6	244	4
Total	541		5,932	

Source: *HIV/AIDS Surveillance Report*, July 1990. Atlanta, GA: Centers for Disease, 1–18.

HIV positive students contracted the virus while still in high school.

Hein (1989) has categorized degrees of risk among adolescents and suggested relevant interventions. One group of adolescents is not at risk for HIV infection (young, virginal, not intravenous drug users). Educational issues for them would focus on "worried well" issues, need for information about the safety of casual-contact behaviors, and support for decision making about their sexual activities. A second group includes sexually active teenagers who have not yet been infected with HIV. Members of this group will need information about how to "know" their partners, ways of assessing their patterns of sexual activity, and use of contraceptives—especially condoms. The third group consists of teenagers who are at risk for HIV infection because they have been exposed to infected individuals. Many members of this group are likely to be black or Hispanic, and issues for them include how to make decisions about HIV testing, knowledge of their partner's antibody status, using barrier methods of contraception, and reconsidering patterns of sexual behavior.

Although the data on AIDS in young people is still sparse, as of June 1990 a total of 541 cases in 13-to-19-year-olds had been reported to the CDC, and another 5,932 cases among 20-to-24-year-olds. Table 8.2 portrays the exposure categories for 13-to-19- and 20-to-24-year-olds. Compared to adult cases, adolescent and young adult cases are less likely to be a result of male homosexual or bisexual contact or intravenous drug use, and are more likely to be a result of hemophilia or coagulation disorders and heterosexual contact. It is very important to note that although only 5 percent of the adult cases are due to heterosexual contact, 12 percent of the 13-to-19-year-old cases and 9 percent of the 20-to-24-year-old cases were attributed to heterosexual exposure.

In particular, runaways and homeless youth appear to be particularly vulnerable to the virus because they often resort to prostitution to earn money. In particular, gay teenagers may be at very high risk (Remafedi, 1988), because their partners may be older (and more likely to be HIV infected themselves), and more anonymous (thus limiting the ability to "know" one's partner). Miller, Turner, and Moses (1990), in their review of AIDS and adolescents, note that one survey of homeless youths in New York City found about 6.5 percent to be HIV positive (almost 9% of the 18-to-23-year-olds), while a Los Angeles study found only 0.16 percent to be HIV positive, suggesting that many regional differences exist with respect to the infection rate among adolescent runaways. Over time, if the virus takes hold in areas with a low incidence of HIV, the percentage of HIV infected youths will probably increase.

Intoxication and sexuality

Alcohol and other drugs often play an important role in sexuality; indeed, the SWI (Sex While Intoxicated) phenomenon (Hochhauser, 1988/89) may be a major component of adolescent—and adult—sexuality. Sexual experiences can be highly stressful, and alcohol or other drugs may be used as a way of reducing such stress. Researchers assume that alcohol may function in several ways to promote sexuality:

- as a disinhibitor. In small amounts, alcohol seems to reduce the inhibitions that a person has in a more sober condition. When a person's inhibitions are reduced, she or he may be able to say and do things that would not otherwise be the case. As inhibitions are decreased, sexual activity may increase. In extreme cases of intoxication, date rape may be the ultimate result.

- as justification for sex. One may be able to convince oneself (or one's partner, or parents, or physician) that he or she was so intoxicated as to have been simply taken advantage of by the partner. Some evidence suggests that alcohol may play an important role in homosexual sexual activity (Molgaard et al., 1988), suggesting that successful prevention programs may have to focus on alcohol and drug use as well as on sexual issues.

One of the common AIDS prevention recommendations is for sexual partners to talk with each other about their sexual history. Given that sexuality among adolescents is often full of anxiety and fear of rejection, and is done "spontaneously," the fear of discussing one's sexual history with a partner may be highly stressful. If so, alcohol or other drugs may be used as a way of reducing such stress.

THE ROLE OF LOVE

As noted by Hochhauser (1990), much of the research on AIDS has emphasized the sexual transmission of the disease, describing risky sexual behaviors, suggesting safer sex activities, comparing the epidemiology of AIDS to gonorrhea and syphillis, and so on. Unfortunately, changing human sexual behavior has never been as simple as just telling people to change, or even how to change. The CDC operates on the traditional public health model for infectious disease control and is the primary agency for AIDS prevention, education, and behavioral change (Turner, Miller, and Moses, 1989). They note that when the AIDS epidemic began in 1981, CDC had fewer than 40 behavioral scientists, and until the spring of 1988, they had added only one behavioral scientist to work on AIDS issues. Given the absence of a behavioral perspective on AIDS, it should not be too surprising that CDC's recommendations for behavioral change are not always based on an understanding of basic psychological principles and human behavior.

A brief literature review

There is no shortage of materials on AIDS; literally hundreds of books and probably thousands of articles have been written since 1981. However, a review of a number of relevant publications (Institute of Medicine, 1988; Turner, Miller, and Moses, 1989; Corless and Pittman-Lindeman, 1988; Dessaint, Kerby, and McLean, 1988; Schinazi and Nahmias, 1988; Miller, Turner, and Moses, 1990) failed to find the category of "love" either in the index or in the table of contents. The only area in which love is mentioned in the context of AIDS is in reference to the treatment of people with AIDS and their need to be treated kindly, compassionately, and with "love." No literature was found that mentioned love as a potentially significant factor in understanding the AIDS phenomenon.

Perhaps this omission of love is because of the homophobia surrounding AIDS and because of the perception (conscious or subconscious) on the part of some researchers and writers that gays are capable only of "promiscuous sex," not of a long-term, loving relationship. As more heterosexual cases of AIDS are reported, the role of love will probably be emphasized much more than it has been in the past, although Masters, Johnson, and Kolodny (1988) did not refer to love in their book on heterosexual behavior and AIDS.

Conversely, in a review of research on love (Sternberg and Barnes, 1988), no references to sexually transmitted diseases could be found. Apparently researchers interested in sex have no interest in love, and researchers interested in love have no interest in sexually transmitted disease. Such findings are consistent with Money's (1973) observation:

> "If you look up most of the books on sex education and check the index, you will find that time and time again the word love never appears. There is no chapter on love. There is in fact, practically no mention of love at all. I think there really ought to be two aspects of sex education. One we might call sex education and the other should be called love education." (pp. 411–412)

Intimacy and sexual behavior

Sexual behavior, be it heterosexual or homosexual, does not occur in a vacuum. Sternberg (1988) has developed a "triangular theory of love" consisting of (1) intimacy, (2) passion, and (3) commitment, which can be combined to form eight types of love:

Components	Types of love
1. Intimacy alone	1. Liking
2. Passion alone	2. Infatuation
3. Commitment alone	3. Empty love
4. Intimacy + Passion	4. Romantic love
5. Intimacy + Commitment	5. Companionate love
6. Passion + Commitment	6. Fatuous love
7. Intimacy + Passion + Commitment	7. Consummate love
8. Absence of components	8. Nonlove

Recognizing the importance of love in human development, straightforward recommendations for safer sex or abstinence should be expected to have a significant impact on intimacy or passion or commitment, and as a result, on the relationship itself. For example, if a couple is afraid that talking about their sexual pasts to each other will hinder intimacy, a relationship based on intimacy and passion (romantic love) could become a relationship based on passion alone (infatuation).

If one partner learns that the other partner has had other sexual partners, the "commitment" component could be weakened. If one or both partners believe that condoms seriously interfere with sexual pleasure, the "passion" component could be weakened. If couples are embarrassed about discussing sex with each other, the "intimacy" component could be weakened. Recommendations for changes in sexual behavior, if suggested and implemented without an understanding of the impact of the changes upon a couple's own type of love, will probably be ineffective. If a couple believes that safer sex (e.g.,

using condoms) will affect the passion of the relationship, will they be willing to use condoms? Although individual health may be maintained by practicing safer sex, what is the price that may be paid in the relationship?

Love and safer sex: self-fulfillment vs. safety

From Maslow's perspective on self-actualization, safer sex recommendations not only would affect basic safety needs, but higher needs of belongingness, esteem, and self-fulfillment as well. For those individuals who have attained higher levels of achievement or who aspire to higher levels, safer sex admonitions may be perceived as being counterproductive. If a person has experienced the satisfaction of his or her need for love, self-esteem, and self-actualization through a loving and sexual relationship, would that person be willing to become sexually abstinent if such abstinence meant that one's safety needs would be met, but one's psychological and self-actualization needs would remain unmet? Will recommendations for abstinence or safer sex keep people physically healthy, but at the potential expense of their psychological health and development? Unless such humanistic issues become part of the discussion of AIDS, simplistic recommendations may have little impact on sexual behavior.

ORGANIZATIONAL ISSUES

AIDS prevention programs do not occur in isolation; many of the programs are school based (elementary, secondary, and postsecondary) and must be developed within the context of an educational organization. As described by Keeling (1989), however, we may not be prepared to deal with HIV infection among young people. He notes that

> "We still hear debate about what language and concepts are appropriately deleted in our classrooms; which realities of human behavior

we had best omit from discussion; what educational messages about sexual behavior will be least offensive and controversial; what we can safely sell in our vending machines; and what platitudes we will speak to placate an outraged parent, alumnus, or trustee.'' (pp. B1–B2)

Abstractly, we deal with prevention programs; concretely, the issue is one of life and death.

SUMMARY

Although different professionals (physicians, public health specialists, behavioral scientists, etc.) have different perspectives on prevention, virtually all have identified education and information as an AIDS prevention strategy. However, many of these recommendations lack any theoretical basis as a rationale for behavior change. To be effective, educationally based programs will need some underlying theory (e.g., ''Bloom's Taxonomy of Educational Objectives'') to guide them.

Educational programs are often effective in changing knowledge and attitudes, but less effective in changing behavior. Many assume that if knowledge is increased and attitudes are changed, behaviors will change as well. Research has shown, however, that sometimes behaviors change first, then attitudes. Scare tactics will not work, because the fearful consequences are in the distant future, medical cures or treatment may be discovered, adolescents often rebel against authority figures (who try to scare them), there is no theoretical model for scare tactics, and misperceptions of risk may occur under fearful conditions.

On the other hand, self-efficacy (the belief that one is a competent person with some mastery over the environment) may be an important objective in school-based prevention programs. Other relevant components include knowing someone with AIDS, being sensitive to multicultural issues and values, incorporating a developmental perspective (e.g., Erikson's psychosocial development perspective or Kohlberg and Gilligan's theories of moral development).

Although much research on AIDS has emphasized the sexual transmission of the virus, ''love'' has not been incorporated into the understanding of human sexual behavior or effective prevention programs. Sternberg's triangular theory of love (intimacy, passion, and commitment) provides a framework for understanding the role of love in human behavior, and a perspective for evaluating the impact of ''safer sex'' recommendations.

REFERENCES

Bandura, A. (1986) *Social foundations of thought and action. A social-cognitive theory.* Englewood Cliffs, NJ: Prentice-Hall.

Baum, A., and Nesselhof, S. E. A. (1988) Psychological research and the prevention, etiology, and treatment of AIDS. *American Psychologist,* 43 (11), 900–906.

Bauman, L. H., and Siegel, K. (1987) Misperception among gay men of the risk for AIDS associated with their sexual behavior. *Journal of Applied Social Psychology,* 17 (3), 329–350.

Becker, M. H., and Joseph, J. G. (1988) AIDS and behavioral change to reduce risk: A review. *American Journal of Public Health,* 78 (4), 394–410.

Biemiller, L. (1989) An average of 2 students in 1,000 found infected with AIDS-linked virus. *Chronicle of Higher Education,* May 24, 1989, p. A30.

Bloom, B. S., ed. (1986) *Taxonomy of educational objectives. Book 1: Cognitive domain.* New York: Longman.

Booth, W. (1987) Another muzzle for AIDS education? *Science,* 238, 1036.

Booth, W. (1988) Social engineers confront AIDS. *Science,* 242, 1237–1238.

Brooks-Gunn, J., Boyer, C. B., and Hein, K. (1988) Preventing HIV infection and AIDS in children and adolescents: Behavioral research and intervention strategies. *American Psychologist,* 43 (11), 958–964.

Centers for Disease Control (1988) *Sexually transmitted disease statistics 1987. Issue #136.* Atlanta, GA: U.S. Department of Health and Human Services.

Centers for Disease Control (1990) *HIV/AIDS Surveillance Report.* June, 1990; 1–18.

Corless, I. B., and Pittman-Lindeman, M. (1988) *AIDS: Principles, practices, & politics.* Washington, DC: Hemisphere Publishing.

Dawson, D. A., and Thornberry, O. T. (1988) AIDS knowledge and attitudes for December 1987. Provisional data from the National Health Interview Survey. *Advance Data from Vital and Health Statistics.* No. 153. DHHS Pub. No. (PHS) 88–1250. Public Health Service. Hyattsville, MD.

Dessaint, A. Y., Kerby, J. L., and McLean, B. E., eds. (1988) *AIDS Abstracts of the psychological and behavioral literature, 1983–1988.* Washington, DC: American Psychological Association.

Gilligan, C. (1982) *In a different voice.* Cambridge, MA: Harvard University Press.

Hahn, R. A., and Castro, K. G. (1989) The health and health care status of Latino populations in the U.S.; a brief review. In O. Martiniz-Mara, D. M. Shin, and H. E. Banks, eds. *Latinos and AIDS. A national strategy symposium.* Los Angeles, CA: Center for Interdisciplinary Research in Immunology and Disease (CIRID).

Hardy, A. M. (1990) AIDS knowledge and attitudes for October–December 1989. Provisional data from the National Health Interview Survey. *Advance Data from Vital and Health Statistics. No. 186.* DHHS Pub. No. (PHS) 90–1250. Hyattsville, MD: Public Health Service.

Hein, K. (1989) Commentary on adolescent acquired immunodeficiency syndrome: The next wave of the human immunodeficiency virus epidemic? *Journal of Pediatrics,* 114 (1), 144–149.

Hochhauser, M. (1988/89). Adolescents and AIDS. *Adolescent Counselor,* 1 (5), 45–49.

Hochhauser, M. (1990) Love: The missing variable in AIDS research. Boston, MA: *American Psychological Association Convention,* August 1990.

Institute of Medicine (1988) *Confronting AIDS: Update 1988.* Washington, DC: National Academy Press.

Keeling, R. (1989) We are not socially, politically, or economically prepared to cope with the spread of AIDS among young Americans. *Chronicle of Higher Education,* September 20, 1989, p. B1–B2.

Leventhal, H., Prohaska, T. R., and Hirschman, R. S. (1985) Preventive health behavior across the life span. In J. C. Rosen, and L. J. Solomon, eds. *Prevention in health psychology.* Hanover, NH: University Press of New England.

Living Webster Encyclopedia Dictionary of the English Language. (1975) Chicago, IL: English Language Institute of America.

Masters, W. H., Johnson, V. E., and Kolodny, R. C. (1988) *Crisis: Heterosexual behavior in the age of AIDS.* New York: Grove Press.

Mays, V. M., and Cochran, S. D. (1988) Issues in the perception of AIDS risk reduction activities by black and Hispanic/Latina women. *American Psychologist,* 43 (11), 949–957.

Miller, H. G., Turner, C. F., and Moses, L. E., eds. (1990) *AIDS. The second decade.* Washington, DC: National Academy Press.

Miller, P. H. (1989) *Theories of developmental psychology. 2nd ed.* New York: W. H. Freeman.

Molgaard, C. A., Nakamura, C., Hovell, M., and Elder, J. P. (1988) Assessing alcoholism as a risk factor for Acquired Immunodeficiency Syndrome (AIDS). *Social Science and Medicine,* 27 (11), 1147–1152.

Money, J. (1973) Pornography in the home: A topic in medical education. In J. Zubin and J. Money, eds. *Contemporary sexual behavior. Critical issues in the 1970s.* Baltimore, MD: Johns Hopkins University Press.

Peterson, J. L., and Marin, G. (1988) Issues in the prevention of AIDS among black and Hispanic men. *American Psychologist,* 43 (11), 871–877.

Remafedi, G. J. (1988) Preventing the sexual transmission of AIDS during adolescence. *Journal of Adolescent Health Care,* 9 (2), 139–143.

Schinazi, R. F., and Nahmias, A. J., eds. (1988) *AIDS in children, adolescents and heterosexual adults: An interdisciplinary approach to prevention.* New York: Elsevier.

Seligman, M. E. P. (1975) *Helplessness: On depression, development and death.* San Francisco: W. H. Freeman & Co.

Siegel, K., and Gibson, W. C. (1988) Barriers to the modification of sexual behavior among heterosexuals at risk for acquired immunodeficiency syndrome. *New York State Journal of Medicine,* 88 (2), 66–70.

Sternberg, R. J. (1988) Triangulating love. In R. H. Sternberg and M. L. Barnes, eds. *The psychology of love.* New Haven: Yale University Press.

Sternberg, R. H., and Barnes, M. L., eds. (1988) *The psychology of love.* New Haven: Yale University Press.

Turner, C. F., Miller, H. G., and Moses, L. E., eds. (1989) *AIDS: Sexual behavior and intravenous drug use.* Washington, DC: National Academy Press.

Winett, R. A. (1986) *Information and behavior: Systems of influence.* Hillsdale, NJ: Lawrence Erlbaum Associates.

The Response of Schools

9

"Nothing is more terrible than activity without insight."

THOMAS CARLYLE

"School cook dies of AIDS: he chopped green beans and roast beef"

NEW YORK POST, SEPTEMBER 12, 1985

"Aids child bites classmate, now both are doomed"

WEEKLY WORLD NEWS, NOVEMBER 12, 1985

"Now no one is safe from AIDS."

LIFE, JULY 1985

HYSTERIA ABOUT AIDS

These hysterical media reports, as noted by Lamers (1988) highlight the role that schools will find themselves playing in the next few decades. Not only will schools have primary responsibility for educating young people on the "facts about AIDS," but they will simultaneously be confronted with issues regarding the "hysteria about AIDS" from students, staff, parents, and community residents. Moreover, several epidemiological and treatment trends suggest that the school systems will not only be encountering more people who are HIV positive or who have been diagnosed with AIDS, but they will also be given more legal responsibility for developing AIDS education programs.

As the virus continues to spread, some students in high school, or even junior high, in some areas, will become HIV positive as a result of sexual or needle-sharing activities. As HIV antibody testing becomes more commonplace and more acceptable, more students will find out their antibody status. By June 1990, the CDC had reported a total of 2,900 AIDS cases diagnosed in young people aged 19 or younger (CDC, 1990). Since AIDS cases represent only about 14 percent of those who are infected with HIV, there may be as many as 21,000 children and adolescents who are carrying the virus.

Many believe that AIDS is primarily a disease of urban areas such as New York City and San Francisco. That belief is often based on the reported number of AIDS cases from particular cities or geographic areas. However, as noted by Hoffman and fellow researchers (1989), the geographic distribution of AIDS is different from the geographic distribution of HIV infection. In a study of HIV antibody tests and AIDS cases in Colorado, these researchers found that the geographic distribution of people who were HIV positive was considerably more widespread than the distribution for AIDS cases. Another study of HIV infection in low-prevalence areas of the United States (Gardner et al., 1989) concluded that HIV infection has spread outside the original urban areas of the epidemic. HIV transmission has been occurring among both black and white adolescents and young adults across all regions of the United States; however, since AIDS cases are reported to CDC and HIV positive cases are not, our national data base (and our national perception) is based on AIDS cases rather than on HIV positive cases.

Given the average 10-year time lag between HIV infection and diagnosis with AIDS, some counties may have many HIV positive residents years before their first AIDS case is diagnosed. Thus, many schools in suburban or rural areas will probably have to cope with issues of HIV infection before they will have to deal with AIDS.

Young people are at considerable risk for contracting HIV from risky sexual behaviors. Turner, Miller, and Moses (1989) have noted that

- by age 19, 83 percent of young men and 74 percent of young women have tried sexual intercourse,
- about half of all teenagers do not use contraception the first time they engage in sexual intercourse,
- except for homosexual men and prostitutes, teenage girls have the highest rates of gonorrhea and chlamydia of any age or sex group.

Second, the number of babies born to HIV infected mothers will increase. Most of those children have a rather gloomy prognosis at present and are not likely to live beyond a few years, at best. However, as treatment for AIDS (such as AZT) becomes more sophisticated and more accessible, the life span of such babies will probably increase. Thus, schools will face an increased number of HIV infected students from the top down (high school and below) and from the bottom up (kindergarten and above). As of June 1990, CDC had reported 1,962 AIDS cases in children under the age of 5 and 418 cases in children between the ages of 5 and 12 (CDC, 1990).

Third, there will probably be some infected school employees, be they teachers, maintenance staff, administrators, or others. Not only will the school system have to deal with AIDS issues from an educational standpoint, but from an organizational and management perspective as well. Far too often, however, the response of most organizations has been to do nothing until a crisis develops, at which point the likelihood of doing the wrong thing seems to increase drastically.

POLICIES REGARDING NONDISCRIMINATION

Federal and state laws with respect to discrimination as it applies to AIDS-related conditions have been changing over the past few years. At the present time, people with AIDS are considered by federal law (Public Law 94–142) to be "handicapped" and are entitled to the rights and protections given to other handicapped individuals.

Although most of the literature dealing with AIDS education has focused on the provision of generic health education programs, the requirement that public schools provide education to all students regardless of their handicap means that some unique AIDS education programs will have to be developed for the school to be in compliance with federal law. As students with developmental disabilities become mainstreamed into the public school system, AIDS education programs will have to be adapted to meet their special needs.

Jacobs and fellow researchers (1989) have described some of the unique features of providing AIDS education to developmentally disabled individuals. For example, information is presented as simply and concretely as possible; instead of discussing the differences between lubricated and nonlubricated condoms, only lubricated condoms are discussed and distributed. Discussions of water-based or oil-based lubricants are avoided—trainees are encouraged only to use water-based lubricants.

Lawsuits, even with no legal merit at all, can be filed by almost anyone. At the very least, the defendant will have to provide for a defense, often at considerable personal or organizational expense. From a risk-management standpoint, it seems only prudent that school districts have in place appropriate antidiscrimination policies and procedures (Fraser, 1989), and that staff are aware of such procedures. On the one hand, having such procedures in place may reduce the likelihood of a lawsuit; on the other hand, as some lawyers have argued, having a policy in place binds the organization to that policy and may give the impression of increased culpability if the policy is not heeded.

Indeed, this is a point that should be well taken. Some employees may not agree with a school district's policy; they may treat HIV infected students and staff in ways that are totally inconsistent with such policies. The policy may not necessarily result in the desired behavior change on the part of those employees who are prejudiced towards people with AIDS. As we cannot expect information about AIDS to necessarily result in behavior change among people at risk for contracting the virus, so we should not be deluded into thinking that simply putting a policy into place will eliminate discrimination in the workplace.

An effective series of policies will need to be developed, including issues of student attendance, staff employment, evaluation of students and staff, confidentiality, testing, infection control, and training (Fraser, 1989). If not already in place, such policies should be developed, with input from a variety of constituencies; administrators, teachers, students, parents, union representatives, lawyers, religious leaders, and others. AIDS has become such a highly charged issue that one can anticipate the possibility of community reaction to an AIDS policy if a policy is made public; it's much easier to get community support while the policy is being developed than after a crisis has developed.

Not everyone will agree with all policies, but they will have had an opportunity to express their viewpoint. An understanding of federal and state law is crucial. Most people realize that they do not have to agree with every law, but that they will still obey the laws. If they do disagree with state or federal law, they have the opportunity of working through the political process to change the law via the legislative process. Schools and their employees are not in a position to selectively obey or disobey laws based on personal preferences or prejudices.

POLICIES REGARDING INFECTION CONTROL

Infection control policies should already be in place for communicable diseases; most schools probably have some plan in place if there is an outbreak of measles, chicken pox, or the flu. In addition, policies will be necessary to deal not only with the rational fear of AIDS, but the irrational fear as well.

Fraser (1989) provides a suggested policy for infection control procedures and addresses issues such as recommended methods for cleaning up body fluids, risk of HIV transmission through exposure to blood at school, staff training, and use of rubber gloves.

From a rational standpoint, schools need to be concerned about the possible transmission of disease via blood or other body fluids. New York City, for example, has made latex gloves available for all teachers, in the event that they have to clean up after a child who has been sick in class and perhaps vomited. If the school system includes students who have not yet been completely toilet trained, there may be a need for some barrier protection for those staff members who may have to clean up bowel or bladder accidents.

There has been at least one case of HIV transmission presumably due to sharing of a needle and syringe for the injection of steroids by a high school athlete. Some contact sports can be bloody; staff who work closely with injured students should be well informed about the possible risks they might encounter, and they should have appropriate equipment for dealing with such bloody injuries.

From an irrational standpoint, many people still believe that HIV can be transmitted via casual contact, despite all the evidence to the contrary. In particular, those individuals with less than a 12th-grade education seem to be the most misinformed about AIDS, and their hysteria level may be relatively high. When afraid, people may make inappropriate decisions. In an attempt to prevent such decisions from being made, schools will have to provide not only informational programs to existing employees (via staff in-services) and to new employees (as part of the new employee orientation), but develop policies and procedures that take into account the fears of some employees. This does not mean that the hysteria has to be taken seriously, but that standards of behavior can be built into school policies so that all employees understand what is considered acceptable and unacceptable behavior.

Many unions are concerned about workplace hazards, including toxic substances and unsafe working conditions. In responding to these concerns, the Occupational Safety and Health Administration and Department of Labor will be developing standards for the workplace with respect to the occupational risk that employees may face from Hepatitis B and HIV. Although they may be reluctant to admit it, the vast majority of employees are at far more risk of contracting HIV from their personal behaviors (sexual and/or drug using) than they are from occupational exposure. However, it may be more socially acceptable to "come down with AIDS" by blaming it on the job than it is to admit that one has engaged in personally risky behaviors that may be unacceptable to one's family, peer group, and co-workers.

Some parents will be concerned for the health of their children who may be attending school with another student who is HIV positive; in particular, parents may be fearful of the HIV positive student biting their child, with the transmission of HIV being the outcome. Despite all evidence to the contrary (the virus is not transmitted that way), the fear that parents express is real and cannot (and should not) be casually dismissed. A plan should be in place that anticipates such problems, and responses should be well thought out in advance. Deciding how to respond after parents picket the school in front of the local media is not an effective way of preventing a crisis.

Box 9

Teaching about AIDS

Although there is no cure for AIDS, there is no shortage of information about the disease. Most of the information is accurate, but some is not. Consequently, because AIDS is such an emotionally charged issue, it is crucial that the information being presented to students, staff, parents, and the community be as accurate as possible. Many of the questions about AIDS are complex and cannot be answered with a simple *yes* or *no;* it takes someone with a comprehensive command of the topic to be able to respond accurately and to say "I don't know" when the information is just not available for a particular question. Competent and well-informed staff are necessary both for internal curriculum development and staff education, as well as external community relations.

What is being done?

Schumacher (1989) has analyzed HIV/AIDS education on a state-by-state basis. Her findings are valuable because they provide a national perspective on AIDS education and point out how much more needs to be done, despite the seemingly unanimous calls for AIDS education. She found the following:

* By May 1989, only 28 states and the District of Columbia required HIV/AIDS education; of these 29
  — 12 require it to be in their comprehensive health education program,
  — 7 require it as a part of family life education, sex education, human growth and development, or parenting,
  — 3 require it to be added to a communicable disease requirement,

  — 1 adds it to an STD requirement,
  — 7 have no context for HIV/AIDS education,
  — 2 states require HIV/AIDS education, but students are not required by the state to receive such education,
  — 1 state requires written parental permission for student attendance.

* Level of education was variable:
  — 17 states required HIV education to begin in K–5,
  — 7 states required it to begin in the middle grades,
  — 1 state required it to begin in high school,
  — 4 states did not require a specific grade level.

* Content of the HIV/AIDS education was inconsistent from state-to-state:
  — 20 required that prevention be taught,
  — 18 required that abstinence be emphasized,
  — 10 described specific elements (self-esteem, decision making, peer pressure, etc.),
  — 7 required discussion of avoidance of sharing IV drugs and needles,
  — 3 required discussion on condom use (recommended or unreliable),
  — 2 required discussion of homosexuality.

Fraser found that of those states with policies (21), most required the state education agency, or the state health agency to have the responsibility for developing resource materials, curriculum guidelines, and outcomes measures.

A Coordinated K–12 Curriculum

Surgeon General Koop recommended in 1986 in his influential booklet "Surgeon General's Report on Acquired Immune Deficiency Syndrome" that

> "Education about AIDS should start in early elementary school and at home so that children can grow up knowing the behavior to avoid to protect themselves from exposure to the AIDS virus." (p. 5)

Many people believed (or wanted to believe) that such education meant that second graders would be taught about condoms, anal sex, and intravenous drug use. That was not what Koop suggested at all. (Somehow his point about education at home was missed by many.) Information about AIDS is complex, involving infection control, an understanding of viruses, multicultural issues, behavior change, and history of disease. Koop's point was that vital information can be taught at appropriate age levels.

Consequently, a coordinated curriculum is a good way of weaving information about AIDS into an existing process. This may be easier said than done. As noted by Owens (1985), health in elementary school may be taught by "fitting it in whenever you can," typically being incorporated into the science curriculum. Certainly not every course need focus on AIDS issues, but there are opportunities to increase student's awareness of AIDS in a variety of ways: discussing the geographical distribution of the disease; comparing AIDS with other diseases; different ways of mathematically calculating the incidence of the disease; political aspects of the disease; and biological advances and treatments. Such educational opportunities should not be expected to result in any individual behavior change, but they might help students to understand the complexity of this issue and respond to AIDS in a more enlightened and less prejudicial fashion.

COMMUNITY INVOLVEMENT

Despite what seemed to be public resistance to AIDS education in elementary schools, many parents seem to want their children to be instructed at school regarding AIDS. As of October–December 1989, 38 percent of Americans with children reported that they had not discussed AIDS with any of their 10-to-17-year-old children. Sixty-three percent reported that their children had had instruction at school about AIDS, while 24 percent didn't know whether their children had had such instruction (Hardy, 1990).

Community involvement is desirable and recommended (Kolbe and Jones, 1988; Valdiserri, 1989) but may be difficult to achieve. Parents who want to get involved in AIDS education may be those who are either the most informed or the least informed—many just seem not to consider it a priority, perhaps believing that AIDS is a disease restricted to gay white men and that their children are just not at risk. Nevertheless, if AIDS is going to be incorporated into the K–12 curriculum, having community involvement as early as possible will probably make it more likely that there will be some parental support for middle and senior high school programs. A number of useful strategies have been suggested by Fraser and Mitchell (1988), including

- seeking support from other educators, including professional and national associations,
- gaining political allies, including the governor and influential state legislators,
- cooperating with other agencies and organizations, such as youth and community groups and religious organizations,
- using the media constructively,
- holding public meetings and planning for expected opposition by knowing what the typical arguments against AIDS education will be and having well-prepared responses.

Despite a school's best efforts, there will no doubt be some vocal opposition regarding classroom discussion, class assignments, or textbook coverage of AIDS. Given the controversy in some areas over evolution versus creationism in school textbooks, one can expect that some individuals or groups will protest the schools' AIDS education efforts.

STUDENT OBJECTIVES

Schools probably will not be able to accomplish what they would like to accomplish with respect to AIDS education, nor what parents and community would like. Historical experiences with sex education, drug education, driver education, and so on suggest that the impact of the school may be much less than had been expected. Yet, given an issue as sensitive as AIDS, where else are young people going to get their information? Following the comparison to alcohol and drug abuse prevention programs, the findings from one particularly effective prevention study (Office for Substance Abuse Prevention, 1990), found the following:

Use in Last Month	Prevention Group	Control Group
Alcohol	36%	50%
Cigarettes	24%	32%
Marijuana	14%	20%

One can be either encouraged or discouraged by these findings. Although fewer students used drugs after being involved in the prevention program, it is somewhat distressing that the benefits were not larger. Such findings do show that changes can occur, but such changes are probably smaller than most educators and parents would like.

Another major evaluation of drug prevention program (Project Alert) in junior high school students (Ellickson and Bell, 1990) did find reductions of young adolescents' use of cigarettes and marijuana, although the program was less effective with confirmed smokers and had only short-term effects on adolescent drinking. Such findings on the difficulty of preventing alcohol use and abuse are consistent with Moskowitz's (1989) assessment that "educational programs have been largely ineffective in preventing substance use or abuse" (p. 69). Even in those cases in which some reduction in alcohol and drug use does occur, such changes are often short-lived; the longer the follow-up, the less impact the programs seem to have on alcohol and drug-using behavior. There is little reason to believe that changes in sexual behavior will be much different from changes in drug use.

Cultural issues

Any educational program *must* take into account minority cultural values and perspectives. Mays and Cochran (1989) have identified a number of crucial factors that will affect risk perception by minority women (who may be parents of adolescents, school employees, or even adolescent parents themselves):

1. AIDS is one risk of many. For women who experience violence, poverty, drug abuse, or homelessness, AIDS is simply one more risk competing for their attention. Your priority may not be their priority.

2. AIDS information is often presented by white male experts, not female ethnic minority experts. To reach female minority students and employees, schools must find relevant sources of expertise.

3. Risk-reduction messages of talking about sex with one's partner may be inappropriate for women who come from cultures where one must first establish a relationship with a man. Such discussions would come much later in the relationship—not at the beginning, as is often recommended in AIDS education programs.

4. Rather than emphasizing individual safety as the major motivation for risk-reduction behaviors, emphasize social responsibility,

especially the need for men and women to survive to care for their parents and children. For those cultures with strong family ties, such a family perspective may be more acceptable, and more successful, than an appeal to personal health.

Program evaluation

Realistically, while something can be done, it will probably not be enough (although for some people it will be too much). Realistic objectives need to be thought through. Given all of the other responsibilities that schools are facing (budgets, increased accountability, etc.), it may be difficult to find the time or the expertise for an AIDS component in the K–12 experience. State Departments of Education will probably help set the agenda for most schools in terms of objectives, program outcomes, and evaluation. From the standpoint of learning outcomes, Schumacher (1989) found the following:

- 23 states have developed student learning outcomes for HIV/AIDS education.

Regarding program/curriculum evaluation:

- 11 states address evaluation in their educational policies, including review by the state education department, annual compliance reports, independent evaluations, collection of statistics from each school district, review by the state education and health agencies, submission of a curriculum.

Regarding educational evaluation:

- most states are using all or part of a CDC survey that measures HIV-related knowledge, beliefs, and behaviors,
  - 17 states, 2 territories, and the District of Columbia are using all of the survey questions,
  - 15 states and 2 territories are asking about HIV-related knowledge and beliefs (but not about behaviors),

  - 3 states are asking about HIV-related knowledge, beliefs, and IV drug-using behaviors (but not about sexual behaviors).

The lack of consistent methods for learner outcome evaluation and program evaluation and educational evaluation will make it very difficult to determine whether significant behavioral changes are taking place. It will be virtually impossible to make state-by-state comparisons, because little comparable data will be collected.

Moreover, the reluctance of some states to ask young people about their risky behaviors (perhaps because they believe that asking about behaviors gives tacit approval to them) means that there will be no way of knowing whether the educational programs had an impact other than by tracking the future prevalence and incidence of HIV infection and AIDS diagnoses. Since knowledge may have little impact on actual behaviors, the survey data may show that knowledge and beliefs about risky behaviors have increased; meanwhile, actual behaviors may not be changing at all. An AIDS educational program that does not measure behavioral change may be an educational success, but a behavioral failure.

PERSONNEL OBJECTIVES

While academic educational objectives may be set by state or local school boards, objectives for education for school personnel may be forthcoming from teachers' unions and federal or state regulatory agencies. Many of the objectives (and their implementation) will probably become part of the collective bargaining process, and school districts should anticipate such bargaining efforts and make sure that collective bargaining representatives are well informed about AIDS-related issues.

On the one hand, no one would argue that employees should be well informed about the real and perceived risks in their environment. On the other hand, staff education can be expensive, and, if done in an inappropriate way, highly cost ineffective. Recognizing limited school budgets, some thought should be directed to the costs of complying with federal and state regulations, as well as collective bargaining agreements that may contain an AIDS-related component.

Who should teach AIDS

Given the role of sexuality and drug use in the transmission of HIV, the most likely candidate for teaching about AIDS is the school health educator (who may or may not be prepared to deal with issues of homosexuality, IV drug use, and death). The issue is complex enough that it demands a response by more than just health education, however. For example,

- school nurses/physicians may have an opportunity to discuss risky behaviors with students who get sick at school,
- counselors may have the opportunity to deal with AIDS-related issues in drug prevention programs, or in aftercare programs at school. Those students who are recovering drug users may be at considerable risk, given the possibility of relapse and unsafe sex or drug-using behaviors,
- athletic coaches and trainers can address AIDS-related issues, such as steroid use and the risks of sharing needles.

Staff training: how and where

Information and understanding of AIDS has increased dramatically and will probably continue to do so during the next few decades. Keeping up with the literature would be virtually impossible, even if a full-time effort were made. To maintain a competent knowledge base, a certain amount of continuing education for staff will be necessary. Relevant resources have been described in the appendixes.

In-services can be helpful; staff from state education or health departments can be brought in

to inform staff both from a student educational perspective and from an employee education perspective. Schumacher (1989) identified a variety of activities that are currently in place for staff training:

- regional training workshops, for educational staff, school administrators, and school board members,
- integration of HIV/AIDS information into existing programs (e.g., wellness, prevention),
- incorporating HIV/AIDS information into certification standards,
- development of educational curricula, teachers' guides, resource materials, newsletters, teleconferences, electronic mail.

SUPPORT FOR HIV POSITIVE STUDENTS AND STAFF

Early surveys (Blake and Arkin, 1988) found that in 1985, about half of the people surveyed believed that school employees with AIDS should be taken off the job. Fifteen to 20 percent believed that if a child had AIDS, the child should be kept out of school, while 6 to 20 percent would keep their own child at home.

If AIDS is a priority, it cannot be a silent priority. School policies and procedures, the development of educational programs, and the involvement of key school staff, cannot be accomplished in a silent vacuum. If the decision is made to make AIDS a priority, then the school leaders need to take a public stand on the importance of AIDS education as a life-saving activity. It's important for the students, teachers, employees, and community to know that the school cares for all of its students and employees, regardless of their health status.

Although a variety of policies have been suggested for dealing with students and staff members who are HIV infected (Fraser, 1989), there are a number of human needs that must be addressed that cannot be accomplished through policies and procedures alone.

Counseling needs

Additional counseling services (including crisis counseling) may be necessary for HIV positive students and staff. What may be considered routine decisions by students may take on a completely different perspective if they are HIV positive. For example, whether a student decides to go on to college or not may become an extremely difficult decision if that student is HIV positive. Guidance counselors will probably need to have some familiarity with the health services that are available on typical college and university campuses, because health services may be as important to the HIV positive student as the academic quality of the college or university she or he is considering.

Although every effort should be made to provide confidentiality regarding the identity of students or staff who are HIV infected, in some cases such confidentiality may be breached, either within the school or from outside the school. A policy on confidentiality may help somewhat. However, there is no doubt that some HIV infected individuals will suffer from verbal abuse, physical harassment, or even physical abuse. Not only will HIV infected students and staff need some support from the school system, but those students and staff who may be inflicting such abuse may also benefit from a counseling program that addresses such behaviors straightforwardly (e.g., recognizing homophobia, developing empathy, coping with death).

Counseling needs vary by school. Some schools (for example, those in areas of the Bronx) have far more HIV infected individuals than other schools (for example, those in Fargo, North Dakota). Each school or each school district will have to determine its own needs and how those needs can best be met.

Risk taking after positive HIV test

Depending upon the quality of the pre- and post-test counseling that accompanies the HIV antibody test, a person who tests positive may or may not engage in risky behaviors. In some cases, fear of death can be so profound that suicide may be attempted. In other cases, there may simply be more "acting out" behavior on the part of adolescents, who may not have the coping skills of an adult to deal with the impact of being told that one is HIV positive.

Some unusual behavior may be expected if an adolescent finds out that one of his or her parents is HIV infected, or diagnosed with AIDS. In dealing with problem behavior at school, the role of HIV infection within the family may become as important in contributing to student behavioral problems as child abuse, alcoholism, or sexual abuse.

Increased suicides

Increased suicides and suicide attempts may be a real possibility, especially if the support network for the HIV infected individual is small or nonexistent. It's not uncommon for people to be abandoned by their families when they find out about their HIV status; friends and colleagues may abandon them as well, simply increasing the alienation and isolation of the individual.

Should a suicide take place, schools need to be careful not to foster a climate in which copycat suicides take place. Special memorial programs are probably not a good idea, because it suggests that one can really get attention by killing oneself. Support groups will probably be necessary for students and staff to cope with suicides, and programs for family members may be necessary to help them deal with the concerns that they may have about their own children.

SUPPORT FOR STAFF AND STUDENTS WITH AIDS

Dealing with AIDS means that schools must confront the hysteria that accompanies this disease. For example,

> "In September 1985, the announcement in New York City that a single child with AIDS would enroll in the public schools touched off an angry boycott in two Queens school districts. Parents vowed to "stand in the schoolhouse door" to keep children with AIDS out of school. On the first day of classes, between nine thousand and eleven thousand children stayed home in protest. At the entrance to one school, parents posted a sign saying "Enter at Your Own Risk." Outside another, parents stood by a mock coffin into which they had placed one of their own children. On the coffin they wrote: Is This the City's Next Idea for Our Kids? (Kass, 1987, p. 66)

Staff and students who are diagnosed with AIDS will probably continue to attend and work at school until the disease simply becomes too incapacitating. Support for these students and staff should be the same as for any other students and staff who might have a serious illness. However, because of some of the physical changes that some may go through, such as the skin lesions that develop in Kaposi's sarcoma, other students and staff may find themselves increasingly uncomfortable around the person with AIDS. Such uncomfortable feelings are likely to come from several sources. First, the physical signs of the disease continually emphasize that the infected person has AIDS. For those who have viewed AIDS at a distance through the mass media, such daily reminders may be difficult, especially if the person with AIDS was a popular and well-liked individual. Second, the visible signs, which generally only increase over time, are a reminder of death. Typically, we are not used to dealing with death in young people; for the student who has AIDS, the issue of death in adolescence may be particularly hard to deal with.

HIV POSITIVE PERSONS AND PERSONS WITH AIDS IN CLASS

Students and teachers in a classroom setting should not present any unique problems, although there may be a certain amount of fear on the part of parents that if a young child who is HIV positive engaged in biting behavior, their son or daughter may be placed at some risk of being exposed to HIV. Given appropriate confidentiality measures, few, if any individuals should know the identity of an HIV infected student or teacher.

SUPPORT FOR SURVIVORS

People with AIDS die. Depending on the situation, some support services may be necessary for the survivors of the student or staff member who dies of AIDS. Grief counseling might be a necessary service in some schools. For those schools that are in geographic areas with a high HIV infection rate in the population, many students and staff may be infected with the virus, and the problem becomes one of dealing not with a single, isolated death, but with multiple deaths, perhaps even in a relatively short period of time. Students and staff may find it relatively easy to cope with the first AIDS death; by the second, third, fourth, or tenth death, the ability to cope may be seriously impaired. Certainly the medical literature suggests that health-care providers who treat AIDS patients routinely may experience emotional burnout from the ultimate death of every AIDS patient.

Death response team

A death response team, a group comprised of trained school personnel, may be a valuable resource for coping with the death of a student or staff member. Such death response teams can be brought together on relatively short notice, and a planned course of action can be implemented without much delay. For those communities with a high number of HIV infections, such a team will be a virtual necessity.

SUMMARY

Hysteria was a typical response to students with AIDS in the mid-1980s. Although it may appear that such hysteria was limited to major cities, many smaller communities have not yet had to deal with some of the issues that urban areas confronted five years ago. More and more communities will have to deal with these emotional issues as more HIV infected students and staff become a reality. Data are beginning to show that HIV infection is much broader geographically than are AIDS cases, and that school districts in suburban and rural areas may have to respond to issues related to HIV-seropositive status in students and faculty before they are actually confronted by AIDS.

Issues that schools will have to address include policies regarding non-discrimination (e.g., treating people with AIDS as "handicapped" and providing AIDS education to developmentally disabled students), infection control (e.g., providing both staff training and barrier protection, such as gloves for those who must clean up blood and body fluids), and the development of educational programs for students and employees that are culturally appropriate (e.g., recognizing the need to emphasize family responsibilities over personal health as a prevention strategy for some ethnic groups).

Some states currently require HIV/AIDS education; during the next few years schools will be responsible for developing a coordinated K–12 curriculum, as well as possibly providing AIDS education to the community (as a way of enhancing support for school-based programs and policies). In particular, the school-based programs will require appropriate objectives for knowledge and attitudes; although behavioral objectives should be a part of an AIDS prevention program, political issues and community values may make it impossible to determine whether the program is having a positive or negative impact on students' risk-taking behaviors.

Decisions will be necessary for teaching assignments on AIDS, training of staff (how and where), and providing psychological support for HIV infected students and staff. Support groups may also be necessary for those students or staff who are coping with the AIDS-related illnesses of parents, friends, co-workers, and other students.

REFERENCES

Blake, S. M., and Arkin, E. B. (1988) *AIDS information monitor: A summary of national public opinion surveys on AIDS: 1983 through 1986.* Washington, DC: American National Red Cross.

CDC (1990) *HIV/AIDS Surveillance Report.* June 1990, 1–18.

Ellickson, P. L., and Bell, R. M. (1990) Drug prevention in junior high: A multi-site longitudinal test. *Science,* 247, 1299–1305.

Fraser, K. (1989) *Someone at school has AIDS. A guide to developing policies for students and school staff members who are infected with HIV.* Alexandria, VA: National Association of State Boards of Education.

Fraser, K., and Mitchell, P. (1988) *Effective AIDS education: A policymakers guide.* Alexandria, VA: National Association of State Boards of Education.

Gardner, L. T., Brundage, J. F., Burke, D. S., et al. (1989) Evidence for spread of the Human Immunodeficiency Virus epidemic into low prevalence areas of the United States. *Journal of Acquired Immune Deficiency Syndromes,* 2 (6), 521–532.

Hardy, A. M. (1990) AIDS knowledge and attitudes for October–December 1989. Provisional data from the National Health Interview Survey. *Advance Data from*

Vital and Health Statistics. No. 186. DHHS Pub. No. (PHS) 90–1250. Hyattsville, MD: Public Health Service.

Hoffman, R. E., Valway, S. E., Wolf, F. C., et al. (1989) Comparison of AIDS and HIV antibody surveillance data in Colorado. *Journal of Acquired Immune Deficiency Syndromes.* 2 (2), 194–200.

Jacobs, R., Samowitz, P., Levy, J. M., and Levy, P. H. (1989) Developing an AIDS prevention education program for persons with developmental disabilities. *Mental Retardation,* 27 (4), 233–238.

Kass, F. C. (1987) Schoolchildren with AIDS. In Dalton, H. L., Burris, S., and the Yale AIDS Law Project, eds. *AIDS and the law. A guide for the public.* New Haven: Yale University Press.

Kolbe, L. J., and Jones, J. (1988) School health education to prevent the spread of AIDS. In R. F. Schinazi and Nahmias, A. J., eds. *AIDS in children, adolescents and heterosexual adults: An interdisciplinary approach to prevention.* New York: Elsevier.

Lamers, E. P. (1988) Public schools confront AIDS. In I. B. Corless and Pitman-Lindeman, M., eds. *AIDS: Principles, practices and politics.* Washington, DC: Hemisphere Publishing Co.

Mays, V., and Cochran, S. D. (1988) Issues in the perception of AIDS risk and risk reduction activities by black and Hispanic/Latina women. *American Psychologist,* 43 (11), 949–957.

Moskowitz, J. (1989) The primary prevention of alcohol problems: A critical review of the research literature. *Journal of Studies on Alcohol,* 50 (1), 54–88.

Office for Substance Abuse Prevention (1990) NIDA study evaluates prevention program. *Prevention Pipeline,* 3 (4), 4–5.

Owens, B. S. (1985) Elementary school health education. In H. P. Cleary, J. M. Kichen, and P. G. Ensor, eds. *Advancing health through education.* Palo Alto, CA: Mayfield Publishing Co.

Schumacher, M. (1989) *The National Association of State Boards of Education HIV/AIDS Education Survey. Profiles of state policy actions.* Alexandria, VA: National Association of State Boards of Education.

Turner, C. F., Miller, H. G., and Moses, L. E., eds. (1989) *AIDS. Sexual behavior and intravenous drug use.* Washington, DC: National Academy Press.

Valdiserri, R. O. (1989) *Preventing AIDS. The design of effective programs.* New Brunswick, NJ: Rutgers University Press.

School Strategies

No young man believes he shall ever die.	
WILLIAM HAZLITT	

Certainly policies and procedures are important, as is having a specific information-based curriculum in place so that students can begin learning the basic facts about AIDS at an early age. Nevertheless, there are some fundamental issues that must be addressed in the development of a school-based program, including: (1) theoretical basis for educational programs, (2) school needs, and (3) the impact on school health programs.

THEORETICAL ISSUES

Development of an AIDS education program without an understanding of learning and behavior change principles will have little impact on behavior. Some of the early drug education programs, which did not have a firm theoretical base, often did little to change drug-using behaviors, although knowledge and attitude changes were seen in some programs. Allensworth and Symons (1989) note that:

> "Educators, regardless of their content area, are well-grounded in learning theories. However, these tenets often are overlooked when planning primary prevention and intervention programs for a controversial subject such as AIDS. As a safe response to media attention and community outcry, school programmers frequently gravitate toward emotionally based or "Band-aid" reactive approaches to the problem." (p. 59)

In their recommendation for a theoretically based approach, they specify several important research and theoretical findings that should have an impact on the structure of a prevention program. One of the most important is the recognition of developmental differences: 5-to-7-year-olds value duty and acceptance of rules; 8-to-10-year-olds model their behavior on adult role models; 11-to-13-year-olds respond more to peers; 14-to-16-year-olds may show considerable conflict between parents and peers. Thus, while a "Just say no" approach to drug use or sexual behavior may be effective for very young children who accept rules, that same approach is likely to be ineffective with those adolescents who are rebelling and trying to test the rules.

Results from smoking prevention programs are relevant to this issue. Figure 10.1 shows the importance of different types of health messages for different ages (McCarthy, 1985). Health information that focuses on physical aspects and consequences of cigarette smoking has its greatest im-

pact on 9-year-olds but decreases in importance throughout adolescence. Psychological messages, which have their lowest impact on 9-year-olds, increase substantially throughout the rest of adolescence, while health messages emphasizing social factors peak at about ages 12–14. With this as a theoretical model, an AIDS education program in junior high and high school that emphasized only the physical aspects of the disease would be least likely to have an impact.

Basch (1989) has identified 11 concepts that he believes are important for the design and implementation of AIDS education programs in a school setting. A few of his concepts are worth exploring in some detail.

Building commitment to a goal helps increase motivation to achieve that goal. Basch notes that public commitments to a goal (e.g., in weight-loss programs) can be an important source of

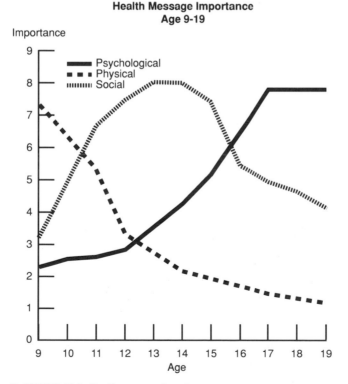

Health Message Importance
Age 9-19

* FIGURE 10.1   Health message importance

motivation. To the extent that students and teachers are willing to make public pledges or behavioral contracts regarding HIV-related issues, such as risky behaviors, a commitment to teaching without prejudice, and so forth, a greater likelihood of success may be achieved. A student may learn the facts about HIV transmission; that is quite different from the student saying (or writing) publicly that he or she will promise to stay abstinent until marriage or will not share needles. A public commitment before parents and peers can help motivate the student toward the desired goal of staying HIV free.

A personal belief in self-efficacy may produce healthier behaviors. AIDS education programs should be planned in such a way as to foster mastery and self-confidence in the learner. To the extent that the student is capable of mastering the material, self-confidence in his or her ability to control behavior may be increased. One of the assumptions in AIDS education seems to be that once the materials are developed and presented to the students, the materials will be mastered equally by all students. Some of the information about AIDS is complicated; some is even contradictory. Not all students will master all of the material at the same rate. Those who do not understand the content may not understand how that information can help them change their behaviors; mastery may mean survival.

ELEMENTARY LEVEL

Student knowledge and ignorance

Most educational programs assume that all of the students need all of the information; typically, educational programs are not developed on the basis of specific areas of ignorance or misinformation. Yet, knowing what students do not know about AIDS can be valuable in designing programs that more effectively meet the student's need—as well as the school's. In an analysis of questions from fifth- and sixth-grade students, Montauk and Scoggin (1989) categorized 400 questions from almost 500 sixth graders and 200 fifth graders. About 40 percent of the questions dealt with transmission concerns, including:

- What if you can't get the condom off?
- If neither partner has AIDS, can they get it with intercourse?
- How can you tell who has it if they aren't honest?
- If a man has AIDS and gives it to a lady (via intercourse), does he still have it?

AIDS education for young children may need to emphasize the ways in which HIV is *not* transmitted (e.g., GAO, 1988) rather than on how it is transmitted. Because young children may not have a thorough understanding of such issues as "casual contact," AIDS education during the elementary grades may be most effective if it provides reassurance that the child is safe and secure. More detailed information about the virus, safer sex, and IV drug use is probably more appropriate in later grades.

Student fears

Very young students probably do not have an accurate understanding of AIDS. There may be significant errors in what they believe to be true about the disease, and such misinterpretations can lead to significant psychological, social, and academic problems. More specifically, fear of AIDS and death can be a serious problem for young children.

Based on their incomplete understanding of AIDS, children may believe that their parents are at risk for the disease, or in some cases, the children may believe that they are susceptible to the disease via casual contact.

Fear (and realty) of parent's death

Based on all of the media coverage about AIDS, some students may be afraid that their parents have contracted the virus and might die, especially if they live in an area where they have been aware of some adults actually dying of AIDS. Or, they may experience the death of an older (or younger) sibling from AIDS. Research literature suggests that the death of a parent or sibling during childhood may produce serious psychological problems later. For example, Krupnick and Solomon (1987) have summarized some of the common observations regarding childhood reaction to such losses:

1. Little is known about the impact of such losses on children under the age of five when a parent or sibling has died,

2. Children may demonstrate lower self-esteem, perhaps because they interpreted the parent's death as desertion because the parent did not love the child, or perhaps because they believe they were responsible for causing the death,

3. Some children may try to imitate the parent or sibling's best traits, perhaps indicating that the grieving process is incomplete; in some cases, the child tries to "replace" a deceased sibling—making it difficult for the child to develop his or her own identity.

Although such findings may not seem to have direct implications for the school setting, the results of the death of a parent or sibling on the educational process cannot be overlooked. Relationships with teachers and other children may be affected, and the ability of the child to learn may be compromised by low self-esteem, psychological depression, school dysfunction, and delinquency. Depending on such factors as age, family support, and quality of caregiving, some children will be more affected by such losses than others and may be considered at "high risk." Since nearly half of the AIDS cases are diagnosed in adults between the ages of 30 and 39, and the

average life span after diagnosis is only a few years, many relatively young parents will die, leaving many young children to survive them.

Coping with illness

Although relatively few children with AIDS (fewer than 2,000 under the age of 12) have been diagnosed, that number will certainly increase during the next few years. Some children will have to cope with their own diagnosis of being HIV positive or being diagnosed with AIDS at an early age. Literature on how children cope with illness (Koocher, 1985) has often focused on a developmental perspective, recognizing that children have different coping styles at different ages. Bibace and Walsh (1980, 1981) describe the following stages:

1. Preoperational period (ages 2–6)
   - Phenomenism: Cause of illness comes from external source (e.g., people get colds from "the sun," or from "God"),
   - Contagion: Cause of illness is located in object or people nearby. Magic may be the explanation of how the illness is contracted (e.g., people get colds when "someone else gets near them"),

2. Concrete operational period (ages 7–12)
   - Contamination: Cause of illness is due to something external that has a harmful aspect to it (e.g., people get colds "when they go outside without a hat"),
   - Internalization: Illness is located more inside the body; the external cause of the illness may be transmitted via inhaling or swallowing (e.g., people get colds from breathing in "bacteria"),

3. Formal operational period (age 12 and beyond)
   - Physiological reasoning: An external cause is seen as causing an internal illness (e.g., people get colds from "viruses"),

• Psychophysiological reasoning: The most sophisticated thinking about illness; child can give physiological explanations of illness, and also be aware of how feelings affect body functions (e.g., people get "heart attacks" by being "nerve wracked").

Depending upon age and developmental level, children may not understand AIDS the same way that adults understand the disease, and as Koocher notes, during periods of crisis, patients may regress to an earlier form of explanation. Adolescents might resort to phenomenism or contagion as a way of coping with AIDS, rather than using physiological explanations.

Burbach and Peterson (1986), in a literature review of children's conception of illness, have pointed out some of the methodological limitations and contradictions in this area of research. Nevertheless, they do support the general contention that older and more cognitively mature children conceptualize illness differently than do younger and less cognitively mature children.

Koocher (1985) suggests five major types of intervention for children and adolescents who have to cope with illness. Not all may be appropriate for classroom-based programs, but some of his insights may be valuable for school nurses, counselors, teachers, and support programs.

1. Anticipation: Anticipating the future can help one deal with it. Children or adolescents with HIV infection or AIDS may be uncertain about their own future, both medically and educationally. To the extent that they can be given ways of coping with future events (e.g., making up classes and exams), they may be better able to cope with the disease.

2. Strategic interventions around expected crisis times may be valuable. Potential stress may be expected upon getting the diagnosis, beginning treatment, side effects of treatment, relapse, and stages of dying. These crises may well affect the child or adolescent at school, in terms of acting-out behavior,

depression, and perhaps even suicide attempts.

3. Patient education, although primarily the responsibility of the child's health-care providers, may require more of a collaborative effort when AIDS is involved. For example, if a child is taking AZT and experiencing side effects from the drug, the school nurse may have to provide some reassurance and education before the child can meet with his or her physician.

4. Enhanced internal control research suggests that if children can be given more control over their illness, they may be better able to cope. Some children and adolescents with AIDS may be given more control over how they administer medication, for example. Collaboration between the patient, parent(s), and medical providers may be essential for such psychological benefits to develop.

5. Open communication patterns can be valuable. Although there is justifiable concern about who should know whether a student is HIV infected, improved communication may help the student cope with the disease. Opening communications must be done carefully and with respect for the child's confidentiality, but confidentiality can develop into secrecy. Such secrecy in other health-care areas (e.g., incest, child abuse, alcohol or drug abuse) can inhibit intervention, treatment, and recovery.

Learning empathy

An important component of learning to deal with such experiences is the development of empathy—the understanding and feeling of what another person is experiencing. Generally, women tend to report themselves as being more empathic than do men, possibly because women are somewhat better than men at reading and interpreting other people's nonverbal cues (Eisenberg and Lennon, 1983), or because women seem to be more aware of emotional reactions. Although empathy will be important for children whose friends die of AIDS, the research on the development of empathy is inconsistent (Radke-Yarrow, Zahn-Waxler, and Chapman, 1983).

As they have noted, part of the confusion stems from the fact that although empathy can be defined cognitively (i.e., recognizing the emotions of another person) or emotionally (i.e., a vicarious emotional arousal and response to another person), both cognitions and emotions combine to affect empathy. Their review concluded that children apparently do not necessarily become more empathic with age. A theory of empathy has yet to be developed, and effective methods for teaching empathy are not yet available.

MIDDLE SCHOOL

What do students know? When do they know it? What do they do? When do they do it?

The effectiveness of an AIDS education program depends, in part, on how much students already know and on how much they need to know to understand both AIDS and their own behaviors. Most surveys have focused on high school or college students, although some of the risky behaviors may begin in middle (or even elementary) school.

A survey of 38,000 Canadian students (King et al., 1989) in grades 7, 9, and 11 and the first year of college assessed knowledge, attitudes, and behavior concerning AIDS. An important part of this survey was that all students were asked all questions, including potentially sensitive questions about sexual experiences. In contrast, a survey developed by the Centers for Disease Control (Kann et al., 1989) also had questions about knowledge, beliefs, and behaviors; however, because of the sensitive nature and political implications of the behavior questions, 15 of 23 education agencies participating in the project chose not to use the behavior items.

Although most people assume that knowledge and attitudes shape behaviors, psychological research has clearly shown that in some situations, behaviors come first, attitudes second. A survey of sexually active adolescents in San Francisco (Kegeles, Adler, and Irwin, 1988) found that although adolescents believed that condoms can prevent STDs and that the adolescents wanted to avoid STDs, such beliefs did not increase either the adolescents' intention to use condoms or their actual use of condoms. Such findings suggest that if young people practice "safer sex," their attitudes regarding "safer sex" will become stronger; if they learn only about "safer sex," their behaviors may well represent "unsafe sex."

Peer influence—public vs. private behaviors

Adolescence is a time when peer influences begin to develop and become an important part of the adolescent's decision-making process. Although peer pressure has often been viewed as a negative factor in an adolescent's life, typically associated with pressures to drink alcohol, use drugs, or become sexually active, peer influence can also produce positive outcomes from the standpoint of role models, social support, and peer education and counseling (NIDA, 1983; Bell and Battjes 1985). For those who desire to go beyond a strict "educational" program to a more intervention-based approach, these studies in substance abuse prevention can provide an excellent theoretical and practical background.

There are many factors that affect a young person's involvement with alcohol, drugs, and sexual behavior. One perspective is to consider these behaviors within the context of the agent (i.e., the drug), the host (i.e., the adolescent), and the environment (i.e., the social context). Figure 10.2 (Kumpfer, 1989) summarizes many of the factors that influence alcohol and drug use.

To the extent that many (or perhaps all) of these variables have an effect on both substance use and sexuality, prevention programs that focus

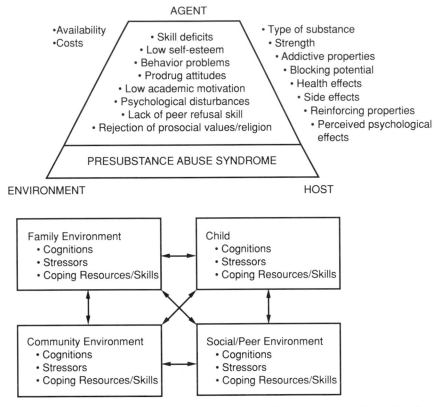

AGENT

•Availability
•Costs

• Skill deficits
• Low self-esteem
• Behavior problems
• Prodrug attitudes
• Low academic motivation
• Psychological disturbances
• Lack of peer refusal skill
• Rejection of prosocial values/religion

• Type of substance
• Strength
• Addictive properties
• Blocking potential
• Health effects
• Side effects
• Reinforcing properties
• Perceived psychological effects

PRESUBSTANCE ABUSE SYNDROME

ENVIRONMENT   HOST

Family Environment
• Cognitions
• Stressors
• Coping Resources/Skills

Child
• Cognitions
• Stressors
• Coping Resources/Skills

Community Environment
• Cognitions
• Stressors
• Coping Resources/Skills

Social/Peer Environment
• Cognitions
• Stressors
• Coping Resources/Skills

• FIGURE 10.2   Vasc (Values/Attitudes, Stressors, Coping Responses) theory of alcohol and drug abuse

on relatively broad factors (e.g., cognitions, stressors, and coping resources) might be expected to have an impact on a variety of behaviors. Although there are major differences between sexual behaviors and drug-using behaviors, some of their contributing factors probably overlap. Consequently, AIDS education need not be considered in isolation from existing school-based prevention programs.

Sex involves two people, a point sometimes omitted when discussing peer influences. One's sexual partner (perhaps one's best friend) is probably the most "equal" of all peers to another adolescent, and may well be able to exert the most influence. Successful drug education programs have been able to use positive peer influences to shape non-drug using behaviors, in part because al-

cohol and drug use among adolescents is generally a public behavior. On the other hand, sexual behavior is generally a private behavior between two adolescents, and the power of peer influence in reducing alcohol or drug use might not be as effective with private sexual behaviors. Although peer expectations may be helpful for establishing a community "norm" for sexual behavior, the fact that sexuality is such a private behavior makes it difficult for the peer group to know whether the sexual behavior has occurred or not, especially if the adolescents do not brag about their sexual activities. Viewed in this way, enhancing one-to-one communication skills between adolescents may be an effective way of shaping sexual behavior to the desired goal (i.e., abstinence or safer sex).

SECONDARY LEVEL

Risky behaviors

Not only are many adolescents sexually active (Turner, Miller, and Moses, 1989), they are also at high risk for sexually transmitted diseases. Unfortunately, much of the data on adolescent sexuality is from 5 to 15 years old. Very few data are available to document changes (if any) in adolescent sexuality since the mid-1980s, when AIDS became a more publicized health issue in the mass media. In addition, adolescents may be at risk from needle sharing when experimenting with drugs (or using steroids), or even alcohol from drug intoxication (which is likely to impair one's judgment for "safer sex"). Risk-taking behavior does tend to put one at risk.

Social skills

One innovative method for AIDS education is the "TEAM PACK" cooperative learning technique (Dorman, Small, and Lee, 1989), which involves two or more student peers working together on a common task. Groups of four students not only teach each other facts and concepts about AIDS, but provide an opportunity for students to express their feelings to each other. In brief, the activity includes sharing questions, answers, and concepts; role playing; and a group process activity.

Role playing

Role playing can be a useful method for helping students, faculty, or staff to deal with issues that produce anxiety. For example, a preliminary study (Ross, Caudle, and Taylor, 1989) of 10th and 11th graders in an Australian high school identified several areas in which students expressed anxiety:

- telling your parents that you have a sexually transmitted disease,

- telling your boyfriend or girlfriend that you have a sexually transmitted disease,
- going to a clinic for an STD or AIDS test,
- telling your parents that you think you have a problem with IV drugs.

All of these situations could be addressed in a role-playing situation, with students given a script to learn and a part to play (e.g., role of a parent). Working through a variety of scenarios throughout a health education class, for example, could help students deal constructively with their anxiety and avoid standard defense mechanisms such as denial.

Safer sex

"Safer sex" is one of the more controversial aspects of AIDS education. Some argue that abstinence is the only message that should be given to adolescents, that any other message is simply immoral. Others argue that not all adolescents will stay abstinent and will therefore need "safer sex" information to protect themselves from HIV. Moreover, if one supports the concept of "safer sex," does that mean that secondary students should just know what "safer sex" means (i.e., cognitions) or should they have the skills to actually practice "safer sex" (i.e., behaviors)? The two are not the same.

Health educators, nurses, teachers, and others who find themselves in conflict with school administrators or vocal members of the community on this issue may choose to develop a referral network for those students who perceive themselves as being at risk. If a health educator cannot teach in the classroom what he or she considers essential "safer sex" knowledge, attitudes, and behavior, a referral to a community organization or agency may be appropriate. Some organizations may be able to discuss and demonstrate "safer sex" practices in a way that simply cannot be done in a classroom setting. Professional discretion is advised.

A person with AIDS (PWA) as a resource

Sometimes students are fearful of HIV infected people or people with AIDS. AIDS education programs can benefit substantially from the involvement of someone who has been affected by the disease. In larger, urban areas, local AIDS organizations often have a speakers' bureau, and someone with AIDS may be willing to talk with the students. If that is not possible, a parent of a person with AIDS may be willing to share his or her experiences with the students.

In particular, if a young person who is HIV positive is willing to talk with the students about his or her own risky behaviors, some students *may* be able to see themselves as being at somewhat higher risk. From the standpoint of prevention, a perception of personal vulnerability is crucial. A peer with AIDS may be able to help increase that perception among students who otherwise would like to deny that they are at risk for AIDS.

IMPACT ON SCHOOL HEALTH AND SCHOOL NURSES

Such efforts will undoubtedly have an impact on school health services in many ways, as school nurses are able to use their expertise in assisting schools in developing AIDS education programs (Nauman, 1989). Not only will health education teachers and nurses be affected by the implementation of specific AIDS education programs in K through 12, but professional roles and expectations may change as well. For example, the roles of the school nurse will be changing as the number of HIV infected students and students with AIDS increases. Brainerd (1989) has outlined three roles of the school nurse that are likely to change:

1. School nurses as planners, to work with community agencies in public education; to work with administrators to adopt policies and procedures; to implement infection-control procedures; to serve as a role model and resource to others.

2. School nurses as managers, to communicate with parents; to meet with health-care providers; to be an advocate for HIV infected students; to protect the HIV infected student's right to privacy.

3. School nurses as change agents, to influence students, staff, and parents regarding risky behaviors; to influence health education programs; to provide health counseling to students who engage in risky behaviors, etc.

Health educators will also find their roles expanding within the context of school health programs. Rienzo and Dorman (1988) have discussed 10 consequences that AIDS are likely to have on the health education profession, including the following:

• the changing of professional preparation programs to help health educators become more comfortable in dealing with human sexuality,

• the development of human sexuality programs that (1) do not promote sexism (assuming that girls are responsible for saying *no*), (2) do not neglect the positive aspects of human sexuality,

• the exploration and development of new ways of presenting health messages,

• the discussion of ethics and values related to AIDS issues.

There is no doubt that AIDS will change school nurses, health educators, and the school health service itself (Adams, Marcontel, and Price, 1988). The common thread throughout these articles is that "business as usual" will not work with AIDS, and that both institutions and individuals will have to change in order to respond to this crisis.

PARENTS AND COMMUNITY

Given the sensitive nature of AIDS education, the need for a collaborative effort among schools, parents, and the community is essential. The ability of the schools to provide an AIDS educational experience that will help young people adopt healthy

Box 10

What Do Schools Need?

Kerr, Allensworth, and Gayle (1989) surveyed teachers, PTA presidents, school administrators, school nurses, school board members, school counselors, and physicians regarding their needs for resources, policies, training, and knowledge. In terms of resources, more than two-thirds reported that they need books, pamphlets, journal articles, films, or videotapes; more than 50 percent need instructional units and individual lesson plans (grades 6–12); more than 40 percent need instructional units and individual lesson plans (grades K–5). Regarding policy needs, the most frequent request (64%) was for confidentiality. More than half need policies regarding the appropriate grade levels for AIDS education, attendance for infected staff, and attendance for infected students, while 44 percent need policies for handling blood and body fluids.

In terms of training update needs, more than 60 percent listed homosexuality, bisexuality, and sexually transmitted diseases; between 50 and 60 percent need updates on risk behaviors for AIDS transmission, IV drug use, death and dying, safer sex practices, and communicating about AIDS with a sexual partner. Information presented, however, is not always information understood. Although not directly focusing on AIDS education issues, Yeaton, Smith, and Rogers (1990) researched the ability of college students to understand media reports of health research. When asked questions about what they had read, students misunderstood about 40 percent of the information, with the error rate generally falling between one-third and one-half for the health articles they studied.

Reaching people at higher risk

Many of the recommendations for AIDS education suggest a "generic" educational format to be taught to all students in virtually the same way, regardless of personal risk factors. However, students are not all the same, and some are obviously at higher risk than others. To address this issue, the General Accounting Office (GAO, 1988) assessed AIDS educational techniques with respect to populations at relatively high risk: IV drug users, minority communities, and youth. Briefly, they have recommended a seven-step AIDS education model, as well as some examples for each step:

A seven-step AIDS education model

1. **Specification of the target group:** Race/ethnicity, community or neighborhood, age bracket, informal communications networks. (A large school district may represent many cultures; the same educational program in each school probably would not be equally effective.)

2. **Identification of characteristics placing the group at risk:** Characteristics of risk behaviors, capabilities, attitudes, health practices, awareness of the health problem. Are there any risks that are more prevalent in the community, such as IV drug use? Do many children come from homes where the native language is not English?

    Goals: Changing characteristics; sidestepping characteristics; accommodating within-group differences. (For some, ethnic identity may be more important than sexual orientation; messages may have to focus on risk behaviors instead of risk groups.)

3. **Selection of media likely to reach the group:** Mass media, personal media, media variety. These include radio, television (feasible in some areas with cable TV), newspapers (including school and community papers), brochures, posters, community leaders, celebrities, health experts, actors, classroom teachers, trained peers.

4. **Determination of factual information to be included:** Risk level, risk-reduction methods, efficacy of risk reduction, models of transmission and nontransmission, medical and biological information, testing and counseling, peer pressure, civil rights issues, etc. Young children may need to learn about modes of nontransmission to reduce unfounded fears. Older children may need to learn about the degree to which one is at risk for HIV, guidelines for risk reduction, and the degree to which following those guidelines can reduce one's risk.

5. **Provision of skills for risk reduction:** Practical skills, verbal and nonverbal interpersonal skills. Some students and staff may need practical skills, such as how to express one's sexuality without being exposed to HIV. Others may need more enhancement of interpersonal skills, such as discussing sexuality.

6. **Provision of motivators for risk reduction:** Negative motivators, tangible and symbolic positive motivators. Some positive motivators may help change behaviors; they might include public commitments to risk reduction, prizes for scoring well on AIDS knowledge tests, or showing students that group norms do not support risky behaviors.

7. **Specification of intended outcomes:** Cognitive, including awareness of the problem, knowledge, attitudes. For young children, this might mean becoming more knowledgeable about the health threat of AIDS; for older children, it might mean having more favorable attitudes about people who are HIV positive or who have AIDS.

Behavioral goals: Risk prevention, risk reduction or elimination, maintenance of risk reduction. While risk prevention (e.g., abstinence) would be the behavioral outcome for people not engaged in risky behavior, risk reduction (e.g., condom use) would be the behavioral outcome for those who have begun risky behaviors.

behaviors will be a result of the willingness of the parents and community to support a program that may have some controversial components.

As mentioned previously, political considerations affected the willingness of some states to use the entire CDC survey to assess knowledge, beliefs, and behavior among adolescents. Behavioral questions were likely to be omitted because of possible controversy that might jeopardize the entire survey. Such concerns are a possibility; however, Miller and Downer (1988) found that when they asked parents for consent for their child to participate in an AIDS education study (December 1986), no parents prevented their children from participating. If the goal is a successful program, such a program may first have to be "sold" to the community.

The survey of educational professionals by Kerr, Allensworth, and Gayle (1989) found some discrepancies in who should be responsible for teaching HIV education, with teachers ranked first (36%), parents second (27%), and school nurses third (26%), although such opinions were closely ranked with one's professional affiliation (i.e., the National Education Association ranked teachers first, the National Association of School Nurses ranked nurses first, and the PTA presidents ranked parents first). In possible conflict with that ranking is a position paper by the Coalition of National Health Education Organizations, which recommends that parents have the major responsibility for AIDS education. Meanwhile, the National Health Interview Survey for October–December 1989 (Hardy, 1990) has found that 39 percent of the population reported never having discussed AIDS with a friend or relative; of those respondents with children, 38 percent had not discussed AIDS with any of their children aged 10–17; 13 percent reported that their children did not have instruction about AIDS at school, while 24 percent did not know whether their children had AIDS education; 31 percent reported knowing "little" or "nothing" about AIDS. Parent education may be a worthy goal, but the data suggest that many parents either do not know very much about AIDS or are not willing to have such discussions with their children.

Recommendations have been made that HIV education be determined locally and in conformance with parental and community values (Black and Jones, 1988). Politically and administratively, that position makes sense; however, DiClemente (1989) has suggested that a centralized, standardized HIV prevention program should be implemented, so that a basic core curriculum is available for each student. One rationale for such standard-

ization is that it would ensure that those students who moved from a low-incidence area of HIV infection to a high-incidence area would be as well informed as possible. Given the number of students who move each year, there may be some merit to that argument. For example, a student in a rural school system who does not receive much information about AIDS might be at some risk if his or her family moves to an area of the country (or world) with a high rate of HIV infection. Risky behaviors that were not dangerous in a rural area could become fatal behaviors in an urban area.

Although many surveys have been administered to students as a way of assessing their knowledge and attitudes about AIDS, similar data on parents (or communities) has not yet been collected. Who represents parental and community values: parents, clergy, businesspeople, health-care providers? Often, the "community" values that are communicated to the schools are the values of those who are most vocal—often a numerical minority. Before assuming that a community will oppose particular components of an AIDS education curriculum, one should objectively collect information from key members of the community to make sure that the reality doesn't contradict the perception.

SUMMARY

Generally, in developing a school-based program, schools must address (1) the theoretical basis for the educational programs, (2) school needs, and (3) the impact on school health programs. At the elementary level, issues of student knowledge and ignorance are important influences of program content: Don't teach the students what they know; teach them what they don't know. Student fears (of their own, their parent's, or friend's health), their ability to cope with illness, and their ability to show empathy to fellow students are factors that

should be addressed not only in prevention programs, but in providing support to those students who are directly experiencing HIV infection in themselves, their family, their friends, and their teachers.

In middle school and junior high, peer influences become an important part of the adolescent's life. They may use alcohol and other drugs, and some students may have their first sexual experience with a member of the same or opposite sex. Learning how to communicate and how to resist inappropriate peer pressure should be important components of any prevention program at this level.

At the secondary level, substance use and sexual behaviors may be less experimental and more common, at least for some students. For those students who may be at higher risk, peer education, role playing, and specific information about safer sex may provide the necessary skills to reduce their risk-taking behaviors.

Prevention programs will affect both health educators and school nurses, perhaps expanding their traditional roles into more creative roles in both the school and the community. Given the sensitive nature of AIDS education, collaboration among schools, parents, and the community will be essential if such programs are to seriously address the life-and-death issues of AIDS.

REFERENCES

Adams, R. M., Marcontel, M., and Price, A. L. (1988) The impact of AIDS on school health services. *Journal of School Health,* 58 (8), 341–343.

Allensworth, D. D., and Symons, C. W. (1989) A theoretical approach to school-based HIV prevention. *Journal of School Health,* 59 (2), 59–65.

Basch, C. E. (1989) Preventing AIDS through education: Concepts, strategies, and research priorities. *Journal of School Health,* 59 (7), 296–300.

Bell, C. S., and Battjes, R. (1985) *Prevention research: Deterring drug abuse among children and adolescents. NIDA Research Monograph 63.* Rockville, MD: National Institute on Drug Abuse.

Bibace, R., and Walsh, M. E. (1980) Development of children's conceptions of illness. *Pediatrics,* 66 (6), 912–917.

Bibace, R., and Walsh, M. E., eds. (1981) *Children's conceptions of health, illness and bodily functions.* San Francisco: Jossey-Bass.

Black, J. L., and Jones, L. H. (1988) HIV infection: Educational programs and policies for school personnel. *Journal of School Health,* 58 (8), 317–322.

Brainerd, E. F. (1989) HIV in the school setting: the school nurse's role. *Journal of School Health,* 59 (7), 316–317.

Burbach, D. J., and Peterson, L. (1986) Children's concepts of physical illness: A review and critique of the cognitive-developmental model. *Health Psychology,* 5 (3), 307–325.

Coalition of National Health Education Organizations (1988). Instruction about AIDS within the school curriculum. *Journal of School Health,* 58 (8), 323.

DiClemente, R. J. (1989) Prevention of Human Immunodeficiency Virus among adolescents. *AIDS Education and Prevention,* 1 (1), 70–78.

Dorman, S. M., Small, P. A., and Lee, D. D. (1989) A cooperative learning technique for AIDS education. *Journal of School Health,* 59 (7), 314–315.

Eisenberg, N., and Lennon, R. (1983) Sex differences in empathy and related capacities. *Psychological Bulletin,* 94, 100–131.

GAO (1988) *AIDS education. Reaching populations at higher risk.* Washington, DC: U.S. General Accounting Office.

Hardy, A. M. (1990) AIDS knowledge and attitudes for October–December 1989. Provisional data from the National Health Interview Survey. *Advance Data from Vital and Health Statistics of the National Center for Health Statistics.* No. 186. DHHS Publication No. (PHS) 90–1250. Hyattsville, MD: National Center for Health Statistics.

Kann, L., Nelson, G. D., Jones, J. T., and Kolbe, L. J. (1989) Establishing a system of complementary school-based surveys, to annually assess HIV-related knowledge, beliefs, and behaviors among adolescents. *Journal of School Health,* 59 (2), 55–58.

Kegeles, S. M., Adler, N. E., and Irwin, C. E. (1988) Sexually active adolescents and condoms: Changes over one year in knowledge, attitudes and use. *American Journal of Public Health,* 78 (4), 460–461.

Kerr, D. L., Allensworth, D. D., and Gayle, J. A. (1989) The ASHA National HIV needs assessment of health and education professionals. *Journal of School Health,* 59 (7), 301–307.

King, A. J., Beezley, R. P., Warren, W. K., et al. (1989) Highlights from the Canada youth and AIDS study. *Journal of School Health,* 59 (4), 139–145.

Koocher, G. P. (1985) Promoting coping with illness in childhood. In J. C. Rosen and L. J. Solmon, eds. *Prevention in health psychology.* Hanover, NH: University Press of New England.

Krupnick, J. L., and Solomon, F. (1987) Death of a parent or sibling during childhood. In J. Bloom-Feschbach, S. Bloom-Feschbach, and Associates. *The psychology of separation and loss.* San Francisco: Jossey-Bass.

Kumpfer, K. L. (1989) Prevention of alcohol and drug abuse: a critical review of risk factors and prevention strategies. In D. Shaffer, I. Philips, and N. B. Enzer, eds. *Prevention of mental disorders, alcohol and other drug use in children and adolescents. OSAP Prevention Monograph-2.* Rockville, MD: Office for Substance Abuse Prevention.

McCarthy, W. J. (1985) The cognitive developmental model and other alternatives to the social skills deficit model of smoking onset. In C. S. Bell and R. Battjes, eds. *Prevention research: deterring drug abuse among children and adolescents. NIDA Research Monograph 63.* Rockville, MD: National Institute on Drug Abuse.

Miller, L., and Downer, A. (1988) AIDS: What you and your friends need to know—A lesson plan for adolescents. *Journal of School Health,* 58 (4), 137–141.

Montauk, S. L., and Scoggin, D. M. (1989) AIDS: Questions from fifth and sixth grade students. *Journal of School Health,* 59 (7), 291–295.

Nauman, L. A. (1989) School nursing and AIDS education. *Journal of School Health,* 59 (7), 312–313.

NIDA. (1983) *Adolescent peer pressure. Theory, correlates, and program implications for drug abuse prevention.* Rockville, MD: National Institute on Drug Abuse.

Radke-Yarrow, M., Zahn-Waxler, C., and Chapman, M. (1983) Children's prosocial dispositions and behavior. In P. H. Mussen, ed. *Handbook of child psychology. (4th ed.) Volume IV: Socialization, personality and social development.* New York: John Wiley & Sons.

Rienzo, B. A., and Dorman, S. M. (1988) Ten consequences of the AIDS crisis for the health education profession. *Journal of School Health,* 58 (8), 335–338.

Ross, M. W., Caudle, C., and Taylor, J. (1989) A preliminary study of social issues in AIDS prevention among adolescents. *Journal of School Health,* 59 (7), 308–311.

Turner, C. F., Miller, H. G., and Moses, L. E., eds. (1989) *AIDS. Sexual behavior and intravenous drug use.* Washington, DC: National Academy Press.

Yeaton, W. H., Smith, D., and Rogers, K. (1990) Evaluating understanding of popular press reports of health research. *Health Education Quarterly,* 17 (2), 223–234.

11 Ethics and Values

> *Morality is simply the attitude we adopt*
> *towards people we personally dislike.*
> OSCAR WILDE

AIDS is a disease of contradictions; of public health and private behaviors, of religious morality and religious compassion, of medical confidentiality and medical disclosure, of voluntary behavior change and mandatory behavior change. None of these conflicts is likely to be resolved any time soon. At best, they can be described and discussed in some detail so that each individual can make an independent decision about this disease, and how one's personal perspective can affect organizational decisions.

AIDS and immorality

Some people have viewed AIDS within a religious framework and have argued that the disease is brought on by biblically described "immoral" be-

haviors. Interpreted in this way, AIDS has been described as a punishment from God for specific acts of immorality—homosexual behaviors. Thus, the person with AIDS (or at least that person who contracted the virus via homosexual behaviors) is seen as deserving of the disease. Meanwhile, the person who has contracted the virus via a blood transfusion, for example, may be described as an "innocent victim" of the disease. Some people deserve the disease, some people don't. At the Gay and Lesbian Pride March in New York City in June 1990, one protester had a sign of Jesus preaching the words, "I shall not allow science to find a cure for AIDS" (Tierney, 1990).

Within most religious perspectives, the only type of effective prevention is sexual abstinence until marriage and avoidance of all drug using behaviors that might transmit the virus. Homosexual behavior is to be avoided under all circumstances. Educational programs are expected to promote this view, and any educational programs that describe "safer sex" or even imply that homosexual behavior is an acceptable form of behavior are considered unacceptable.

Such issues highlight the conflict between individual morality and public health education. Public schools are supported by tax dollars from many segments of the general public: heterosexuals, homosexuals, lesbians, drug users, drug abstainers, atheists, agnostics, religious believers, Christians, Jews, Moslems, Native Americans, African Americans, Hispanics, whites, and many other groups. To what extent is it appropriate to impose one set of moral values (e.g., those values of the political party currently in power) upon those individuals who do not subscribe to that particular set of values?

Not everyone believes, for example, that premarital sex is to be completely avoided and that sexual activity should not occur until marriage. What about those individuals who choose not to marry? Should those individuals be expected to live a life of abstinence? If a man or woman chooses not to marry, should that person be given information about "safer sex," or should that person simply be expected to avoid all sexual activity outside a committed marriage, and not be given any information that could save his or her life? What is the public responsibility to educate those individuals whose beliefs or behaviors are different from those of the majority?

Trafford (1988) has described "fundamentalist medicine," the combining of medicine and morality to address a variety of health-care problems such as alcoholism, drug abuse, and AIDS. Such an approach, she argues, tends to justify victim blaming (sick people are responsible for being sick), reducing medical benefits (so as not to pay for "lifestyle" diseases), and setting public policy based on a particular version of "morality." In the short term, such policies may seem to be effective; people with AIDS can be blamed for

having contracted HIV, corporate medical benefits may be denied to employees with AIDS, and educational programs may be based on an inexpensive "Just say no" philosophy.

In the long term, however, people who are not educated about how to protect themselves from the virus will be more likely to contract the disease. If their employer does not provide healthcare treatment for AIDS, they will resort to treatment at public hospitals, and as more and more people develop AIDS via IV drug use, heterosexual activity, and perhaps blood transfusions, blaming the victim will seem less and less appropriate.

Kayal (1985) has suggested that such victim blaming will take place when the cause of a disease (such as AIDS) is (1) framed in a "moral" perspective, and (2) the illness affects religiously stigmatized and legally proscribed minorities such as gay and bisexual men or intravenous drug users. To what extent will such victim blaming reduce the future spread of the virus or help family members cope with the disease? For example, suppose you are teaching an adolescent whose father has been diagnosed with AIDS; what psychological and emotional impact will an educational program have that emphasizes the immorality of the people who contract the HIV and their responsibility for their own illness? What will it do to a child to hear that his father is essentially an "immoral" person, who deserves to die because of his own inappropriate behaviors?

Conversely, what is the impact on an adult parent of an adolescent or young adult child who is dying of AIDS; will the parents be better able to cope with the impending death of their son by believing that he was an immoral person who got what he deserved for behaving in "immoral" ways? Interpreting AIDS exclusively in the context of morality tends to blame the victim and reduce our capacity for compassion and humanity not only for those who have been diagnosed with AIDS, but for those young people who need to be educated in life-saving behaviors.

Compassion

Compassion is defined in one dictionary as a sympathetic emotion created by the misfortunes of another, accompanied by a desire to help; pity; mercy. *(Living Webster Encyclopedic Dictionary of the English Language,* 1975)

Many authors, including those with strong religious convictions, have commented on the need for compassion in the treatment of people with AIDS; there is a growing body of literature on this issue (Brown, 1988; Hedges, 1989). However, such compassion is often available only to those who are dying of the disease; compassion has generally not been applied to young people who are still healthy. The dictionary definition of compassion emphasizes the misfortunes of another; one can certainly sympathize with the misfortunes of a person with AIDS.

On another level, however, ignorance can also be viewed as a "misfortune of another," and compassion for those who are ill informed about AIDS might be a useful part of any AIDS education program. Sometimes people forget that AIDS is truly a life-and-death issue, and moralistic arguments that essentially justify the death of people who are "different" in their sexual orientations or in their risk-taking behaviors will do little to prevent future AIDS cases and future deaths. As Camus (1948) so eloquently stated in his classic work *The Plague:*

> "All I maintain is that on this earth there are pestilences and there are victims, and it's up to us, so far as possible, not to join forces with the pestilences." (p. 236)

BLAMING THE VICTIM

Consider your attitude if you found out that someone you know contracted HIV because she engaged in unprotected sex. "What a fool," you might say, "How could she be so stupid as to do that?" you might ask. "Wasn't she listening to all of the information about AIDS for the last decade?" you might ask. On the other hand, consider your attitude if you found that a close friend had been killed in an automobile accident. "Too bad," you might say. "I wonder if the other driver was drinking," you might say. Would you wonder if your friend was wearing a seat belt? Both condoms and seat belts can save lives; on the one hand, it may be difficult to understand how someone could have sex without a condom in the age of AIDS. On the other hand, we seldom think about why someone won't wear a seat belt in the age of accidents. In both cases, the result is the same (death), the behavior is the same (not using available protection), but our attitudes may be vastly different. In one case, we blame the victim; in the other, we blame external circumstances.

The classic work on blaming the victim is Ryan's (1976) book, *Blaming the Victim.* Although AIDS was not known at that time, some of his observations regarding victim blaming in other contexts are relevant to current AIDS issues. His primary contention is that the victim is blamed when "defects" are found in him or her, with such "defects" justifying unequal treatment. In other words, defective people do not deserve the same treatment as do people without such defects.

Change the victim

First, the deficiency is within the person, or in Ryan's terms, the victim. AIDS is due to high risk "groups" such as gay and bisexual men and intravenous drug users behaving in "immoral" ways. To prevent future AIDS cases, change the victim. Recommendations for mandatory testing and quarantine, for example, are directed specifically and exclusively to the person with the disease. This approach assumes that if the people with the disease can be changed, society itself will not have to change. Rather than examining the public policies that affect homosexuals (e.g., in many states homosexual behavior is illegal) or intravenous drug users (e.g., in many states sterile syringes are not legally available), simply try to change the victim.

Identify those who are "different"

A second strategy is to "look sympathetically at those who 'have' the problem in question, to separate them out and define them in some way as a special group that is *different* from the population in general. . . . The Different Ones are seen as less competent, less skilled, less knowing—in short, less human." (Ryan, 1976, pp. 9–10)

By identifying people who are HIV positive or who have AIDS, they can be set apart from the rest of the "general" population, and because they have engaged in "risky" behaviors, they can be viewed as less competent, less knowing, and less human. Violence towards people with AIDS can be justified if people with AIDS are not considered part of the general population, if they are viewed as being less human than the rest of us. If people's identify as human beings can be reduced by a simple label (e.g., gay, drug user, prostitute), they can be treated or mistreated as the majority sees fit. Because some believe that AIDS began in Central Africa, some European countries have been requiring HIV antibody tests for visitors from those Central African countries, but not from visitors from the United States. (More AIDS cases have been reported in the United States than from any other country.)

Blame the "deviant"

Third, we believe that "those deviant individuals" are the source of the particular problem under investigation. People who engage in behaviors that are different from our behaviors are labeled as being "deviant"; once such labels are applied, the "deviants" can be segregated from the rest of the population (perhaps through massive quarantine-isolation) and "fixed" according to the standards of the general population. Is it possible to address the disproportionate number of AIDS cases in African Americans and Hispanics without also addressing issues of poverty, racism, discrimination, and lack of medical coverage? AIDS does not exist in a vacuum, and to believe that it does will virtually guarantee the ultimate failure of education and prevention efforts.

In this victim-blaming philosophy, the problem of AIDS is a problem of "them," not of "us." By blaming "deviant" people with AIDS for contracting the disease through their "deviant" behavior, programs of mandatory HIV testing and quarantine-isolation can be justified. Moreover, if only "deviant" people get AIDS, there is no need to provide public education about AIDS, since only those people who are "deviant" will get the disease, and if they do, they deserve what they get. Ultimately, the status quo is justified, and education need not really change in response to the AIDS crisis. As long as AIDS is viewed as a disease of "deviants" and "outcasts," there is no need to change the social circumstances that might be significant contributors to this disease. When AIDS is viewed as a disease of "us" and not just "them," then the need for change becomes clear, since the risk is more visible and closer to home.

The stigma of AIDS

In their analysis of public reactions to AIDS, Herek and Glunt (1988) described "AIDS-related stigma"—those marks of shame or discredit that are directed at people perceived to be infected with HIV. They argue that AIDS-related stigma is a social reaction to a fatal illness that has been most commonly found in people who are already targets of prejudice. In their review of illness and stigma, they note several characteristics of AIDS that make it a stigmatized disease: (1) it is sexually transmitted and it is fatal, (2) people with HIV can be blamed for causing the disease, and (3) the symptoms of the disease can be visible (i.e., Kaposi's sarcoma, wasting syndrome, etc.). When combined with the denial of death, many people find it easier to cope with this disease by psychologically distancing themselves from those with the disease. To the extent that people with AIDS can be categorized in ways that help separate them from others, they can be stigmatized by blame, denial, and avoidance, and they can be viewed as deserving to die.

Such issues, although not always articulated, will become a part of the discussion regarding the content of school-based AIDS education programs. Indeed, there are probably some school administrators, school board members, and teachers who would rather stigmatize people with AIDS than develop an effective AIDS prevention program. In some ways, AIDS education in the 1990s may be where alcohol and drug education was in the 1950s. At that time, alcoholism was considered to be a moral weakness; it was only when the disease concept of alcoholism became more acceptable that serious prevention efforts began. Unless public health issues can be separated from moral issues with respect to AIDS education, the actual ability of school-based AIDS education programs to prevent future cases of AIDS will be very minimal.

MORALITY VS. MORAL DEVELOPMENT

While moral arguments may be attractive in their appeal to a simplistic response to the AIDS crisis, research is abundantly clear that moral choices do not simply occur as a result of specific instruction, but develop over time in somewhat of a sequential fashion. A 16-year-old probably does not think the way that a 36-year-old thinks about moral choices. Emphasizing an absolute standard for behavior simply ignores the reality that many adolescents are in a period of experimentation; indeed, the stronger the sanctions against particular behaviors, the more likely some adolescents are to engage in that behavior as a form of risk-taking behavior or rebellion against adult-imposed rules of conduct. By the time they reach adulthood, a certain amount of risk taking (e.g., in one's job) and rebellion

(e.g., challenging the political opposition) is essential for the development of an adult character.

Strict emphasis on an absolute moral standard of behavior (as defined by adults) may have little impact on the development of moral behavior in adolescents and may ultimately prove to be counterproductive. To develop a system that would effectively prohibit young people from experimenting with sexual behaviors and alcohol and drug use would place demands on a free society that probably would not be acceptable either constitutionally or politically. Young people sometimes make bad decisions; telling them not to make such decisions will probably be ineffective for many.

Damon (1988) has summarized some of the crucial differences between what he has characterized as seven myths about moral development and what is known about childhood morality based upon scientific research observation (pp. 116–118):

Myth 1: Children are naturally good, but they become morally corrupted when they are exposed to the wrong social influences.

Damon 1: Because they participate in social relationships, children do encounter classic moral issues such as fairness, honesty, kindness, and obedience. Moral awareness does not need to be imposed from the "outside," because it develops from "inside" a child's normal social experience.

Myth 2: Children are born with immoral tendencies; moral sensibilities must be imposed upon them against their will from the outside.

Damon 2: A child's moral awareness is shaped both by positive emotional reactions (such as empathy) that support compassion, and negative emotions (such as fear, guilt, and shame) that support obedience and rule following. Natural feelings of love and attachment toward parents help the child develop future respect for authority.

Myth 3:   The parent is solely responsible for the child's moral development.

Damon 3:   Relations with parents, teachers, and other adults introduce the child to important standards and rules of behavior. The most positive method for developing moral judgment is an "authoritative" relationship between adults and children in which firm demands are made of the child, while at the same time there are clear communications between parents and children regarding the reasons for such demands

Myth 4:   Little can be done about the child's moral character, because the child's personality is formed through congenital factors that are largely beyond anyone's control.

Damon 4:   Peer relationships introduce children to standards of sharing, cooperation, and fairness. Children learn how to interact with others, and their peer relationships may enhance the child's growing moral awareness and helping behaviors.

Myth 5:   Children's peers are a negative influence on their moral judgment.

Damon 5:   Different social experiences produce differences in children's moral orientation. For example, girls tend to orient more towards the morality of care for others, and boys toward the morality of rules and justice.

Such differences in moral orientation might account in part for the different perceptions toward people with AIDS, with males often tending to be more homophobic and less accepting of homosexual behavior, while females tend to be more accepting of homosexuality and perhaps even more willing to provide care to a person with AIDS. In many family situations where a son has developed AIDS, it is not uncommon for the father to completely reject his son—perhaps responding

to a morality of rules, while the mother may even move in with the son to help take care of him—perhaps responding to the morality of care.

Gilligan and Wiggins (1987) have also addressed these two moral orientations of care and justice; in particular, they note the difficulty in presuming a single standard of morality (typically male), which makes it difficult to discuss sex differences in morality with one group (typically male) being "more moral" and one group (typically female) being considered "less moral." Separate moralities of justice and care, however, simply permits identification of differences in moral orientation, not necessarily deficiencies in moral orientation.

Myth 6:   Children need to be shielded from television, film, or music that suggests poor moral values.

Myth 7:   Moral education means telling children about the value held by our society and the virtues expected of them.

Damon 6 and 7:   Moral growth in school is subject to the same developmental processes as moral growth in other situations. Lessons and lectures about morality are likely to have little impact on a child's developing sense of morality, while their active involvement with other children and adults is likely to have much more of an impact.

The above comparisons suggest that differences in the perception of moral development will have a profound effect on the content of AIDS education and the messages that are communicated (either overtly or covertly) to the students. Based on the myths of moral development, AIDS education would:

1.   Emphasize the negative impact of social influences such as peers, television, and music. Implied in this message is that your friends are not good for you and that peer pressure is to be resisted.

2. impose moral standards upon them from the outside (e.g., parents, teachers, and other authority figures) to reduce their natural immoral tendencies toward experimentation and rebellion.

3. encourage the learning of morality by telling children about the societal values and the virtues that are expected of them by society (such as sexual abstinence, not engaging in homosexual behaviors). Learning morality would not be very different from learning history or arithmetic.

On the other hand, using Damon's characterization of moral development during childhood, an AIDS education program would:

1. Emphasize the positive impact of social influences, such as peers, as related to sharing, cooperation, fairness, and honesty. Peer pressure can be a positive force in a child's development, not just a negative influence.

2. develop moral standards based on the recognition of different social experiences, gender differences, ethnic and cultural backgrounds, and the active involvement with other children and adults. Rigid lessons about morality will not have as much of an influence on behavior as will active behavioral experiences. Morality can be learned but not taught.

3. recognize the importance of relationships between the developing child and parents, teachers, and other adults. Standards of behavior are likely to develop on the basis of an ''authoritative'' relationship between a child and an adult, not on the basis of concrete moral standards.

EDUCATION AND THE LAW

Regardless of one's personal beliefs, both federal and state law will determine what type of educational services are to be provided for children who are HIV infected, and what type of personnel decisions are appropriate for staff who are HIV infected. Dickens (1988) has reviewed many of the legal rights and duties that may be encountered in the AIDS epidemic. From an educational standpoint, he identified several potential legal conflicts:

School-aged children who are HIV infected (and their parents) may invoke the right of the child to be educated on the basis of compulsory school attendance laws. However, resistance to such education may come from those who invoke public health laws on contagious or infectious diseases.

Or, parents can argue that a child's right to an education cannot be met if the public school provides isolated education (e.g., isolating the child at school, or perhaps providing a home tutor), since a major part of a child's education is peer socialization. Educational malpractice suits could be filed if the child does not have an opportunity for a classroom education, especially if the child has not achieved basic literacy or other skills.

Such potential conflicts raise issues that may not have been fully discussed in the context of education. During the past few years, considerable debate has taken place in the medical community regarding the obligation of physicians to treat patients with AIDS (Emanuel, 1988). Although the risks to a physician who cares for AIDS patients are considerably more serious than for a teacher who merely instructs an HIV infected student, there are a few issues that probably should be discussed in the educational setting:

1. Are public school teachers obligated to teach students who are either HIV infected or diagnosed with AIDS? Although the law may mandate equal educational opportunities, are there conditions under which a teacher may believe that he or she cannot provide equal education to all students? Under what conditions (if any) can a teacher refuse to teach a student? What are the relationships among

public, professional, and private responsibilities?

2. What occupational risks are acceptable (or unacceptable) for teachers, coaches, trainers, school nurses, etc.? How is AIDS similar to or different from other health problems (e.g., polio) with which the educational profession has had to cope?

Striking an appropriate balance between all affected parties is difficult. Certainly the student who is HIV infected and his or her parents will be concerned about the quality of the child's public education; on the other hand, the parents of children who are not HIV infected may express concern about the risks that their children will be taking by attending school with HIV infected children (Davis, 1987).

WHO TEACHES ABOUT AIDS

To say that AIDS is a value-laden topic would be a gross understatement. Given the import of such values, who should be responsible for teaching about AIDS? What are the criteria for an AIDS educator in a public school; should AIDS simply be incorporated into existing health classes in the hope that the health educator is competent to teach about AIDS? Or should there be some standards for the assignment of AIDS education, based on such factors as content competencies, an interest in the topic, or a willingness to take on the political and personal challenges of the community?

Private schools, and those that have a particular religious affiliation, may have a rather different set of criteria for teaching about AIDS, if the decision is made to teach about AIDS at all. Because private and religious schools serve a more well-defined constituency, they may not have the responsibilities of the public school system. Consequently, AIDS education may be less of a priority than in the public sector, and the content of that education may be much more proscribed, because of the religious orientation of the particular school.

MALE VS. FEMALE PERSPECTIVES

AIDS has been viewed largely as a disease of men, both because of the high number of gay and bisexual men who have been diagnosed with AIDS, and the general perception of IV drug users as being male. Nevertheless, females currently comprise about 10 percent of the total reported AIDS cases. Bell (1989) has identified some of the ethical issues regarding women and AIDS, for example, condom use and women. On the one hand, condoms have been recommended as a method for preventing the spread of HIV, and a considerable amount of information about condoms has been presented both to males and to females. However, effective condom use may be offset by the unwillingness of many men to use condoms, the expectation in some cultures that women will give in to sex upon demand, and the recognized ineffectiveness of condoms in preventing pregnancy. A woman's perspective on what constitutes acceptable sex may be quite different from a male's perspective. Like birth control, "safer sex" may become the primary responsibility of the woman.

HIV ANTIBODY TESTING: VALUES AND ETHICS

Some have argued that mandatory HIV antibody testing should be put into place as a way of identifying those individuals who are carrying the virus. Recent developments, however, suggest that the effectiveness of any kind of testing (mandatory or voluntary) may be subject to question.

AZT has been approved by the Food and Drug Administration for the treatment of AIDS; it is the only anti-viral drug thus far federally approved for such use. Consequently, many have called for mass HIV antibody testing to take place, not only in hopes that more people will learn their HIV status, but to identify people early in the stage of HIV infection so that they may be started on AZT treatment as soon as possible. However,

Box 11

Private Beliefs, Public Responsibilities

One area of potential conflict is the relationship between one's private beliefs and one's public responsibilities. Surgeon General Koop emphasized many times in his public statements that he kept his personal beliefs separate from his public responsibilities. Can a "public" employee impose his or her values on other members of the public who do not share those same values? Walters (1988) has suggested that:

> "Imaginative public education will be moral education in the sense that it helps the hearer to see clearly the possible effects of his or her behavior on others. One possible approach to such education involves the use of ethical if-then statements such as the following. "We have discussed the pros and cons of engaging in behavior X. If you choose to do X, then, in order to avoid harming others, you should adopt measures A, B, and C." Fortunately, many of the measures that protect others are also self-protective. Thus, public educators can simultaneously appeal to both the self-interested and altruistic sentiments of the audiences. (p. 597)

Suppose that if-then statement is translated into "We have discussed the pros and cons of engaging in receptive anal intercourse with another male. If you choose to engage in receptive anal intercourse, then, in order to avoid harming others, you should reduce the number of sexual partners that you have, use a condom every time you have anal intercourse, and discuss safer sex practices with your partner." Is that a message that administrators, teachers, parents, and students will find acceptable?

Whose standards?

Reliance upon a single moral standard ignores the differences that exist in American culture; the same beliefs are not equally shared by everyone. Reliance upon one set of standards may well alienate those individuals who do not share those standards; such conflicts are apparent not only with respect to AIDS, but to issues such as abortion and prayer in the school. While a strong set of standards may reinforce the beliefs of those individuals who believe in those particular standards, such an imposition may have little, if any, impact upon those individuals who have a different set of standards.

Suppose that a public official, a superintendent of schools, or a school board member, strongly believes that adolescents in a publicly funded school should not be given specific information about "safer sex" behavior, because such information is contradictory to his or her personal beliefs, even if such information could save lives. Do publicly elected officials, or publicly supported employees have an educational responsibility to all students, or only to those students whose behaviors and values are consistent with their own?

Personal conflicts

Moreover, what are the choices for a public employee who finds himself or herself personally in conflict with administrative decisions? Should that employee compromise his or her values to keep a job? Should that employee ignore educational recommendations from a superior? Should that employee try to sabotage the educational efforts in order to not compromise personal values? Over the next few years, such issues will probably have to be discussed publicly, for example, in forums in which parents and school personnel discuss the direction in which AIDS education will progress. No doubt such issues will have a strong impact on the decision of who is competent to teach sex education that addresses AIDS issues.

there are some risks in addition to the benefits of such testing.

A report by Benenson and fellow researchers (1989) of a pilot study of possible sources of incorrect laboratory reports of HIV antibody testing found that some laboratories reported an HIV-positive blood sample as being "indeterminate"; other labs provided incorrect or misleading information to physicians as to the results of the blood test, and the interpretation of such results. Such misinformation may have serious consequences, since between 23 and 32 million HIV antibody tests were performed in 1988 (Drotman and Valdiserri, 1989). It may matter little if the tests (ELISA and Western Blot) are accurate, but the results and interpretation to the physician are confusing or misleading.

If physicians can be occasionally misled by the reports from a testing laboratory, adding another layer (i.e., parents, teachers, staff) into the communication network may mean additional confusion. If an issue of HIV antibody status arises in an educational setting with regard to a "need-to-know" situation, every effort must be made to ensure that the information flow is as accurate as possible—in both directions. If a school nurse needs to know that a particular student is HIV positive, extra effort must be made to ensure that the information that the testing lab gives to the physician who gives it to the parents who give it to the school nurse doesn't lose anything from speaker to listener.

CONFIDENTIALITY VS. DISCLOSURE

Because of the fear surrounding HIV transmission, the issue of confidentiality of HIV test results (or even AIDS diagnosis) has been widely discussed. Despite the fact that many people would like to know who is infected with the virus (e.g., among students, teachers, administrators), such information is still considered confidential medical information, as is any other kind of information that might be found in a medical record.

The general public still believes that HIV infected people in some professions should not be allowed to keep working, even if they are well enough to do their jobs (Gerbert et al., 1989):

Occupation	Percentage Believing That Person Should Not Keep Working
• Cook	55%
• Nurse	50%
• Schoolteacher	23%
• Bus driver	8%

Maintaining confidentiality may be particularly difficult in small school districts, where there may be few physicians and where one's personal life may be known by many, many people. Larger communities may offer the advantage of anonymity of one's health status; although the standard of care demands that health-care providers not disclose health information inappropriately, the health-care literature is full of cases of individuals whose health status was inappropriately made public.

Should it become publicly known, for example, that a teacher is HIV positive, some members of the community may try to have that teacher fired, and may succeed in that effort if they are influential enough with the school board. Indeed, some school board members may believe that a teacher who is HIV positive *should* be fired. Such organizational decisions are no less a "moral" issue than are the moral issues surrounding HIV infection.

SUMMARY

AIDS has been interpreted by some as a disease from God, as a punishment for biblically proscribed "immoral" behaviors. Within this religious perspective, the only type of effective prevention is sexual abstinence until marriage, and avoidance of all drug-using behaviors that might transmit the virus; "safer sex" and "safer drug use" should not be taught in the schools. Such issues highlight the conflict between individual morality and public health education, which is supported by tax dollars from many different types of people. Such conflicts will affect schools, which are supported by public funds but may be expected to teach only one set of values.

"Blaming the victim" may be a common response to AIDS. Ryan's work on this topic suggests that victim blaming occurs when a particular deficiency is assigned to a victim who must be changed (i.e., isolating gay men who are HIV positive), when people are identified as being "different" (i.e., such differences cause them to be seen as less competent or less human), and when those different people can be labeled as "deviant" (i.e., AIDS is a disease of "them," not of "us"). Blaming the victim can justify the status quo, so that there is no need to change the social circumstances (e.g., poverty, racism, discrimination, lack of health care) that might be contributing to this disease.

Morality is not the same as moral development. Although many would argue that young people need a clear set of morals, research on moral development shows that moral behavior is much more complex than mere insistence upon an absolute moral standard of behavior in young people. Moreover, research has shown different moral orientations between males (a morality of rules and justice) and females (a morality of caring).

REFERENCES

Bell, N. K. (1989) AIDS and women: Remaining ethical issues. *AIDS Education and Prevention,* 1 (1), 22–30.

Benenson, A. S., Peddecord, K. M., Hofherr, L. K., et al. (1989) Reporting the results of Human Immunodeficiency Virus testing. *Journal of the American Medical Association,* 262 (24), 3435–3438.

Brown, B. (1988) Creative acceptance: An ethics for AIDS. In I. B. Corless, and M. Pittman-Lindeman, eds. *AIDS: Principles, practices, and politics.* Washington, DC: Hemisphere Publishing Corp.

Camus, A. (1948) *The plague.* New York: Vintage Books.

Damon, W. (1988) *The moral child. Nurturing children's natural moral growth.* New York: Free Press.

Davis, D. S. (1987) Children with AIDS in the public schools: The ethical issues. *Journal of Medical Humanities and Bioethics,* 8 (2), 101–109.

Dickens, B. M. (1988) Legal rights and duties in the AIDS epidemic. *Science,* 239, 580–585.

Drotman, D. P., and Valdiserri, R. O. (1989) Are Human Immunodeficiency Virus Test results clear to clinicians? *Journal of the American Medical Association,* 262 (24), 3465–3466.

Emanuel, E. J. (1988) Do physicians have an obligation to treat patients with AIDS? *New England Journal of Medicine,* 318 (25), 1686–1690.

Gerbert, B., Maguire, B. T., Hulley, S. B., and Coates, T. J. (1989) Physicians and Acquired Immunodeficiency Syndrome. *Journal of the American Medical Association,* 262 (14), 1969–1972.

Gilligan, C., and Wiggins, G. (1987) In J. Kagan and S. Lamb, eds. *The emergence of morality in young children.* Chicago, IL: University of Chicago Press.

Hedges, J. (1989) Freedom for compassion: Children and AIDS. *Interaction: The AIDS National Interfaith Network Newsletter,* 1 (1), 2–3.

Herek, G. M., and Glunt, E. K. (1988) An epidemic of stigma: Public reactions to AIDS. *American Psychologist,* 43 (11), 886–891.

Kayal, P. M. (1985) "Morals," medicine, and the AIDS epidemic. *Journal of Religion and Health,* 243 (3), 218–238.

Living Webster encyclopedic dictionary of the English language. (1975) Chicago, IL: English Language Institute of America.

Ryan, W. (1976) *Blaming the victim.* New York: Vintage Books.

Tierney, J. (1990) Throngs cheer gay and lesbian march. *New York Times,* June 25, 1990, p. A12.

Trafford, A. (1988) Fundamentalist medicine blames the ill for being ill. *Minneapolis Star Tribune,* December 21, p. 21a.

Walters, L. (1988) Ethical issues in the prevention and treatment of HIV infection and AIDS. *Science,* 239, 587–603.

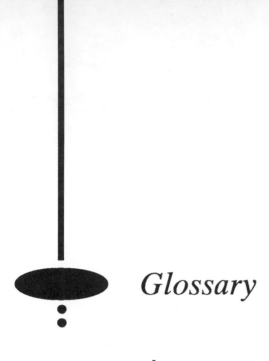

Glossary

Acquired Immune Deficiency Syndrome: the severe set of symptoms and opportunistic infections resulting from being infected with HIV (Human Immunodeficiency Virus).

AIDS-Related Complex (ARC):   a variety of symptoms that occurred in some patients who were infected with HIV, but did not meet the CDC diagnosis for AIDS. ARC included swollen glands, weight loss, fever, diarrhea, etc., but it was not certain that a patient with ARC would develop AIDS. This term is no longer used; HIV infection is the preferred description for these symptoms.

Amyl nitrite: an inhalable substance (''popper'') that dilates the blood vessels and was believed by gay men to prolong or intensify an orgasm. Some researchers thought that such substances might be a cofactor for AIDS.

Antibodies: proteins in the blood that the body produces when it is invaded with foreign molecules. The antibodies work with other parts of the immune system to eliminate infectious microorganisms from the body. Antibodies to HIV are measured with the ELISA and Western Blot antibody tests.

Antigens: substances that, when introduced into the body, produces a specific antibody.

Asymptomatic: having no symptoms.

Attitude: a belief or feeling that may predispose a person to respond in a particular way to people or experiences.

Autologous transfusion: a blood transfusion in which a patient donates his or her own blood several weeks before elective surgery, and then receives that blood (if needed) during surgery. Such transfusions may not be feasible for emergency surgical procedures, because it may take hours to thaw the frozen blood.

Bisexual: a sexual orientation in which a person has sexual contact with both men and women.

Case-control studies: a research design for public health studies that matches people with a disease (cases) with people who do not have that disease (controls). Subjects in case-control studies are often matched on the basis of age, race, sex, socioeconomic status, occupation, and other factors so that comparisons can be made between the two groups. If all extraneous conditions have been controlled, differences between people with the disease and those without the disease can be detected.

Casual contact: routine daily interactions between HIV infected people and others, at work, home, or in school. Such contact does not include intimate sexual contact or IV drug using behaviors.

Cofactor: a factor other than the basic cause of a disease that increases the likelihood of developing that disease. Some inhalants that were used by gay men to heighten sexual experiences were initially thought to be contaminated with substances that made it easier to develop AIDS.

Dementia: chronic intellectual impairment that affects one's ability to function socially or occupationally. It usually causes problems with memory and thinking; it is often irreversible.

ELISA: Enzyme-Linked ImmunoSorbent Assay, a blood test that is used to detect antibodies to HIV.

Empathy: the ability to understand and feel what another person feels.

Endemic: a disease that is commonly found in and specific to certain peoples, a locale, or a region. (See **epidemic**.)

Epidemic: an outbreak of a disease at a rate higher than normally expected. (See **endemic**.)

Epidemiology: the discipline of identifying the patterns of disease and the factors (time, place, people) that influence those patterns.

False negative: a negative test result for a condition that is, in fact, present. A false negative for the HIV antibody test would report that a person does not have HIV antibodies, when in fact, the person does have such antibodies.

False positive: a positive test result for a condition that is, in fact, not present. A false positive for the HIV antibody test would report that a person does have HIV antibodies, when in fact, the person does not have such antibodies.

Hemophilia: a rare, hereditary bleeding disorder in males. Hemophilia is inherited through the mother (who carries the gene for the disease but does not suffer from it) and is an inability to make one or more of the proteins that are necessary for blood to clot.

HIV (Human Immunodeficiency Virus): the name given to the virus believed to cause AIDS. It was agreed upon in 1986 as a way of facilitating communication among researchers, who were using three different terms for the virus.

HIV-1: the name that many researchers are using for the original HIV, to distinguish it from HIV-2.

HIV-2: a genetic variation of the HIV-1 virus, which has been detected in a few countries in Western Africa and Latin America. It is not known whether HIV-2 causes AIDS as reliably as does HIV-1.

Homophobia: an irrational fear of someone who is homosexual, either gay or lesbian. In extreme cases, homophobia results in physical or verbal violence directed at gays or lesbians.

Immune system: the body's natural system of defense, in which specialized cells in the blood and other body fluids function to eliminate disease-producing microorganisms and other foreign substances that have invaded the body.

Immunosuppressed: a condition of the body in which the immune system does not function normally. It can be caused by illnesses or certain drugs.

Incidence: the number of new cases of a disease occurring in a given population over a specific time period.

Incubation period: the latent stage of an infectious disease between the time of infection and the appearance of symptoms.

Intimacy: the ability to form close, loving relationships. In Erik Erikson's theory, intimacy is the major developmental task of early adulthood.

Intravenous: injected into a vein via a needle and syringe.

Kaposi's sarcoma (KS): a cancer or tumor of the blood or walls of the lymph nodes, usually showing up as blue-violet or brown skin blotches or raised bumps. Prior to AIDS, it was fairly rare in the United States, where it was most often found in men over age 50, usually of Mediterranean background. KS due to AIDS is much more severe than the typical (non-AIDS) form of the disease.

Learned helplessness: passive resignation, or even depression, that occurs when a person has been unable to avoid unpredictable and uncontrollable aversive experiences.

Modeling: the process of observing and imitating a behavior.

Opportunistic infections: an infection caused by a microorganism that would not cause such a disease in persons with a normally functioning immune system. Many of the infections found in AIDS patients are opportunistic in nature and are not likely to occur in people with healthy immune systems.

Persistent generalized lymphadenopathy (PGL):   a condition of persistent, generalized swelling of the glands, not due to any current illness.

Pneumocystis carinii pneumonia **(PCP):**   an infection of the lungs. PCP is the most common opportunistic infection found in AIDS patients. PCP can be fatal. It is caused by a parasite that can be destroyed by a healthy immune system, but not by a weakened immune system.

Prejudice: an unjustified attitude toward a group and its members. Prejudice usually involves stereotyped beliefs, negative feelings, and a tendency toward discriminatory behaviors.

Prevalence: the total number of people in a population with a disease at a given time. Prevalence is usually described as the percentage of people with a disease.

PWA: Person With AIDS.

Quarantine-isolation: Quarantine refers to the separation of people from others for a period of time to determine whether they will become ill. If they become ill, they are then isolated.

Reliability: the extent to which a survey or questionnaire yields consistent results.

Retrovirus: a class of viruses that contain genetic material and have the ability to insert this genetic material into a cell, such as a T-4 lymphocyte cell in the immune system. HIV, a retrovirus, can insert its genetic material into immune system cells. When those immune cells reproduce, the new cells are defective, because HIV has changed their genetic structure.

Role: a set of expectations about one's social position. These expectations help define how a person should behave in that social position.

Self-efficacy: a belief that one is competent and effective.

Self-esteem: one's feelings of low or high self-worth.

Sensitivity: the percentage of people who test positive who do, in fact, have the condition for which they are being tested. (See **specificity**.)

Seroconversion: refers to the initial development of antibodies to a specific antigen. In HIV infection, seroconversion refers to the body's development of antibodies to the HIV antigen. When these antibodies have developed and are measured through the ELISA and Western Blot, the person is said to have seroconverted.

Serologic: pertaining to blood.

Seronegative: In HIV antibody testing, the condition in which antibodies to HIV are not found in the blood.

Seropositive: In HIV antibody testing, the condition in which antibodies to HIV are found in the blood.

Sexual orientation: a person's sexual attraction toward members of one's own sex (homosexual orientation) or the other sex (heterosexual orientation). Sexual orientation is not a matter of free choice, and it is not easily changed.

Shooting galleries: locations, such as abandoned buildings, where intravenous drug users gather to administer illicit drugs, often sharing needles, syringes, and other equipment with each other.

Specificity: the percentage of people who test negative who, in fact, do not have the condition for which they are being tested. (See **sensitivity**.)

Stereotype: a generalized (sometimes overgeneralized) belief about a group of people. It is often based on age, race, religion, ethnic background, gender, occupation, or other common characteristics.

Syndrome: a pattern of symptoms or signs that characterize a particular disease. They may show up one at a time or simultaneously.

T-cells: cells that mature in the thymus gland. They are found mainly in the blood and lymph organs. T-cells have a variety of functions within the immune system.

Validity: the extent to which a survey or questionnaire measures what it was designed to measure.

Western Blot (WB):   a blood test that requires the identification of antibodies to specific HIV protein molecules. The WB is thought to be more specific than the ELISA test and is often used as a confirmatory test on blood samples found to be repeatedly reactive on ELISA tests. The Western Blot is considerably more expensive than the ELISA, and more difficult to perform and interpret.

APPENDIX I   *Information*
                    Sources

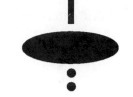

> *Knowledge is of two kinds. We know a*
> *subject ourselves, or we know where we*
> *can find information upon it.*
>   SAMUEL JOHNSON

AGENCIES FOR FURTHER INFORMATION

I. FEDERAL:

National AIDS Hotlines
(800) 342-AIDS (English)
(800) 344-SIDA (Spanish)

**National AIDS Information
Clearinghouse**
P. O. Box 6003
Rockville, MD 20850
(800) 458-5231

**U.S. Centers for Disease
Control**
1600 Clifton Road, NE
Atlanta, GA 30333
(404) 639-3131

U.S. Department of Education
400 Maryland Avenue, SW
Washington, DC 20202
(202) 732-3120

II. NATIONAL ORGANIZATIONS:

AIDS Action Council
729 8th Street SE: Suite 200
Washington, DC 20003
(202) 547-3101

AIDS Information Exchange
U.S. Conference of Mayors
1620 Eye Street NW
Washington, DC 20006
(202) 293-7330

AIDS National Interfaith
Network
475 Riverside Drive: 10th Floor
New York, NY 10015
(212) 870-2100

American Alliance for
Health, Physical Education,
Recreation & Dance
1900 Association Drive
Reston, VA 22091
(703) 476-3480

American Civil Liberties
Union
AIDS-Related Discrimination
Unit
132 West 43rd Street
New York, NY 10036
(212) 944-9800 Ext. 545

American College Health
Association
1300 Piccard Drive: #200
Rockville, MD 20850
(301) 963-1100

American Foundation for
AIDS Research
(AmFAR)—New York Office
1515 Broadway: Suite 3601
New York, NY 10036
(212) 719-0033

American Foundation for
AIDS Research
(AmFAR)—Los Angeles Office
5900 Wilshire Blvd.
2nd Floor—East Satellite
Los Angeles, CA 90036
(213) 857-5900

American Hospital Association
840 North Lake Shore Drive
Chicago, IL 60611
(312) 280-6000

American Psychological
Association
1200 Seventeenth Street, NW
Washington, DC 20036
(202) 955-7600

American Public Health
Association
1015 Fifteenth Street, NW
Washington, DC 20005
(202) 789-5600

American Red Cross
1730 E Street, NW
Washington, DC 20006
(202) 639-3223

American School Health Association
P. O. Box 13827
Research Triangle Park, NC 27709
(919) 361-2742

Gay Men's Health Crisis
132 West 24th Street:
P. O. Box 274
New York, NY 10011
(212) 807-6655

Health Education Resource Organization (HERO)
101 West Read Street:
Suite 812
Baltimore, MD 21201
(301) 685-1180

Institute for the Protection of Lesbian and Gay Youth
401 West Street
New York, NY 10014
(212) 633-8920

Lambda Legal Defense and Education Fund
666 Broadway: 12th Floor
New York, NY 10012
(212) 995-8585

Metropolitan Life Insurance Company
One Madison Avenue
New York, NY 10010
(212) 578-7273

National Association of People with AIDS
P. O. Box 65472
Washington, DC 20335
(202) 483-7979

National Association of School Nurses
P. O. Box 1300
Scarborough, ME 04074
(207) 883-2117

National Association of Social Workers
7981 Eastern Avenue: 4th Floor
Silver Spring, MD 20910
(301) 565-0333

National Association of State Boards of Education
1012 Cameron Street
Alexandria, VA 22314
(703) 684-4000

National Education Association
Health Information Network
100 Colony Square: Suite 200
Atlanta, GA 30361
(404) 875-8819

National Hemophilia Foundation
110 Green Street
Soho Building: #406
New York, NY 10012
(212) 219-8180

**National Leadership Coalition
on AIDS**
1150 17th Street NW: #202
Washington, DC 20036
(202) 429-0930

**San Francisco AIDS
Foundation**
333 Valencia Street: 4th Floor
San Francisco, CA 94103
(415) 864-4376

**National Parents and
Teachers Association**
700 North Rush Street
Chicago, IL 60611-2571
(312) 787-0977

**Sex Information and
Education Council of the U.S.
(SIECUS)**
32 Washington Place: #52
New York, NY 10003
(212) 673-3850

III. STATE HEALTH AND EDUCATION DEPARTMENTS

State health and education departments can be a valuable source of information, not only to determine AIDS direction for your own state, but to identify similarities or differences in other states.

State	Health Department	Education Department
Alabama	(205) 261-5017	(205) 261-5240
Alaska	(907) 561-4406	(907) 465-2841
Arizona	(602) 230-5808	(602) 255-3051
Arkansas	(501) 661-2153	(501) 682-4395
California	(916) 323-7415	(916) 322-4018
Colorado	(303) 331-8320	(303) 866-6664
Connecticut	(203) 566-1157	(203) 566-3461
Delaware	(302) 736-5617	(302) 736-4886
District of Columbia	(202) 673-3679	(202) 724-4008
Florida	(904) 488-0900	(904) 488-7835
Georgia	(404) 894-5304	(404) 656-2415
Hawaii	(808) 735-5304	(808) 548-2360
Idaho	(208) 344-5941	(208) 334-2281
Illinois	(217) 524-5983	(217) 782-6601
Indiana	(317) 633-0851	(317) 269-9611
Iowa	(515) 281-4938	(515) 281-4804

Kansas	(913) 296-5587	(913) 296-6716
Kentucky	(502) 564-4478	(502) 564-2106
Louisiana	(504) 568-7525	(504) 342-5824
Maine	(207) 289-3591	(207) 289-5918
Maryland	(301) 225-5013	(301) 333-2489
Massachusetts	(617) 727-0368	(617) 770-7593
Michigan	(517) 335-8371	(517) 373-2589
Minnesota	(612) 623-5414	(612) 296-2414
Mississippi	(601) 960-7725	(601) 359-3768
Missouri	(314) 751-6438	(314) 751-6762
Montana	(406) 444-2544	(406) 444-4434
Nebraska	(402) 471-2937	(402) 471-4334
Nevada	(702) 885-4800	(702) 885-3136
New Hampshire	(603) 271-4490	(603) 271-2452
New Jersey	(609) 292-7232	(609) 984-1890
New Mexico	(505) 827-0006	(505) 827-6516
New York	(518) 473-7238	(518) 474-1491
North Carolina	(919) 733-7301	(919) 733-3906
North Dakota	(701) 224-2378	(701) 224-2514
Ohio	(614) 466-5480	(614) 466-2211
Oklahoma	(405) 271-4636	(405) 521-3361
Oregon	(503) 229-5792	(503) 378-4327
Pennsylvania	(717) 787-6436	(717) 787-9862
Rhode Island	(401) 277-2362	(401) 277-2638
South Carolina	(803) 734-5000	(803) 734-8378
South Dakota	(605) 773-3364	(605) 773-4699
Tennessee	(615) 741-7387	(615) 741-7856
Texas	(512) 458-7207	(512) 463-9501
Utah	(801) 538-6191	(801) 538-7780
Vermont	(802) 863-7240	(802) 828-3111
Virginia	(804) 786-6267	(804) 225-2866
Washington	(206) 753-0222	(206) 753-2744
West Virginia	(304) 348-5358	(304) 348-8830
Wisconsin	(608) 266-9853	(608) 266-8857
Wyoming	(307) 777-5800	(307) 777-6216
Puerto Rico	(809) 754-8118	(809) 753-0989
Virgin Islands	(809) 773-1059	(809) 774-4976

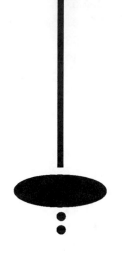

ANNOTATED BIBLIOGRAPHY

> *New opinions are always suspected, and usually opposed, without any other reason but because they are not already common.*
>
> JOHN LOCKE

SOURCEBOOKS

Learning AIDS: An Information Resources Directory (2nd ed.)
American Foundation for AIDS Research
1515 Broadway: Suite 3601
New York, NY 10036
(800) 521-8810

This is a comprehensive review of more than 1,700 AIDS educational materials in a variety of formats (e.g., books, brochures, videos, instructional programs). It can serve as a reference for educators, health-care providers, program directors, and others interested in available educational resources on AIDS.

The AIDS/HIV Record Directory
Key AIDS/HIV Program Officials in Federal, State, County and City Governments (2nd ed.)
BioData Publishers
P. O. Box 66020
Washington, DC 20035
(202) 393-2437

This directory lists key personnel, addresses, and phone numbers in a variety of AIDS related agencies, including federal agencies, independent agencies, state, county and city governments, and international organizations.

AIDS Information Source
Book: 2nd edition 1989–1990
H. R. Malinowsky and
G. Perry, editors
Oryx Press
2214 North Central at Encanto
Phoenix, AZ 85004-1483
(800) 457-6799

An alphabetical list of national and community-based AIDS education organizations by state and type of organization. Includes an extensive bibliography and subject index.

AIDS: Looking
Forward/Looking Back
Carolyn Patierno
SIECUS
32 Washington Place: #52
New York, NY 10003
(212) 673-3850

An annotated bibliography of AIDS-related resources.

Women and AIDS: An
Annotated Bibliography
NOVA Research Company
4720 Montgomery Lane: #210
Bethesda, MD 20814
(301) 986-1891

Addresses prevention of AIDS among female sexual partners of IV drug users. The book covers resources for project staff, client education, and posters.

Evaluative publications

AIDS Bibliography Series:
AIDS 1989
David Tyckoson
Oryx Press
2214 N. Central at Encanto
Phoenix, AZ 85004-1483
(800) 457-6799

A selection of annotated and evaluated articles on medical and health-care issues, hemophilia, women, children, and minorities, vaccines, the workplace, and insurance.

How Effective Is Aids
Education? (June 1988)
Health Program
Office of Technology
Assessment
U.S. Congress
Washington, DC 20510-8025

A summary of what is known about the effectiveness of AIDS education, documentation of AIDS education programs being funded by federal agencies, and some suggestions for developing more effective programs.

AIDS Education: Reaching
Populations at Higher Risk
(September 1988)
United States General
Accounting Office
Washington, DC 20548

This publication addresses two questions: (1) What lessons regarding the design of effective health education can be learned from previous public-health research? and (2) How can these lessons be applied to the education of populations at relatively high risk for AIDS? A seven-step model of health education is suggested.

School-based information from

Health Information Network
100 Colony Square: #200
Atlanta, GA 30361
(404) 875-8819

**Responding to HIV and AIDS
(1989)**

This is a 34-page handbook developed for the National Education Association concerning the HIV epidemic. It contains sections on basic information on HIV and AIDS, the HIV antibody test, guidelines for handling blood and other body fluids in schools, the need for care and compassion, saying goodbye to someone you love, and information about AIDS hotlines and state HIV education liaisons.

**National Association of State
Boards of Education (NASBE)**
1012 Cameron Street
Alexandria, VA 22314
(703) 684-4000

**Effective AIDS Education: A
Policymaker's Guide (1988)**

A NASBE booklet summarizing the need for prevention education, methods of providing effective AIDS prevention, and strategies for developing a comprehensive state leadership role.

**HIV/AIDS Education Survey
(1989)**

This 139-page book is a NASBE analysis of state policies regarding HIV/AIDS education for elementary and secondary school students. Information is presented for each state regarding HIV/AIDS education requirements, state health education requirements, state funding levels, surveillance, and evaluation.

**Someone at School Has AIDS.
A Guide to Developing
Policies for Students and
School Staff Members Who
Are Infected with HIV (1989)**

This 35-page NASBE booklet assesses policies and procedures for evaluating students or staff members who are infected with HIV, and addresses confidentiality issues, testing, techniques for infection control and training, etc.

Parent/youth programs

**National AIDS Information
and Education Program
(NAIEP)**
Centers for Disease Control
1600 Clifton Road
Atlanta, GA 30333
(800) 342-AIDS
(800) 458-5231

Information about the ''America Responds to AIDS'' campaign, including an ''AIDS Prevention Guide'' to help parents, clergy, and civic and youth group leaders to talk with young people about how to prevent HIV infection.

VIDEOTAPES

Audience: Elementary school

"A Is for AIDS," 1988
(15 minutes)
An animated character, Dr. Andy Answer, explains the basic facts about AIDS to three youngsters. Viewers learn about HIV, how it can and cannot be transmitted, and how the immune system is affected. Viewers are introduced to two children who have AIDS, and learn about the feelings that these people experience as well as that it is all right to attend school and play with children who have AIDS.
Perennial Education
930 Pitner
Evanston, IL 60202
(800) 323-9084

"Food for Thought," 1988
(11 minutes)
DRAC, the grandson of Dracula, learns that his food supply may be tainted. Two of his friends teach him how HIV can and cannot be transmitted. Ways of avoiding high-risk behavior are discussed, with the emphasis on IV drug transmission. A teacher's guide contains objectives, masters for activities, and lesson plans.
Odyssey in Learning
Three Bankers Drive
Washington Crossing, PA 18977
(215) 493-1675

"I Have AIDS—A Teenager's
Story" (30 minutes)
This 30-minute television special addresses questions that elementary schoolchildren have about AIDS. Ryan White, 16 years old, meets with students in their Manhattan classroom and answers their questions. The program contains animation

and a model of HIV to ensure that complex information is communicated clearly.
School Services Department
Children's Television Workshop
One Lincoln Plaza
New York, NY 10023
(212) 595-3456, ext. 535

Audience: Middle school/junior high school

"ABC's of STDs," 1989 (20
minutes)
This video provides basic information about STDs in simple language and in a nonthreatening style. It identifies the most common STDs, how they are transmitted, symptoms, and what to do if infected. The video also describes how to communicate with one's sexual partners.
Polymorph Films
118 South Street
Boston, MA 02111
(800) 223-5107

"AIDS—Answers for Young
People," 1987 (20 minutes)
Questions about AIDS from a seventh-grade class are answered by teenage peer counselors, a health educator, a physician, a 12-year-old adolescent with hemophilia, and several other people with AIDS. Animation is used to describe how the virus attacks the immune system and how the virus is transmitted via IV drug use and unprotected sex.
Churchill Films
662 N. Robertson Blvd.
Los Angeles, CA 90069
(213) 657-5110

"AIDS: Taking Action,"
1988 (30 minutes)
This is a discussion of AIDS with a recent high school graduate who returns to discuss AIDS with

younger students. A 14-page teaching guide is available for students of different maturity levels in junior high and includes sections on information, learning projects, and action projects.

All Media Productions,
Educational Division
1424 Lake Drive SE: Suite 222
Grand Rapids, MI 49506

**"AIDS: What Everyone
Needs to Know," 1985
(18 minutes)**
This video provides basic information about AIDS—the immune system, the virus, methods of transmission, and high-risk behaviors and how they can be avoided.

Churchill Films
662 N. Robertson Blvd.
Los Angeles, CA 90069-9990
(213) 657-5110

**"A Letter from Brian," 1987
(29 minutes)**
This drama deals with high school–aged youths, and the psychosocial and psychosexual issues surrounding AIDS (American Red Cross).

**"Answers About AIDS,"
1987 (16 minutes)**
Surgeon General Koop discusses AIDS in a classroom setting: handout materials include pre- and posttest discussion questions for the instructor (American Red Cross).

**"Don't Forget Sherrie," 1987
(20 minutes)**
This drama focuses on a group of urban teenagers who are responding to the spread of HIV and are questioning their own values and behavior. The

video is aimed at African-American youth (American Red Cross).

American Red Cross
1730 E Street, NW
Washington, DC 20006
(202) 639-3223

**"Face to Face with AIDS,"
1988 (29 minutes)**
This video makes the connection between high-risk behaviors and HIV transmission; it is aimed at Hispanic youth.

Select Media, Inc.
74 Varick Street, #305
New York, NY 10013-1909
(212) 431-8923

**"Smart Talk," 1988
(13 minutes)**
This video describes the common myths about STDs, including AIDS, and emphasizes the importance of prompt medical treatment. Abstinence is strongly recommended, and adolescents talk about delaying sexual activity.

Intermedia
1600 Dexter Avenue N.
Seattle, WA 98109
(206) 282-7262

**"The Subject is AIDS," 1987
(23 minutes)**
A revised version of "Sex, Drugs and AIDS" includes a revision of two scenes and an introduction by Surgeon General Koop. The video places more emphasis on abstinence.

ODN Productions
74 Varick Street: Suite 304
New York, NY 10013
(212) 431-8923

Audience: High school

"AIDS," 1987 (20 minutes)
Actress Ally Sheedy hosts a program in which doctors and health educators answer high school students' questions about AIDS. The video recommends abstinence but also discusses safer sex practices.

Walt Disney Educational Media
Company
c/o Coronot/MTI Film & Video
108 Wilmot Road
Deerfield, IL 60015
(312) 940-1260

"AIDS: Learn for Your Life," 1987 (30 minutes)
A recent high school graduate discusses AIDS issues, prevention, and risk-reduction techniques, with questions answered by medical experts. A curriculum guide (role-playing activities, report topics, etc.) offers information on AIDS and lesson plans.

All Media Productions
Educational Division
1424 Lake Drive, SE: Suite 222
Grand Rapids, MI 49506

"AIDS: Can I Get It?" 1987 (20 minutes)
Interviews with experts, people with AIDS, and people on the streets address both myths and facts about AIDS. Topics include HIV transmission, effect of HIV on the immune system, and safety of the blood supply. Both safe and unsafe sexual practices are discussed, along with HIV antibody testing and treatment with AZT for people with AIDS.

Light Video Television
21 Highland Circle
Needham Heights, MA 02194
(617) 449-7770

"All of Us and AIDS," 1988 (30 minutes)
This video is about adolescents who are making a video on AIDS prevention in their own style and language. The video focuses on sexual decision making, including abstinence and safer sex, and shows a diverse perspective of adolescent values.

Network Publication
P.O. Box 1830
Santa Cruz, CA 95061-1830
(408) 438-4080

"National AIDS Awareness Test," 1987 (120 minutes)
This is a 55-question test on AIDS; answers are based on the latest (1987) medical research.

Video Publishing House
1011 East Touhy Avenue: #580
Des Plaines, IL 60018
(800) 824-8889

"Sex, Drugs and AIDS," 1986 (18 minutes)
Narrated by actress Rae Dawn Chong, this video is a frank and open discussion about risky sexual practices, condom use, and drugs. The video addresses casual and sexual contact, unsafe behavior, and a humane approach to people with AIDS.

Select Media
74 Varick Street: Suite 305
New York, NY 10013
(212) 431-8923

"The AIDS Movie," 1986
(26 minutes)
This video focuses on the impact of AIDS on high school-aged adolescents. A health educator talks to a high school class, with interviews of three people with AIDS interspersed in his talk. The people with AIDS describe their personal experiences and warn against risky behaviors.

Durrin Films/New Day Films
1748 Kalorama Road, NW
Washington, DC 20009
(202) 387-6700

"What You Should Know—Young People and AIDS," 1988 (18 minutes)
This video addresses basic questions that young people have about AIDS (e.g., what is AIDS; who can get AIDS; how can you protect yourself). Additional materials (booklets, posters and leader's guide) are available.

Channing L. Bete Co.
200 State Road
South Deerfield, MA 01373
(413) 665-7611

Audience: College/Adult

"AIDS: Changing the Rules," 1987 (30 minutes)
Basic facts about AIDS are presented by Ron Reagan (former President Reagan's son), model Beverly Johnson and Salsa star Ruben Blades. Basic facts are described, along with three women discussing their attitudes about condoms and a segment on people with AIDS. (Version with Spanish subtitles is available.)

San Francisco AIDS Foundation
333 Valencia Street: PO Box 6182
San Francisco, CA 94101-6182
(415) 864-4376

"The Best Defense"
This is a multiracial video dealing with IV drug use and methods for cleaning one's works. Condom use is demonstrated, and a couple discusses the use of condoms in their relationship.

Intermedia
1600 Dexter Avenue, N.
Seattle, WA 98109
(206) 282-7262

Audience: African Americans

"Black People Get AIDS, too," 1987 (22 minutes)
Facts about AIDS and its impact on the black community are provided in several formats (e.g., orally, in vignettes, in charts). Topics include high-risk behaviors, HIV antibody testing, condoms, and cleaning of needles.

Multicultural Prevention
Resource Center
1540 Market Street: Suite 320
San Francisco, CA 94102
(415) 861-2142

"Seriously Fresh," 1989
Focuses on four black friends and how they deal with their friend's AIDS-related illness. Topics include family relations, drug use, safer sex, homosexuality, acceptance, and support. Deals with emotional issues of fear, rejection, confusion, anger, and other reactions to AIDS, and uses humor to make its point.

AIDSfilms
50 West 34th Street: #6B6
New York, NY 10001
(212) 629-6288

"Til Death Do Us Part,"
1988 (16 minutes)
AIDS information is presented to black youths via music, poetry, rap, and dance, and focuses on basic facts about AIDS, women at risk, and IV drug use. A discussion guide is available.

Durrin Films/New Day Films
1748 Kalorama Road, NW
Washington, DC 20009
(202) 387-6700

Audience: Latinos

"Ojos Que No Ven (Eyes
That Fail to See)"
(52 minutes)
A humorous Mexican soap opera is used to present AIDS awareness information for the Latino community. Topics include homosexuality, drug use, and methods for cleaning needles and syringes.

Instituto Familiar de la Raza
Latino AIDS Project
2515 24th Street: #2
San Francisco, CA 94110
(415) 647-5450

"VIDA," 1989
The story of a young woman who struggles to deal with AIDS in a friend, as well as her inability to talk about AIDS with another friend. The two friends discuss condom use, negotiating skills, and self-empowerment.

AIDSfilms
50 West 34th Street: #6B6
New York, NY 10001
(212) 629-6288

Audience: Native Americans

"Her Giveaway: A Spiritual
Journal with AIDS," 1988
(20 minutes)
This is the story of Carole LeFavor, an American Indian woman with AIDS and of those who are close to her. Basic information about HIV risk reduction is provided, as well as a discussion of AIDS within the context of Native American culture.

American Indian AIDS
Task Force
c/o Indian Affairs Council
127 University Avenue
St. Paul, MN 55155
(612) 296-3611

EDUCATIONAL MATERIALS

Elementary Sources:

"AIDS—What You Should
Know." Teacher and student
editions, 1988
Linda Meeks and Philip Heit
A 27-page booklet for fifth through eighth graders with basic information about AIDS. Risky behaviors and risky situations are identified. The teacher edition includes teaching strategies, review activities, and transparency masters for each section.

Merrill Wellness Series
Merrill Publishing Company
Columbus, OH 43116

"AIDS: What You Need to
Know," 1989
AIDS booklet for students (grades 4 through 6) and answers for teachers.

Weekly Reader Subscription
Office
4343 Equity Drive
Columbus, OH 43228

**"Children and the AIDS
Virus—A Book for Children,
Parents and Teachers," 1989**
Rosemarie Hausberr
A 48-page booklet that explains the facts about
HIV and AIDS. Many black-and-white photographs and large print for younger children.

Clarion Books
52 Vanderbilt Avenue
New York, NY 10017
(212) 972-1190

"Does AIDS Hurt?"
Marcia Quackenbush and
Sylvia Villarreal
Basic information, stories and suggestions for
teachers, parents, and care providers or children to
age 10. Includes goals for teachers, sexuality issues, responding to questions, and developmental
stages.

Network Publications
ETR Associates
P.O. Box 1830
Santa Cruz, CA 95061-1830
(408) 438-4080

**"Terry and Friends Present
AIDS Education," 1988**
Contains a teacher's guide for K–3 and 4–6
   Terry, the friendly dragon, helps you be AIDS
   smart, a study guide and activity book for the
   grade school child (1987)
A 15-page booklet for mid-elementary students
describes the immune system as a suit of armor,
summarizes how HIV cannot be caught, and

describes ways that the immune system can be
protected through hand washing and vaccines. Map
puzzles and picture-find activities are included.

Creative Graphics
P.O. Box 381
Mt. Vernon, OH 43050

Middle/Secondary Sources

**"AIDS, Trading Fears for
Facts: A Guide for Young
People," 1989**
Karen Hein and Theresa Foy
Digeronimo
A 196-page book for young people, providing
basic facts about AIDS, relationships between sex,
drugs and AIDS, HIV antibody testing, and treatment issues.

Consumer Reports Books
Consumers Union
Mt. Vernon, NY 10553

**"AIDS: What Teens Need to
Know"**
A 32-page booklet for grades 7–9 includes information about HIV, the immune system, and how
the virus is transmitted.

Weekly Reader Subscription
Office
4343 Equity Drive
Columbus, OH 43228

**"AIDS, What We Need to
Know," 1988**
N. Bartel and J. Orlando
An extensive program for grades 7–9 (Level I) and
grades 9–12 (Level II) includes a 70-page
workbook for students, as well as lesson plans,

transparency masters, student activities, and other aids for teachers.

Pro-ed
5341 Industrial Oaks Blvd.
Austin, TX 78735

**"AIDS: What Young Adults
Should Know," 1987**
William Yarber
Written for high school students, this summarizes AIDS issues and includes handouts, worksheets, and pre- and posttests.

American Alliance for Health,
Physical Education,
Recreation & Dance
1900 Association Drive
Reston, VA 22091

**"AIDS: Understanding and
Prevention," Teacher and
student editions, 1988**
Linda Meeks and Philip Heit
This is a detailed, 27-page booklet about AIDS and the immune system—it emphasizes prevention and decision making. The teacher's guide includes performance objectives, teaching strategies, and teacher and student masters.

Merrill Wellness Series
Merrill Publishing Company
Columbus, OH 43216

**"An Educational Package on
AIDS," 1988**
This package uses the cognitive-interactive approach to teaching about AIDS for administrators and teachers in grades 9–12. It includes an administrator's guide, teacher's guide, video ("Choice: Learning about AIDS"), student booklet, and parent booklet.

Customer Service
Representative
National Safety Council
P.O. Box 11933
Chicago, IL 60611
(800) 621-7619

**"Educator's Guide to AIDS
and Other STDs," 1987**
Stephen Sroke and Leonard Calabrese
This instructor's guide (with student handouts and activities) is based on a behavioral approach to prevention with a communicable disease perspective. The emphasis is on abstinence, responsible sexuality, and drug-use prevention. It has been adapted for younger teens and religious groups.

Health Education Consultants
1284 Manor Park
Lakewood, OH 44107
(216) 521-1766

"Looking into AIDS," 1989
A middle-school curriculum focusing on self-esteem, assertiveness skills, and IV drug use. Includes an instructor's guide (with worksheets, learning opportunities, and ways to implement an AIDS curriculum) and student handbook.

Phi Delta Kappa
P.O. Box 789
Bloomington, IN 47402-0789
(812) 339-1156

"Teaching AIDS, A Resource Guide on the Acquired Immunodeficiency Syndrome," 1988
Marcia Quackenbush and
Pamela Sargent
This book includes basic information about AIDS, as well as teaching plans for high school students on such topics as public response to AIDS, civil rights issues involving AIDS, epidemics and AIDS, and STDs and AIDS. Revisions include information about condoms, abstinence and 35 pages of resources.

Network Publications
ETR Associates
P.O. Box 1830
Santa Cruz, CA 95061-1830
(408) 438-4080

"The Kids on the Block," 1988
An AIDS prevention program for grades 5 and higher, designed to complement an existing sex education or family life education program.

KIDS on the Block, Inc.
9385-C Gerwig Lane
Columbia, MD 21406
(301) 290-9095

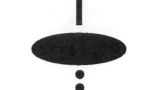

APPENDIX III

SCHOOL EDUCATION GUIDELINES

> *There's always an easy solution to every human problem—neat, plausible and wrong.*
>
> H. L. MENCKEN

Easy solutions to AIDS do not exist. Consequently, the Centers for Disease Control have developed guidelines for effective school health education programs to prevent the spread of HIV and subsequent AIDS cases. Although these guidelines may not be feasible for all schools, they do provide a framework that can be adapted by individual school districts.

As with infection-control guidelines, the school education guidelines can be helpful in explaining the rationale of school-based AIDS education programs to teachers, staff, parents, and members of the community.

Guidelines for Effective School Health Education To Prevent the Spread of AIDS*

INTRODUCTION

Since the first cases of acquired immunodeficiency syndrome (AIDS) were reported in the United States in 1981, the human immunodeficiency virus (HIV) that causes AIDS and other HIV-related diseases has precipitated an epidemic unprecedented in modern history. Because the virus is transmitted almost exclusively by behavior that individuals can

*MMWR, Morbidity and Mortality Weekly Report. Printed and distributed by the Massachusetts Medical Society, publishers of *The New England Journal of Medicine*, January 29, 1988/Vol. 37/No. S-2.

modify, educational programs to influence relevant behavior can be effective in preventing the spread of HIV (1–5).

The guidelines below have been developed to help school personnel and others plan, implement, and evaluate educational efforts to prevent unnecessary morbidity and mortality associated with AIDS and other HIV-related illnesses. The guidelines incorporate principles for AIDS education that were developed by the President's Domestic Policy Council and approved by the President in 1987 (see Appendix I).

The guidelines provide information that should be considered by persons who are responsible for planning and implementing appropriate and effective strategies to teach young people about how to avoid HIV infection. These guidelines should not be construed as rules, but rather as a source of guidance. Although they specifically were developed to help **school personnel,** personnel from other organizations should consider these guidelines in planning and carrying out effective education about AIDS for youth who do **not** attend school and who may be at high risk of becoming infected. As they deliberate about the need for and content of AIDS education, educators, parents, and other concerned members of the community should consider the prevalence of behavior that increases the risk of HIV infection among young people in their communities. Information about the nature of the AIDS epidemic, and the extent to which young people engage in behavior that increases the risk of HIV infection, is presented in Appendix II.

Information contained in this document was developed by CDC in consultation with individuals appointed to represent the following organizations:

American Academy of Pediatrics

American Association of School Administrators

American Public Health Association

American School Health Association

Association for the Advancement of Health Education

Association of State and Territorial Health Officers

Council of Chief State School Officers

National Congress of Parents and Teachers

National Council of Churches

National Education Association

National School Boards Association

Society of State Directors of Health, Physical Education, Recreation and Dance

U.S. Department of Education

U.S. Food and Drug Administration

U.S. Office of Disease Prevention and Health Promotion

Consultants included a director of health education for a state department of education, a director of curriculum and instruction for a local education department, a health education teacher, a director of school health programs for a local school district, a director of a state health department, a deputy director of a local health department, and an expert in child and adolescent development.

PLANNING AND IMPLEMENTING EFFECTIVE SCHOOL HEALTH EDUCATION ABOUT AIDS

The Nation's public and private schools have the capacity and responsibility to help assure that young people understand the nature of the AIDS epidemic and the specific actions they can take to prevent HIV infection, especially during their adolescence and young adulthood. The specific scope and content of AIDS education in schools should be locally determined and should be consistent with parental and community values.

Because AIDS is a fatal disease and because educating young people about becoming infected through sexual contact can be controversial, school systems should obtain broad community participation to ensure that school health education policies and programs to prevent the spread of AIDS are locally determined and are consistent with community values.

The development of school district policies on AIDS education can be an important first step in developing an AIDS education program. In each community, representatives of the school board, parents, school administrators and faculty, school health services, local medical societies, the local health department, students, minority groups, religious organizations, and other relevant organizations can be involved in developing policies for school health education to prevent the spread of AIDS. The process of policy development can enable these representatives to resolve various perspectives and opinions, to establish a commitment for implementing and maintaining AIDS education programs, and to establish standards for AIDS education program activities and materials. Many communities already have school health councils that include representatives from the aforementioned groups. Such councils facilitate the development of a broad base of community expertise and input, and they enhance the coordination of various activities within the comprehensive school health program (6).

AIDS education programs should be developed to address the needs and the developmental levels of students and of school-age youth who do not attend school, and to address specific needs of minorities, persons for whom English is not the primary language, and persons with visual or hearing impairments or other learning disabilities. Plans for addressing students' questions or concerns about AIDS at the early elementary grades, as well as for providing effective school health education about AIDS at each grade from late elementary/middle school through junior high/senior high school, including educational materials to be used, should be reviewed by representatives of the school board, appropriate school administrators, teachers, and parents before being implemented.

Education about AIDS may be most appropriate and effective when carried out within a more comprehensive school health education program that establishes a foundation for understanding the relationships between personal behavior and health (7–9). For example, education about AIDS may be more effective when students at appropriate ages are more knowledgeable about sexually transmitted diseases, drug abuse, and community health. It may also have greater impact when they have opportunities to develop such qualities as decision-making and communication skills, resistance to persuasion, and a sense of self-efficacy and self-esteem. However, education about AIDS should be provided as rapidly as possible, even if it is taught initially as a separate subject.

State departments of education and health should work together to help local departments of education and health throughout the state collaboratively accomplish effective school health education about AIDS. Although all schools in a state should provide effective education about AIDS, priority should be given to areas with the highest reported incidence of AIDS cases.

PREPARATION OF EDUCATION PERSONNEL

A team of representatives including the local school board, parent-teachers associations, school administrators, school physicians, school nurses, teachers, educational support personnel, school counselors, and other relevant school personnel should receive general training about a) the nature of the AIDS epidemic and means of controlling its spread, b) the role of the school in providing education to prevent transmission of HIV, c) methods and materials to accomplish effective programs of school health education about AIDS, and d) school policies for students and staff who may be infected. In addition, a team of school personnel responsible for teaching about AIDS should receive more specific training about AIDS education. All school personnel, especially those who teach about AIDS, periodically should receive continuing education about AIDS to assure that they have the most current information about means of controlling the epidemic, including up-to-date information about the most effective health education interventions available. State and local departments of education and health, as well as colleges of education, should assure that such in-service training is made available to all schools in the state as soon as possible and that continuing in-service and pre-service training is subsequently provided. The local school board should assure that release time is provided to enable school personnel to receive such in-service training.

PROGRAMS TAUGHT BY QUALIFIED TEACHERS

In the elementary grades, students generally have one regular classroom teacher. In these grades, education about AIDS should be provided by the regular classroom teacher because that person ideally should be trained and experienced in child development, age-appropriate teaching methods, child health, and elementary health education methods and materials. In addition, the elementary teacher usually is sensitive to normal variations in child development and aptitudes within a class. In the secondary grades, students generally have a different teacher for each subject. In these grades, the secondary school health education teacher preferably should provide education about AIDS, because a qualified health education teacher will have training and experience in adolescent development, age-appropriate teaching methods, adolescent health, and secondary school health education methods and materials (including methods and materials for teaching about such topics as human sexuality, communicable diseases, and drug abuse). In secondary schools that do not have a qualified health education teacher, faculty with similar training and good rapport with stu-

dents should be trained specifically to provide effective AIDS education.

PURPOSE OF EFFECTIVE EDUCATION ABOUT AIDS

The principal purpose of education about AIDS is to prevent HIV infection. The content of AIDS education should be developed with the active involvement of parents and should address the broad range of behavior exhibited by young people. Educational programs should assure that young people acquire the knowledge and skills they will need to adopt and maintain types of behavior that virtually eliminate their risk of becoming infected.

School systems should make programs available that will enable and encourage young people who **have not** engaged in sexual intercourse and who **have not** used illicit drugs to continue to—

- Abstain from sexual intercourse until they are ready to establish a mutually monogamous relationship within the context of marriage;
- Refrain from using or injecting illicit drugs.

For young people who **have** engaged in sexual intercourse or who **have** injected illicit drugs, school programs should enable and encourage them to—

- Stop engaging in sexual intercourse until they are ready to establish a mutually monogamous relationship within the context of marriage;
- Stop using or injecting illicit drugs.

Despite all efforts, some young people may remain unwilling to adopt behavior that would virtually eliminate their risk of becoming infected. Therefore, school systems, in consultation with parents and health officials, should provide AIDS education programs that address preventive types of behavior that should be practiced by persons with an increased risk of acquiring HIV infection. These include:

- Avoiding sexual intercourse with anyone who is known to be infected, who is at risk of being infected, or whose HIV infection status is not known;
- Using a latex condom with spermicide if they engage in sexual intercourse;
- Seeking treatment if addicted to illicit drugs;
- Not sharing needles or other injection equipment;
- Seeking HIV counseling and testing if HIV infection is suspected.

State and local education and health agencies should work together to assess the prevalence of these types of risk behavior, and their determinants, over time.

CONTENT

Although information about the biology of the AIDS virus, the signs and symptoms of AIDS, and the social and economic costs of the epidemic might be of interest, such information is not the essential knowledge that students must acquire in order to prevent becoming infected with HIV. Similarly, a single film, lecture, or school assembly about AIDS will not be sufficient to assure that students develop the complex understanding and skills they will need to avoid becoming infected.

Schools should assure that students receive at least the essential information about AIDS, as summarized in sequence in the following pages, for each of three grade-level ranges. The exact grades at which students receive this essential information should be determined locally, in accord with community and parental values, and thus may vary from community to community. Because essential information for students at higher grades requires an understanding of information essential for students at lower grades, secondary school personnel will need to assure that students understand basic concepts before teaching more advanced information. Schools simultaneously should assure that students have opportunities to learn about emotion-

al and social factors that influence types of behavior associated with HIV transmission.

Early elementary school

Education about AIDS for students in early elementary grades principally should be designed to allay excessive fears of the epidemic and of becoming infected.

> *AIDS is a disease that is causing some adults to get very sick, but it does not commonly affect children.*
> *AIDS is very hard to get. You cannot get it just by being near or touching someone who has it.*
> *Scientists all over the world are working hard to find a way to stop people from getting AIDS and to cure those who have it.*

Late elementary/middle school

Education about AIDS for students in late elementary/middle school grades should be designed with consideration for the following information.

> *Viruses are living organisms too small to be seen by the unaided eye.*
> *Viruses can be transmitted from an infected person to an uninfected person through various means.*
> *Some viruses cause disease among people.*
> *Persons who are infected with some viruses that cause disease may not have any signs or symptoms of disease.*
> *AIDS (an abbreviation for acquired immunodeficiency syndrome) is caused by a virus that weakens the ability of infected individuals to fight off disease.*
> *People who have AIDS often develop a rare type of severe pneumonia, a cancer called Kaposi's sarcoma, and certain other dis-*

eases that healthy people normally do not get.

About 1 to 1.5 million of the total population of approximately 240 million Americans currently are infected with the AIDS virus and consequently are capable of infecting others.

People who are infected with the AIDS virus live in every state in the United States and in most other countries of the world. Infected people live in cities as well as in suburbs, small towns, and rural areas. Although most infected people are adults, teenagers can also become infected. Females as well as males are infected. People of every race are infected, including whites, blacks, Hispanics, Native Americans, and Asian/Pacific Islanders.

The AIDS virus can be transmitted by sexual contact with an infected person; by using needles and other injection equipment that an infected person has used; and from an infected mother to her infant before or during birth.

A small number of doctors, nurses, and other medical personnel have been infected when they were directly exposed to infected blood.

It sometimes takes several years after becoming infected with the AIDS virus before symptoms of the disease appear. Thus, people who are infected with the virus can infect other people—event though the people who transmit the infection do not feel or look sick.

Most infected people who develop symptoms of AIDS only live about 2 years after their symptoms are diagnosed.

The AIDS virus cannot be caught by touching someone who is infected, by being in the same room with an infected person, or by donating blood.

Junior high/senior high school

Education about AIDS for students in junior high/senior high school grades should be developed and presented taking into consideration the following information.

The virus that causes AIDS, and other health problems, is called human immunodeficiency virus, or HIV.

The risk of becoming infected with HIV can be virtually eliminated by not engaging in sexual activities and by not using illegal intravenous drugs.

Sexual transmission of HIV is not a threat to those uninfected individuals who engage in mutually monogamous sexual relations.

HIV may be transmitted in any of the following ways: a) by sexual contact with an infected person (penis/vagina, penis/rectum, mouth/vagina, mouth/penis, mouth/rectum); b) by using needles or other injection equipment that an infected person has used; c) from an infected mother to her infant before or during birth.

A small number of doctors, nurses, and other medical personnel have been infected when they were directly exposed to infected blood.

The following are at increased risk of having the virus that causes AIDS and consequently of being infectious: a) persons with clinical or laboratory evidence of infection; b) males who have had sexual intercourse with other males; c) persons who have injected illegal drugs; d) persons who have had numerous sexual partners, including male or female prostitutes; e) persons who received blood clotting products before 1985; f) sex partners of infected persons or persons at increased risk; and g) infants born to infected mothers.

The risk of becoming infected is increased by having a sexual partner who is at increased risk of having contracted the AIDS virus (as identified previously), practicing sexual behavior that results in the exchange of body fluids (i.e., semen, vaginal secretions, blood), and using unsterile needles or paraphernalia to inject drugs.

Although no transmission from deep, open-mouth (i.e., ''French'') kissing has been documented, such kissing theoretically could transmit HIV from an infected to an uninfected person through direct exposure of mucous membranes to infected blood or saliva.

In the past, medical use of blood, such as transfusing blood and treating hemophiliacs with blood clotting products, has caused some people to become infected with HIV. However, since 1985 all donated blood has been tested to determine whether it is infected with HIV; moreover, all blood clotting products have been made from screened plasma and have been heated to destroy any HIV that might remain in the concentrate. Thus, the risk of becoming infected with HIV from blood transfusions and from blood clotting products is virtually eliminated. Cases of HIV infection caused by these medical uses of blood will continue to be diagnosed, however, among people who were infected by these means before 1985.

Persons who continue to engage in sexual intercourse with persons who are at increased risk or whose infection status is unknown should use a latex condom (not natural membrane) to reduce the likelihood of becoming infected. The latex condom must be applied properly and used from start to finish for every sexual act. Although a latex condom does not provide 100% protection—

because it is possible for the condom to leak, break, or slip off—it provides the best protection for people who do not maintain a mutually monogamous relationship with an uninfected partner. Additional protection may be obtained by using spermicides that seem active against HIV and other sexually transmitted organisms in conjunction with condoms.

Behavior that prevents exposure to HIV also may prevent unintended pregnancies and exposure to the organisms that cause Chlamydia infection, gonorrhea, herpes, human papillomavirus, and syphilis.

Persons who believe they may be infected with the AIDS virus should take precautions not to infect others and to seek counseling and antibody testing to determine whether they are infected. If persons are not infected, counseling and testing can relieve unnecessary anxiety and reinforce the need to adopt or continue practices that reduce the risk of infection. If persons are infected, they should: a) take precautions to protect sexual partners from becoming infected; b) advise previous and current sexual or drug-use partners to receive counseling and testing; c) take precautions against becoming pregnant; and d) seek medical care and counseling about other medical problems that may result from a weakened immunologic system.

More detailed information about AIDS, including information about how to obtain counseling and testing for HIV, can be obtained by telephoning the AIDS National Hotline (toll free) at 800-342-2437; the Sexually Transmitted Diseases National Hotline (toll free) at 800-227-8922; or the appropriate state or local health department (the telephone number of which can be obtained by calling the local information operator).

CURRICULUM TIME AND RESOURCES

Schools should allocate sufficient personnel time and resources to assure that policies and programs are developed and implemented with appropriate community involvement, curricula are well-planned and sequential, teachers are well-trained, and up-to-date teaching methods and materials about AIDS are available. In addition, it is crucial that sufficient classroom time be provided at **each** grade level to assure that students acquire essential knowledge appropriate for that grade level, and have time to ask questions and discuss issues raised by the information presented.

PROGRAM ASSESSMENT

The criteria recommended in the foregoing "Guidelines for Effective School Health Education To Prevent the Spread of AIDS" are summarized in the following nine assessment criteria. Local school boards and administrators can assess the extent to which their programs are consistent with these guidelines by determining the extent to which their programs meet each point shown below. Personnel in state departments of education and health also can use these criteria to monitor the extent to which schools in the state are providing effective health education about AIDS.

1. To what extent are parents, teachers, students, and appropriate community representatives involved in developing, implementing, and assessing AIDS education policies and programs?
2. To what extent is the program included as an important part of a more comprehensive school health education program?
3. To what extent is the program taught by regular classroom teachers in elementary grades and by qualified health education teachers or other similarly trained personnel in secondary grades?

4. To what extent is the program designed to help students acquire essential knowledge to prevent HIV infection at each appropriate grade?
5. To what extent does the program describe the benefits of abstinence for young people and mutually monogamous relationships within the context of marriage for adults?
6. To what extent is the program designed to help teenage students avoid specific types of behavior that increase the risk of becoming infected with HIV?
7. To what extent is adequate training about AIDS provided for school administrators, teachers, nurses, and counselors—especially those who teach about AIDS?
8. To what extent are sufficient program development time, classroom time, and educational materials provided for education about AIDS?
9. To what extent are the processes and outcomes of AIDS education being monitored and periodically assessed?

REFERENCES

1. US Public Health Service. Coolfont report: a PHS plan for prevention and control of AIDS and the AIDS virus. Public Health Rep 1986; 101:341.
2. Institute of Medicine. National Academy of Sciences. Confronting AIDS: directions for public health, health care, and research. Washington, DC: National Academy Press, 1986.
3. US Department of Health and Human Services, Public Health Service. Surgeon General's report on acquired immune deficiency syndrome. Washington, DC: US Department of Health and Human Services, 1986.
4. US Public Health Service. AIDS: information/education plan to prevent and control AIDS in the United States, March 1987. Washington, DC: US Department of Health and Human Services, 1987.
5. US Department of Education. AIDS and the education of our children, a guide for parents and

teachers. Washington, DC: US Department of Education, 1987.

6. Kolbe, LJ., Iverson, DC. Integrating school and community efforts to promote health: strategies, policies, and methods. Int J Health Educ 1983; 2:40–47.
7. Noak M. Recommendations for school health education. Denver: Education Commission of the States, 1982.
8. Comprehensive school health education as defined by the national professional school health education organizations. J Sch Health 1984; 54:312–315.
9. Allensworth D, Kolbe L. (eds). The comprehensive school health program: exploring an expanded concept. J Sch Health 1987; 57:402–76.

Appendix I

THE PRESIDENT'S DOMESTIC POLICY COUNCIL'S PRINCIPLES FOR AIDS EDUCATION

The following principles were proposed by the Domestic Policy Council and approved by the President in 1987:

Despite intensive research efforts, prevention is the only effective AIDS control strategy at present. Thus, there should be an aggressive Federal effort in AIDS education.

The scope and content of the school portion of this AIDS education effort should be locally determined and should be consistent with parental values.

The Federal role should focus on developing and conveying accurate health information on AIDS to the educators and others, not mandating a specific school curriculum on this subject, and trusting the American people to use this information in a manner appropriate to their community's needs.

Any health information developed by the Federal Government that will be used for education should encourage responsible sexual behavior—based on fidelity, commit-

ment, and maturity, placing sexuality within the context of marriage.

Any health information provided by the Federal Government that might be used in schools should teach that children should not engage in sex and should be used with the consent and involvement of parents.

Appendix II

THE EXTENT OF AIDS AND INDICATORS OF ADOLESCENT RISK

Since the first cases of acquired immunodeficiency syndrome (AIDS) were reported in the United States in 1981, the human immunodeficiency virus (HIV) that causes AIDS and other HIV-related diseases has precipitated an epidemic unprecedented in modern history. Although in 1985, fewer than 60% of AIDS cases in the United States were reported among persons residing outside New York City and San Francisco, by 1991 more than 80% of the cases will be reported from other localities (1).

It has been estimated that from 1 to 1.5 million persons in the United States are infected with HIV (1), and, because there is no cure, infected persons are potentially capable of infecting others indefinitely. It has been predicted that 20%–30% of individuals currently infected will develop AIDS by the end of 1991 (1). Fifty percent of those diagnosed as having AIDS have not survived for more than about 1.5 years beyond diagnosis, and only about 12% have survived for more than 3 years (2).

By the end of 1987, about 50,000 persons in the United States had been diagnosed as having AIDS, and about 28,000 had died from the disease (2). Blacks and Hispanics, who make up about 12% and 6% of the U.S. population, respectively, disproportionately have contracted 25% and 14% of all reported AIDS cases (3). It has been estimated that during 1991, 74,000 cases of AIDS will be diagnosed, and 54,000 persons will die from the disease. By the end of that year, the total number of deaths caused by AIDS will be about 179,000 (1). In addition, health care and supportive services for the 145,000 persons projected to be living with AIDS in that year will cost our Nation an estimated $8–$10 billion in 1991 alone (1). The World Health Organization projects that by 1991, 50–100 million persons may be infected worldwide (4). The magnitude and seriousness of this epidemic requires a systematic and concerted response from almost every institution in our society.

A vaccine to prevent transmission of the virus is not expected to be developed before the next decade, and its use would not affect the number of persons already infected by that time. A safe and effective antiviral agent to treat those infected is not expected to be available for general use within the next several years. The Centers for Disease Control (5), the National Academy of Sciences (6), the Surgeon General of the United States (7), and the U.S. Department of Education (8) have noted that in the absence of a vaccine or therapy, educating individuals about actions they can take to protect themselves from becoming infected is the most effective means available for controlling the epidemic. Because the virus is transmitted almost exclusively as a result of behavior individuals can modify (e.g., by having sexual contact with an infected person or by sharing intravenous drug paraphernalia with an infected person), educational programs designed to influence relevant types of behavior can be effective in controlling the epidemic.

A significant number of teenagers engage in behavior that increases their risk of becoming infected with HIV. The percentage of metropolitan teenage girls who had ever had sexual intercourse increased from 30%–45% between 1971 and 1982. The average age at first intercourse for females remained at approximately 16.2 years between 1971 and 1979 (9). The average proportion of never-married teenagers who have ever had intercourse increases with age from 14 through 19 years. In 1982, the percentage of never-married girls who reported having engaged in sexual intercourse was as follows: approximately 6% among 14-year-olds (10), 18% among 15-year-olds, 29% among 16-year-olds, 40% among 17-year-olds, 54% among 18-year-olds, and 66% among 19-year-olds (11). Among never-married boys living in metropolitan areas, the percentage who reported having engaged in sexual intercourse was as follows: 24% among 14-year-olds, 35% among 15-year-olds, 45% among 16-year-olds, 56% among 17-year-olds, 66% among 18-year-olds, and 78% among 19-year-olds (9, 12). Rates of sexual experience (e.g., percentage having had intercourse) are higher for black teenagers than for white teenagers at every age and for both sexes (11, 12).

Male homosexual intercourse is an important risk factor for HIV infection. In one survey conducted in 1973, 5% of 13- to 15-year-old boys and 17% of 16- to 19-year-old boys reported having had at least one homosexual experience. Of those who reported having had such an experience, most (56%) indicated that the first homosexual experience had occurred when they were 11 or 12 years old. Two percent reported that they currently engaged in homosexual activity (13).

Another indicator of high-risk behavior among teenagers is the number of cases of sexually transmitted diseases they contract. Approximately 2.5 million teenagers are affected with a sexually transmitted disease each year (14).

Some teenagers also are at risk of becoming infected with HIV through illicit intravenous drug use. Findings from a national survey conducted in 1986 of nearly 130 high schools indicated that although overall illicit drug use seems to be declining slowly among high school seniors, about 1% of seniors reported having used heroin and 13% reported having used cocaine within the previous year (15). The number of seniors who injected each of these drugs is not known.

Only 1% of all the persons diagnosed as having AIDS have been under age 20 (2); most persons in this group had been infected by transfusion or perinatal transmission. However, about

21% of all the persons diagnosed as having AIDS have been 20–29 years of age. Given the long incubation period between HIV infection and symptoms that lead to AIDS diagnosis (3 to 5 years or more), some fraction of those in the 20- to 29-year-age group diagnosed as having AIDS were probably infected while they were still teenagers.

Among military recruits screened in the period October 1985–December 1986, the HIV seroprevalence rate for persons 17–20 years of age (0.6/1,000) was about half the rate for recruits in all age groups (1.5/1,000) (16). These data have lead some to conclude that teenagers and young adults have an appreciable risk of infection and that the risk may be relatively constant and cumulative (17).

Reducing the risk of HIV infection among teenagers is important not only for their well-being but also for the children they might produce. The birth rate for U.S. teenagers is among the highest in the developed world (18); in 1984, this group accounted for more than 1 million pregnancies. During that year the rate of pregnancy among sexually active teenage girls 15–19 years of age was 233/1,000 girls (19).

Although teenagers are at risk of becoming infected with and transmitting the AIDS virus as they become sexually active, studies have shown that they do not believe they are likely to become infected (20, 21). Indeed, a random sample of 860 teenagers (ages 16–19) in Massachusetts revealed that, although 70% reported they were sexually active (having sexual intercourse or other sexual contact), only 15% of this group reported changing their sexual behavior because of concern about contracting AIDS. Only 20% of those who changed their behavior selected effective methods such as abstinence or use of condoms (20). Most teenagers indicated that they want more information about AIDS (20, 21).

Most adult Americans recognize the early age at which youth need to be advised about how to protect themselves from becoming infected with HIV and recognize that the schools can play an important role in providing such education. When asked in a November 1986 nationwide poll whether children should be taught about AIDS in school, 83% of Americans agreed, 10% disagreed, and 7% were not sure (22). According to information gathered by the United States Conference of Mayors in December of 1986, 40 of the Nation's 73 largest school districts were providing education about AIDS, and 24 more were planning such education (23). Of the districts that offered AIDS education, 63% provided it in 7th grade, 60% provided it in 9th grade, and 90% provided it in 10th grade. Ninety-eight percent provided medical facts about AIDS, 78% mentioned abstinence as a means of avoiding infection, and 70% addressed the issues of avoiding high-risk sexual activities, selecting sexual partners, and using condoms. Data collected by the National Association of State Boards of Education in the summer of 1987 indicated that a) 15 states had mandated comprehensive school health education; eight had mandated AIDS education; b) 12 had legislation pending on AIDS education, and six had state board of education actions pending; c) 17 had developed curricula for AIDS education, and seven more were developing such materials; and d) 40 had developed policies on admitting students with AIDS to school (24).

The Nation's system of public and private schools has a strategic role to play in assuring that young people understand the nature of the epidemic they face and the specific actions they can take to protect themselves from becoming infected—especially during their adolescence and young adulthood. In 1984, 98% of 14- and 15-year-olds, 92% of 16- and 17-year-olds, and 50% of 18- and 19-year-olds were in school (25). In that same year, about 615,000 14- to 17-year-olds and 1.1 million 18- to 19-year-olds were not enrolled in school and had not completed high school (26).

REFERENCES

1. US Public Health Service. Coolfont report: a PHS plan for prevention and control of AIDS and the AIDS virus. Public Health Rep 1986; 101:341.

2. CDC. Acquired immunodeficiency syndrome (AIDS) weekly surveillance report—United States. Cases reported to CDC. December 28, 1987.

3. CDC. Acquired immunodeficiency syndrome (AIDS) among blacks and Hispanics—United States. MMWR 1986; 35:655–8, 663–6.

4. World Health Organization. Special program on AIDS: strategies and structure projected needs. Geneva: World Health Organization, 1987.

5. CDC. Results of a Gallup Poll on acquired immunodeficiency syndrome—New York City, United States. MMWR 1985; 34:513–4.

6. Institute of Medicine. National Academy of Sciences. Confronting AIDS: directions for public health, health care, and research. Washington, DC: National Academy Press, 1986.

7. US Department of Health and Human Services, Public Health Service. Surgeon General's report on acquired immune deficiency syndrome. Washington, DC: US Department of Health and Human Services, 1986.

8. US Department of Education. AIDS and the education of our children, a guide for parents and teachers. Washington, DC: US Department of Education, 1987.

9. Zelnick M, Kantner JF. Sexual activity, contraceptive use, and pregnancy among metropolitan-area teenagers: 1971–1979. Fam Plann Perspect 1980; 12:230–7.

10. Hofferth SL, Kahn J, Baldwin W. Premarital sexual activity among United States teenage women over the past three decades. Fam Plann Perspect 1987; 19:46–53.

11. Pratt WF, Mosher WD, Bachrach CA, et al. Understanding US fertility: findings from the National Survey of Family Growth, cycle III. Popul Bull 1984:39:1–42.

12. Teenage pregnancy: the problem that hasn't gone away. Tables and References. New York: The Alan Guttmacher Institute, June 1981.

13. Sorensen RC. Adolescent sexuality in contemporary America. New York, World Publishing, 1973.

14. Division of Sexually Transmitted Diseases, Annual Report, FY 1986. Center for Prevention Services, Centers for Disease Control, US Public Health Service, 1987.

15. Johnston LD, Bachman JG, O'Malley PM. Drug use among American high school students, college, and other young adults: national trends through 1986.

Rockville, Md: National Institute on Drug Abuse, 1987.

16. CDC. Trends in human immunodeficiency virus infection among civilian applicants for military service—United States, October 1985–December 1986. MMWR 1987; 36:273–6.

17. Burke DS, Brundage JF, Herbold JR, et al. Human immunodeficiency virus infections among civilian applicants for United States military service. October 1985 to March 1986. N Engl J Med 1987; 317:131–6.

18. Jones EF, Forrest JD, Goldman N, et al. Teenage pregnancy in developed countries: determinants and policy implications. Fam Plann Perspect 1985; 17:53–63.

19. National Research Council. Risking the future: adolescent sexuality, pregnancy, and childbearing (vol. 1). Washington, DC: National Academy Press, 1987.

20. Strunin L, Hingson R. Acquired immunodeficiency syndrome and adolescents: knowledge, beliefs, attitudes, and behaviors. Pediatrics 1987; 79:825–8.

21. DiClemente RJ, Zorn J, Temoshok L. Adolescents and AIDS: a survey of knowledge, attitudes, and beliefs about AIDS in San Francisco. Am J Public Health 1986; 76:1443–5.

22. Yankelovich Clancy Shulman. Memorandum to all data users from Hal Quinley about Time/Yankelovich Clancy Shulman Poll findings on sex education, November 17, 1986. New York City: Yankelovich Clancy Shulman, 1986.

23. United States Conference of Mayors. Local school districts active in AIDS education. AIDS Information Exchange 1987; 4:1–10.

24. Cashman J. Personal communication on September 8, 1987, about the National Association of State Boards of Education survey of state AIDS-related policies and legislation. Washington, DC: National Association of State Boards of Education.

25. US Department of Commerce, Bureau of the Census. Statistical abstract of the United States, 105th ed. Washington, DC: US Department of Commerce, 1985.

26. US Department of Commerce, Bureau of the Census. School enrollment—social and economic characteristics of students: October 1984: Current Population Reports. Washington, DC: US Department of Commerce, 1985 (Series P-20, No. 404).

APPENDIX IV

HIV/AIDS Surveillance Report (Year-End Edition)

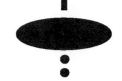

This report was received while the book was in production. In order to provide more recent statistics, we have included it as a separate appendix. There will be some discrepancies between the text and this report.

U.S. AIDS cases reported through December 1990   **Issued January 1991**

Contents

> Acquired immunodeficiency syndrome (AIDS) is a specific group of diseases or conditions which are indicative of severe immunosuppression related to infection with the human immunodeficiency virus (HIV).

U.S. DEPARTMENT OF HEALTH AND HUMAN SERVICES
Public Health Service
Centers for Disease Control
Center for Infectious Diseases
Division of HIV/AIDS

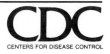

CENTERS FOR DISEASE CONTROL

The *HIV/AIDS Surveillance Report* is published each month by the Division of HIV/AIDS, Center for Infectious Diseases, Centers for Disease Control, Atlanta, GA 30333. An expanded, year-end edition is published each January. All data contained in the *Report* are provisional.

Suggested Citation: Centers for Disease Control. HIV/AIDS Surveillance Report, January 1991: 1-22

Centers for Disease Control ....William L. Roper, M.D., M.P.H.
Director

Gary R. Noble, M.D., M.P.H.
Deputy Director (HIV)

Center for Infectious Diseases ....Frederick A. Murphy, D.V.M., Ph.D.
Director

Division of HIV/AIDS...James W. Curran, M.D., M.P.H.
Director

Surveillance Branch...Ruth L. Berkelman, M.D.
Chief

Reporting and Analysis Section ....Harold Van Patten
Acting Chief

Statistics and Data Management Branch...W. Meade Morgan, Ph.D.
Chief

Xenophon M. Santas
Computer Specialist

Single copies of the *HIV/AIDS Surveillance Report* are available free from the National AIDS Information Clearinghouse, P.O. Box 6003, Rockville, MD 20850. Individuals or organizations can be added to the mailing list by writing to Centers for Disease Control, OD/OPS/MASO, 1/B49, Mailstop A-22, Atlanta, GA 30333. Confidential information, referrals, and educational material on AIDS are available from the National AIDS Hotline: 1-800-342-2437, 1-800-344-7432 (Spanish access), and 1-800-243-7889 (TTY, deaf access).

Figure 1. AIDS annual rates per 100,000 population, for cases reported in 1990, United States

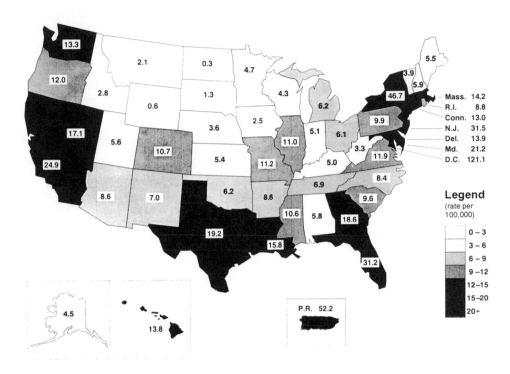

Figure 2. Adult/adolescent and pediatric AIDS cases, reported in 1990, United States

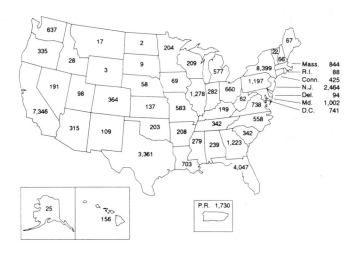

Figure 3. Pediatric AIDS cases, reported in 1990, United States

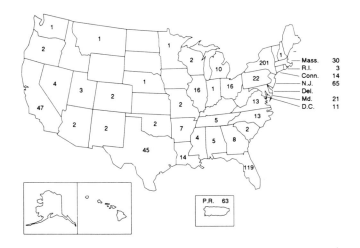

Figure 4. AIDS cases by quarter-year of report, reported January 1982 through December 1990, United States

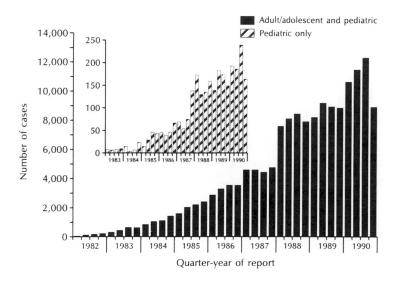

Figure 5. AIDS cases by month of diagnosis, adjusted for reporting delays,[1] January 1982 through September 1990, United States

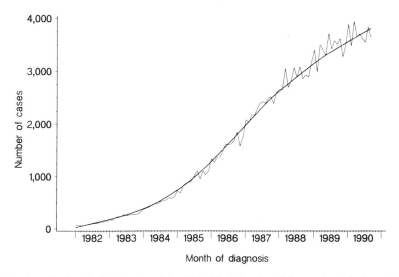

[1]See technical notes for explanation of adjusting and smoothing of data. Adjusted numbers of diagnosed cases for the most recent 3 months are not shown because of the imprecision of these estimates.

Table 1. AIDS cases and annual rates per 100,000 population, by state, reported in 1989 and 1990; and cumulative totals, by state and age group, through December 1990[1]

State of residence	1989 No.	1989 Rate	1990 No.	1990 Rate	Cumulative totals Adults/ adolescents	Cumulative totals Children < 13 years old	Total
Alabama	216	5.2	239	5.8	873	21	894
Alaska	17	3.1	25	4.5	97	2	99
Arizona	332	9.3	315	8.6	1,290	8	1,298
Arkansas	79	3.3	208	8.6	445	10	455
California	6,467	22.4	7,346	24.9	30,462	212	30,674
Colorado	387	11.5	364	10.7	1,585	9	1,594
Connecticut	431	13.3	425	13.0	1,805	63	1,868
Delaware	81	12.1	94	13.9	310	4	314
District of Columbia	496	80.7	741	121.1	2,672	40	2,712
Florida	3,479	27.5	4,047	31.2	13,607	386	13,993
Georgia	1,102	17.1	1,223	18.6	4,226	44	4,270
Hawaii	180	16.1	156	13.8	627	2	629
Idaho	23	2.3	28	2.8	77	2	79
Illinois	1,139	9.8	1,278	11.0	4,661	67	4,728
Indiana	397	7.1	282	5.1	1,007	10	1,017
Iowa	56	2.0	69	2.5	229	3	232
Kansas	114	4.5	137	5.4	442	3	445
Kentucky	114	3.1	189	5.0	500	5	505
Louisiana	508	11.5	703	15.8	2,251	39	2,290
Maine	66	5.4	67	5.5	219	2	221
Maryland	717	15.3	1,002	21.2	3,075	68	3,143
Massachusetts	755	12.8	844	14.2	3,270	72	3,342
Michigan	506	5.5	577	6.2	1,973	32	2,005
Minnesota	176	4.1	204	4.7	823	8	831
Mississippi	165	6.3	279	10.6	650	10	660
Missouri	442	8.6	583	11.2	1,821	12	1,833
Montana	13	1.6	17	2.1	55	1	56
Nebraska	33	2.1	58	3.6	184	2	186
Nevada	181	16.7	191	17.1	626	7	633
New Hampshire	37	3.3	66	5.9	190	5	195
New Jersey	2,230	28.7	2,464	31.5	10,091	280	10,371
New Mexico	94	6.1	109	7.0	346	3	349
New York	6,010	33.5	8,399	46.7	33,694	802	34,496
North Carolina	447	6.8	558	8.4	1,628	36	1,664
North Dakota	8	1.2	2	0.3	20	—	20
Ohio	486	4.5	660	6.1	2,259	40	2,299
Oklahoma	167	5.1	203	6.2	699	11	710
Oregon	228	8.2	335	12.0	1,014	5	1,019
Pennsylvania	1,073	8.9	1,197	9.9	4,362	75	4,437
Rhode Island	88	8.8	88	8.8	372	10	382
South Carolina	331	9.4	342	9.6	1,023	21	1,044
South Dakota	4	0.6	9	1.3	25	—	25
Tennessee	266	5.4	342	6.9	1,092	15	1,107
Texas	2,397	14.0	3,361	19.2	11,320	111	11,431
Utah	74	4.3	98	5.6	331	8	339
Vermont	20	3.6	22	3.9	77	1	78
Virginia	390	6.4	738	11.9	2,018	35	2,053
Washington	499	10.6	637	13.3	2,147	12	2,159
West Virginia	55	2.9	62	3.3	177	2	179
Wisconsin	130	2.7	209	4.3	623	4	627
Wyoming	16	3.3	3	0.6	34	—	34
U.S. total	**33,722**	**13.6**	**41,595**	**16.6**	**153,404**	**2,620**	**156,024**
Guam	1	0.7	2	1.4	8	—	8
Pacific Islands, U.S.	—	—	1	0.5	2	—	2
Puerto Rico	1,478	44.7	1,730	52.2	4,798	162	4,960
Virgin Islands, U.S.	29	25.2	11	9.4	75	4	79
Total	**35,230**	**14.0**	**43,339**	**17.0**	**158,287**	**2,786**	**161,073**

[1]During December 1990, 3,496 cases and 2,265 deaths among adults/adolescents and 52 cases and 18 deaths among children were reported to the CDC.

Table 2. AIDS cases and annual rates per 100,000 population, by metropolitan area with 500,000 or more population, reported in 1989 and 1990; and cumulative totals, by area and age group, through December 1990

Metropolitan area of residence	1989 No.	1989 Rate	1990 No.	1990 Rate	Cumulative totals Adults/ adolescents	Cumulative totals Children <13 years old	Total
Akron, Ohio	23	3.5	29	4.4	106	—	106
Albany-Schenectady, N.Y.	71	8.3	83	9.7	326	3	329
Albuquerque, N.M.	51	10.2	49	9.6	176	1	177
Allentown, Pa.	32	4.7	59	8.6	155	4	159
Anaheim, Calif.	283	12.3	376	16.1	1,319	9	1,328
Atlanta, Ga.	860	30.6	941	32.6	3,237	25	3,262
Austin, Tex.	203	26.2	233	29.1	716	7	723
Bakersfield, Calif.	36	6.7	35	6.4	115	—	115
Baltimore, Md.	477	20.2	647	27.2	1,843	49	1,892
Baton Rouge, La.	51	9.4	59	10.8	192	4	196
Bergen-Passaic, N.J.	210	16.3	350	27.1	1,322	27	1,349
Birmingham, Ala.	75	8.1	74	7.9	279	6	285
Boston, Mass.	586	15.6	604	16.1	2,549	51	2,600
Bridgeport, Conn.	136	16.6	115	14.0	541	20	561
Buffalo, N.Y.	66	6.9	93	9.8	259	2	261
Charleston, S.C.	66	12.7	75	14.1	231	—	231
Charlotte, N.C.	90	8.0	95	8.3	322	7	329
Chicago, Ill.	929	14.9	1,076	17.2	3,945	51	3,996
Cincinnati, Ohio	63	4.3	132	9.0	347	6	353
Cleveland, Ohio	126	6.9	144	7.9	578	10	588
Columbus, Ohio	111	8.2	140	10.2	499	4	503
Dallas, Tex.	540	21.3	794	30.5	2,787	14	2,801
Dayton, Ohio	56	5.9	68	7.2	229	6	235
Denver, Colo.	318	19.1	305	18.0	1,301	5	1,306
Detroit, Mich.	353	8.1	394	9.1	1,377	23	1,400
El Paso, Tex.	33	5.5	32	5.2	106	1	107
Fort Lauderdale, Fla.	615	50.9	846	68.8	2,459	49	2,508
Fort Worth, Tex.	153	11.5	200	14.6	624	8	632
Fresno, Calif.	49	7.8	64	10.0	194	2	196
Gary, Ind.	41	6.7	19	3.1	90	—	90
Grand Rapids, Mich.	27	4.0	35	5.1	103	1	104
Greensboro, N.C.	71	7.6	96	10.2	252	6	258
Greenville, S.C.	39	6.2	41	6.5	125	—	125
Harrisburg, Pa.	48	8.1	34	5.7	159	4	163
Hartford, Conn.	144	12.9	152	13.5	545	15	560
Honolulu, Hawaii	122	14.4	116	13.5	483	2	485
Houston, Tex.	906	27.4	1,368	40.5	4,758	46	4,804
Indianapolis, Ind.	197	15.8	131	10.4	472	3	475
Jacksonville, Fla.	200	21.7	284	30.1	771	25	796
Jersey City, N.J.	311	57.6	354	65.7	1,693	43	1,736
Kansas City, Mo.	239	15.0	290	18.0	991	4	995
Knoxville, Tenn.	22	3.6	31	5.1	111	1	112
Lake County, Ill.	21	4.2	16	3.1	73	2	75
Las Vegas, Nev.	126	19.3	156	23.2	465	7	472
Little Rock, Ark.	31	6.0	82	15.7	181	5	186
Los Angeles, Calif.	2,351	26.9	2,372	26.8	10,762	93	10,855
Louisville, Ky.	45	4.6	73	7.5	206	2	208
Memphis, Tenn.	85	8.6	106	10.6	350	6	356
Miami, Fla.	1,011	55.0	1,060	57.0	4,060	163	4,223
Middlesex, N.J.	194	19.6	165	16.5	800	24	824
Milwaukee, Wis.	72	5.2	115	8.2	353	2	355
Minneapolis-Saint Paul, Minn.	158	6.5	179	7.3	733	6	739
Monmouth-Ocean City, N.J.	184	18.7	201	20.1	655	23	678
Nashville, Tenn.	79	8.0	114	11.4	361	6	367
Nassau-Suffolk, N.Y.	362	13.7	398	15.0	1,610	39	1,649
New Haven, Conn.	111	13.9	130	16.2	570	27	597
New Orleans, La.	313	23.8	390	29.6	1,421	20	1,441
New York, N.Y.	4,976	57.8	7,282	84.3	29,255	728	29,983
Newark, N.J.	956	50.7	985	52.2	4,216	126	4,342
Norfolk, Va.	74	5.3	186	13.0	449	7	456

Table 2. AIDS cases and annual rates per 100,000 population, by metropolitan area with 500,000 or more population, reported in 1989 and 1990; and cumulative totals, by area and age group, through December 1990 — Continued

| Metropolitan area of residence | 1989 | | 1990 | | Cumulative totals | | |
	No.	Rate	No.	Rate	Adults/ adolescents	Children <13 years old	Total
Oakland, Calif.	404	19.8	606	29.3	2,031	14	2,045
Oklahoma City, Okla.	87	8.9	101	10.2	356	—	356
Omaha, Neb.	23	3.7	39	6.2	121	1	122
Orlando, Fla.	160	15.9	262	25.2	734	8	742
Oxnard-Ventura, Calif.	31	4.7	39	5.8	146	—	146
Philadelphia, Pa.	782	15.8	898	18.1	3,305	52	3,357
Phoenix, Ariz.	239	11.4	228	10.6	943	5	948
Pittsburgh, Pa.	157	7.6	135	6.5	552	2	554
Portland, Oreg.	173	14.4	269	22.3	801	2	803
Providence, R.I.	81	8.9	85	9.3	348	9	357
Raleigh-Durham, N.C.	97	13.9	115	16.1	355	10	365
Richmond, Va.	93	10.9	137	15.8	385	7	392
Riverside-San Bernardino, Calif.	256	10.8	280	11.4	1,007	15	1,022
Rochester, N.Y.	63	6.4	83	8.4	346	3	349
Sacramento, Calif.	168	11.8	151	10.4	634	9	643
Saint Louis, Mo.	181	7.3	294	11.8	815	7	822
Salt Lake City, Utah	60	5.5	90	8.2	293	5	298
San Antonio, Tex.	195	14.4	239	17.2	798	12	810
San Diego, Calif.	510	21.0	670	26.8	2,308	19	2,327
San Francisco, Calif.	1,786	111.4	2,124	131.5	9,404	17	9,421
San Jose, Calif.	118	8.1	193	13.2	707	8	715
San Juan, P.R.	875	55.1	1,138	71.3	3,000	106	3,106
Scranton, Pa.	25	3.4	45	6.1	123	3	126
Seattle, Wash.	372	19.6	477	24.8	1,631	10	1,641
Springfield, Mass.	43	7.2	86	14.5	194	10	204
Syracuse, N.Y.	39	6.0	39	6.0	156	5	161
Tacoma, Wash.	38	6.7	40	6.9	139	2	141
Tampa-Saint Petersburg, Fla.	385	18.8	417	19.9	1,528	26	1,554
Toledo, Ohio	23	3.7	38	6.2	111	3	114
Tucson, Ariz.	61	9.4	58	8.8	243	2	245
Tulsa, Okla.	50	6.8	55	7.4	198	3	201
Washington, D.C.	856	22.6	1,293	33.5	4,527	69	4,596
West Palm Beach, Fla.	331	39.0	354	40.3	1,363	52	1,415
Wilmington, Del.	64	11.0	83	14.2	259	3	262
Worcester, Mass.	40	5.9	54	7.9	176	4	180
Metropolitan area subtotal[1]	**29,044**	**19.9**	**36,288**	**24.6**	**135,244**	**2,333**	**137,577**
All other areas	**6,186**	**5.8**	**7,051**	**6.6**	**23,043**	**453**	**23,496**
Total	**35,230**	**14.0**	**43,339**	**17.0**	**158,287**	**2,786**	**161,073**

[1] Includes data from metropolitan areas which have populations of 500,000 or more.

Table 3. AIDS cases by age group, exposure category, and sex, reported in 1989 and 1990; and cumulative totals, by age group and exposure category, through December 1990, United States

Adult/adolescent exposure category	Males 1989 No. (%)	Males 1990 No. (%)	Females 1989 No. (%)	Females 1990 No. (%)	Totals 1989 No. (%)	Totals 1990 No. (%)	Cumulative total[1] No. (%)
Male homosexual/bisexual contact	19.891 (64)	23.738 (63)	—	—	19.891 (58)	23.738 (56)	94.126 (59)
Intravenous (IV) drug use (female and heterosexual male)	6.218 (20)	7.689 (20)	1.871 (51)	2.329 (48)	8.089 (23)	10.018 (24)	34.398 (22)
Male homosexual/bisexual contact and IV drug use	2.214 (7)	2.295 (6)	—	—	2.214 (6)	2.295 (5)	10.557 (7)
Hemophilia/coagulation disorder	283 (1)	329 (1)	6 (0)	11 (0)	289 (1)	340 (1)	1.386 (1)
Heterosexual contact	778 (3)	1.054 (3)	1.232 (34)	1.657 (34)	2.010 (6)	2.711 (6)	8.440 (5)
Sex with IV drug user	390	469	770	1.062	1.160	1.531	4.470
Sex with bisexual male	—	—	109	129	109	129	498
Sex with person with hemophilia	1	2	20	26	21	28	79
Born in Pattern-II[2] country	247	305	132	117	379	422	2.036
Sex with person born in Pattern-II country	19	22	12	22	31	44	130
Sex with transfusion recipient with HIV infection	13	24	22	40	35	64	151
Sex with HIV-infected person, risk not specified	108	232	167	261	275	493	1.076
Receipt of blood transfusion, blood components, or tissue[3]	469 (2)	501 (1)	308 (8)	365 (7)	777 (2)	866 (2)	3.684 (2)
Other/undetermined[4]	1.093 (4)	2.061 (5)	222 (6)	528 (11)	1.315 (4)	2.589 (6)	5.696 (4)
Adult/adolescent subtotal	30.946 (100)	37.667 (100)	3.639 (100)	4.890 (100)	34.585 (100)	42.557 (100)	158.287 (100)

Pediatric (13 years old) exposure category	Males 1989 No. (%)	Males 1990 No. (%)	Females 1989 No. (%)	Females 1990 No. (%)	Totals 1989 No. (%)	Totals 1990 No. (%)	Cumulative total[1] No. (%)
Hemophilia/coagulation disorder	24 (7)	31 (7)	1 (0)	—	25 (4)	31 (4)	139 (5)
Mother with/at risk for HIV infection	282 (84)	342 (82)	283 (92)	339 (92)	565 (88)	681 (87)	2.327 (84)
IV drug use	139	167	123	147	262	314	1.163
Sex with IV drug user	67	75	61	75	128	150	487
Sex with bisexual male	8	3	7	5	15	8	48
Sex with person with hemophilia	—	1	—	1	—	2	9
Born in Pattern-II country	27	20	28	20	55	40	213
Sex with person born in Pattern-II country	1	2	2	4	3	6	12
Sex with transfusion recipient with HIV infection	1	1	5	—	6	1	12
Sex with HIV-infected person, risk not specified	10	15	16	21	26	36	98
Receipt of blood transfusion, blood components, or tissue	4	5	6	7	10	12	47
Has HIV infection, risk not specified	25	53	35	59	60	112	238
Receipt of blood transfusion, blood components, or tissue	25 (7)	26 (6)	15 (5)	13 (4)	40 (6)	39 (5)	252 (9)
Undetermined	5 (1)	16 (4)	10 (3)	15 (4)	15 (2)	31 (4)	68 (2)
Pediatric subtotal	336 (100)	415 (100)	309 (100)	367 (100)	645 (100)	782 (100)	2.786 (100)
Total	31,282	38,082	3,948	5,257	35,230	43,339	161,073

[1] Includes 3 patients known to be infected with human immunodeficiency virus type 2 (HIV-2). See MMWR 1989;38:572-580

[2] See technical notes.

[3] Includes 14 transfusion recipients who received blood screened for HIV antibody, and 1 tissue recipient.

[4] "Other" refers to 3 health-care workers who seroconverted to HIV and developed AIDS after occupational exposure to HIV-infected blood. "Undetermined" refers to patients whose mode of exposure to HIV is unknown. This includes patients under investigation; patients who died, were lost to follow-up, or refused interview; and patients whose mode of exposure to HIV remains undetermined after investigation. See Figure 6.

Table 4.   AIDS cases by age group, exposure category, and race/ethnicity, reported through December 1990, United States

Adult/adolescent exposure category	White, not Hispanic No. (%)	Black, not Hispanic No. (%)	Hispanic No. (%)	Asian/Pacific Islander No. (%)	American Indian/ Alaskan Native No. (%)	Total[4] No. (%)
Male homosexual/bisexual contact	67,049 (76)	15,966 (36)	10,051 (40)	733 (74)	123 (54)	94,126 (59)
Intravenous (IV) drug use (female and heterosexual male)	6,954 (8)	17,232 (39)	10,050 (40)	44 (4)	38 (17)	34,398 (22)
Male homosexual/bisexual contact and IV drug use	6,112 (7)	2,852 (6)	1,526 (6)	21 (2)	30 (13)	10,557 (7)
Hemophilia/coagulation disorder	1,153 (1)	95 (0)	110 (0)	16 (2)	8 (4)	1,386 (1)
Heterosexual contact:	1,799 (2)	5,039 (11)	1,535 (6)	37 (4)	10 (4)	8,440 (5)
Sex with IV drug user	*980*	*2,264*	*1,191*	*16*	*7*	*4,470*
Sex with bisexual male	*274*	*155*	*58*	*9*	*1*	*498*
Sex with person with hemophilia	*68*	*7*	*3*	*1*	*—*	*79*
Born in Pattern-II[1] country	*8*	*2,004*	*16*	*4*	*—*	*2,036*
Sex with person born in Pattern-II country	*41*	*80*	*8*	*—*	*—*	*130*
Sex with transfusion recipient with HIV infection	*96*	*26*	*26*	*1*	*—*	*151*
Sex with HIV-infected person, risk not specified	*332 503*	*233* *6*	*21,076*			
Receipt of blood transfusion, blood components, or tissue[2]	2,580 (3)	638 (1)	380 (2)	70 (7)	6 (3)	3,684 (2)
Other/undetermined[3]	2,093 (2)	2,205 (5)	1,278 (5)	64 (6)	12 (5)	5,696 (4)
Adult/adolescent subtotal	87,740 (100)	44,027 (100)	24,930 (100)	985 (100)	227 (100)	158,287 (100)

Pediatric (<13 years old) exposure category						
Hemophilia/coagulation disorder	95 (16)	18 (1)	23 (3)	3 (25)	—	139 (5)
Mother with/at risk for HIV infection:	366 (61)	1,326 (92)	617 (86)	4 (33)	6 (100)	2,327 (84)
IV drug use	*181*	*657*	*318*	*1*	*2*	*1,163*
Sex with IV drug user	*77*	*211*	*196*	*1*	*1*	*487*
Sex with bisexual male	*18*	*21*	*9*	*—*	*—*	*48*
Sex with person with hemophilia	*6*	*2*	*1*	*—*	*—*	*9*
Born in Pattern-II country	*2*	*209*	*2*	*—*	*—*	*213*
Sex with person born in Pattern-II country	*—*	*11*	*—*	*—*	*—*	*12*
Sex with transfusion recipient with HIV infection	*5*	*3*	*3*	*—*	*—*	*12*
Sex with HIV-infected person, risk not specified	*20*	*46*	*29*	*1*	*1*	*98*
Receipt of blood transfusion, blood components, or tissue	*16*	*19*	*12*	*—*	*—*	*47*
Has HIV infection, risk not specified	*41*	*147*	*47*	*1*	*2*	*238*
Receipt of blood transfusion, blood components, or tissue	133 (22)	56 (4)	58 (8)	5 (42)	—	252 (9)
Undetermined	8 (1)	39 (3)	21 (3)	—	—	68 (2)
Pediatric subtotal	602 (100)	1,439 (100)	719 (100)	12 (100)	6 (100)	2,786 (100)
Total	**88,342**	**45,466**	**25,649**	**997**	**233**	**161,073**

[1] See technical notes.

[2] Includes 14 transfusion recipients who received blood screened for HIV antibody, and 1 tissue recipient.

[3] "Other" refers to 3 health-care workers who seroconverted to HIV and developed AIDS after occupational exposure to HIV-infected blood. "Undetermined" refers to patients whose mode of exposure to HIV is unknown. This includes patients under investigation; patients who died, were lost to follow-up, or refused interview; and patients whose mode of exposure to HIV remains undetermined after investigation. See Figure 6.

[4] Includes 386 persons whose race/ethnicity is unknown.

Table 5. Adult/adolescent AIDS cases by sex, exposure category, and race/ethnicity, reported through December 1990, United States

Male exposure category	White, not Hispanic		Black, not Hispanic		Hispanic		Asian/Pacific Islander		American Indian/ Alaskan Native		Total[4]	
	No.	(%)	No.	(%)	No.	(%)	No.	(%)	No.	(%)	No.	(%)
Male homosexual/bisexual contact	67,049	(80)	15,966	(44)	10,051	(46)	733	(81)	123	(63)	94,126	(66)
Intravenous (IV) drug use (heterosexual)	5,305	(6)	12,676	(35)	8,442	(39)	30	(3)	22	(11)	26,540	(19)
Male homosexual/bisexual contact and IV drug use	6,112	(7)	2,852	(8)	1,526	(7)	21	(2)	30	(15)	10,557	(7)
Hemophilia/coagulation disorder	1,127	(1)	89	(0)	108	(0)	16	(2)	8	(4)	1,352	(1)
Heterosexual contact:	570	(1)	2,442	(7)	340	(2)	9	(1)	2	(1)	3,367	(2)
Sex with IV drug user	*355*		*713*		*212*		*5*		*2*		*1,287*	
Sex with person with hemophilia	*5*		*—*		*1*		*—*		*—*		*6*	
Born in Pattern-II[1] country	*4*		*1,462*		*11*		*3*		*—*		*1,483*	
Sex with person born in Pattern-II country	*34*		*36*		*7*		*—*		*—*		*77*	
Sex with transfusion recipient with HIV infection	*27*		*14*		*7*		*—*		*—*		*49*	
Sex with HIV-infected person, risk not specified	*145*		*217*		*102*		*1*		*—*		*465*	
Receipt of blood transfusion, blood components, or tissue[2]	1,658	(2)	341	(1)	199	(1)	44	(5)	2	(1)	2,252	(2)
Other/undetermined[3]	1,798	(2)	1,624	(5)	1,080	(5)	50	(6)	8	(4)	4,600	(3)
Male subtotal	83,619	(100)	35,990	(100)	21,746	(100)	903	(100)	195	(100)	142,794	(100)

Female exposure category	White, not Hispanic		Black, not Hispanic		Hispanic		Asian/Pacific Islander		American Indian/ Alaskan Native		Total[4]	
IV drug use	1,649	(40)	4,556	(57)	1,608	(51)	14	(17)	16	(50)	7,858	(51)
Hemophilia/coagulation disorder	26	(1)	6	(0)	2	(0)	—		—		34	(0)
Heterosexual contact:	1,229	(30)	2,597	(32)	1,195	(38)	28	(34)	8	(25)	5,073	(33)
Sex with IV drug user	*625*		*1,551*		*979*		*11*		*5*		*3,183*	
Sex with bisexual male	*274*		*155*		*58*		*9*		*1*		*498*	
Sex with person with hemophilia	*63*		*7*		*2*		*1*		*—*		*73*	
Born in Pattern-II country	*4*		*542*		*5*		*1*		*—*		*553*	
Sex with person born in Pattern-II country	*7*		*44*		*1*		*—*		*—*		*53*	
Sex with transfusion recipient with HIV infection	*69*		*12*		*19*		*1*		*—*		*102*	
Sex with HIV-infected person, risk not specified	*187*		*286*		*131*		*5*		*2*		*611*	
Receipt of blood transfusion, blood components, or tissue	922	(22)	297	(4)	181	(6)	26	(32)	4	(13)	1,432	(9)
Other/undetermined	295	(7)	581	(7)	198	(6)	14	(17)	4	(13)	1,096	(7)
Female subtotal	4,121	(100)	8,037	(100)	3,184	(100)	82	(100)	32	(100)	15,493	(100)
Total	**87,740**		**44,027**		**24,930**		**985**		**227**		**158,287**	

[1] See technical notes.
[2] Includes 14 transfusion recipients who received blood screened for HIV antibody, and 1 tissue recipient.
[3] "Other" refers to 3 health-care workers who seroconverted to HIV and developed AIDS after occupational exposure to HIV-infected blood. "Undetermined" refers to patients whose mode of exposure to HIV is unknown. This includes patients under investigation; patients who died, were lost to follow-up, or refused interview; and patients whose mode of exposure to HIV remains undetermined after investigation. See Figure 6.
[4] Includes 341 males and 37 females whose race/ethnicity is unknown.

Table 6.   AIDS cases in adolescents and adults under age 25, by exposure category, reported in 1989 and 1990, and cumulative totals through December 1990, United States

	13-19 years old						20-24 years old					
	1989		1990		Cumulative total		1989		1990		Cumulative total	
Exposure category	No.	(%)	No.	(%)	No.	(%)	No.	(%)	No.	(%)	No.	(%)
Male homosexual/bisexual contact	35	(28)	27	(16)	165	(26)	789	(54)	820	(50)	3,803	(57)
Intravenous (IV) drug use (female and heterosexual male)	18	(14)	15	(9)	70	(11)	271	(19)	292	(18)	1,089	(16)
Male homosexual/bisexual contact and IV drug use	3	(2)	4	(2)	27	(4)	130	(9)	132	(8)	619	(9)
Hemophilia/coagulation disorder	39	(31)	53	(32)	192	(31)	32	(2)	35	(2)	169	(3)
Heterosexual contact:	18	(14)	36	(21)	87	(14)	161	(11)	204	(12)	649	(10)
Sex with IV drug user	*15*		*27*		*58*		*94*		*132*		*371*	
Sex with bisexual male	*1*		*1*		*4*		*12*		*8*		*51*	
Sex with person with hemophilia	*—*		*1*		*1*		*8*		*3*		*15*	
Born in Pattern-II[1] country	*—*		*2*		*13*		*19*		*19*		*109*	
Sex with person born in Pattern-II country	*—*		*—*		*—*		*2*		*5*		*9*	
Sex with transfusion recipient with HIV infection	*—*		*1*		*1*		*1*		*5*		*7*	
Sex with HIV-infected person, risk not specified	*2*		*4*		*10*		*25*		*32*		*87*	
Receipt of blood transfusion, blood components, or tissue	5	(4)	11	(7)	47	(7)	11	(1)	26	(2)	101	(2)
Undetermined[2]	8	(6)	22	(13)	41	(7)	57	(4)	128	(8)	290	(4)
Total	**126**	**(100)**	**168**	**(100)**	**629**	**(100)**	**1,451**	**(100)**	**1,637**	**(100)**	**6,720**	**(100)**

[1] See technical notes.

[2] "Undetermined" refers to patients whose mode of exposure to HIV is unknown. This includes patient under investigation; patients who died, were lost to follow-up, or refused interview; and patients whose mode of exposure to HIV remains undetermined after investigation. See Figure 6.

Table 7.   AIDS cases by age at diagnosis and exposure category, reported through December 1990, United States

Age at diagnosis (years)	Male homosexual/ bisexual contact		IV drug use (female and heterosexual male)		Male homo- sexual/bisexual contact and IV drug use		Hemophilia/ coagulation disorder		Heterosexual contact: sex with person with/at risk for HIV infection	
	No.	(%)	No.	(%)	No.	(%)	No.	(%)	No.	(%)
Under 5	—		—		—		7	(0)	—	
5-12	—		—		—		132	(9)	—	
13-19	165	(0)	70	(0)	27	(0)	192	(13)	74	(1)
20-24	3,803	(4)	1,089	(3)	619	(6)	169	(11)	540	(8)
25-29	15,460	(16)	4,869	(14)	2,210	(21)	218	(14)	1,375	(21)
30-34	22,383	(24)	9,706	(28)	3,158	(30)	205	(13)	1,490	(23)
35-39	20,224	(21)	9,654	(28)	2,472	(23)	168	(11)	1,045	(16)
40-44	13,959	(15)	5,136	(15)	1,198	(11)	118	(8)	655	(10)
45-49	8,483	(9)	2,163	(6)	512	(5)	109	(7)	433	(7)
50-54	4,697	(5)	994	(3)	206	(2)	53	(3)	291	(5)
55-59	2,884	(3)	488	(1)	103	(1)	39	(3)	198	(3)
60-64	1,369	(1)	171	(0)	34	(0)	55	(4)	142	(2)
65 or older	699	(1)	58	(0)	18	(0)	60	(4)	161	(3)
Total	**94,126**	**(100)**	**34,398**	**(100)**	**10,557**	**(100)**	**1,525**	**(100)**	**6,404**	**(100)**

Age at diagnosis (years)	Heterosexual contact: born in Pattern-II[1] country		Receipt of transfusion[2]		Mother with/at risk for HIV infection		Other/ undetermined[3]		Total	
	No.	(%)	No.	(%)	No.	(%)	No.	(%)	No.	(%)
Under 5	—		125	(3)	2,091	(90)	53	(1)	2,276	(1)
5-12	—		127	(3)	236	(10)	15	(0)	510	(0)
13-19	13	(1)	47	(1)	—		41	(1)	629	(0)
20-24	109	(5)	101	(3)	—		290	(5)	6,720	(4)
25-29	476	(23)	232	(6)	—		794	(14)	25,634	(16)
30-34	608	(30)	282	(7)	—		1,063	(18)	38,895	(24)
35-39	407	(20)	301	(8)	—		861	(15)	35,132	(22)
40-44	214	(11)	298	(8)	—		793	(14)	22,371	(14)
45-49	90	(4)	249	(6)	—		579	(10)	12,618	(8)
50-54	55	(3)	275	(7)	—		450	(8)	7,021	(4)
55-59	35	(2)	350	(9)	—		364	(6)	4,461	(3)
60-64	15	(1)	459	(12)	—		229	(4)	2,474	(2)
65 or older	14	(1)	1,090	(28)	—		232	(4)	2,332	(1)
Total	**2,036**	**(100)**	**3,936**	**(100)**	**2,327**	**(100)**	**5,764**	**(100)**	**161,073**	**(100)**

[1] See technical notes.

[2] Includes 14 transfusion recipients who received blood screened for HIV antibody, and 1 tissue recipient.

[3] "Other" refers to 3 health-care workers who seroconverted to HIV and developed AIDS after occupational exposure to HIV-infected blood. "Undetermined" refers to patients whose mode of exposure to HIV is unknown. This includes patients under investigation; patients who died, were lost to follow-up, or refused interview; and patients whose mode of exposure to HIV remains undetermined after investigation. See Figure 6.

Table 8.   AIDS cases by sex, age at diagnosis, and race/ethnicity, reported through December 1990, United States

Males Age at diagnosis (years)	White, not Hispanic		Black, not Hispanic		Hispanic		Asian/Pacific Islander		American Indian/ Alaskan Native		Total[1]	
	No.	(%)	No.	(%)	No.	(%)	No.	(%)	No.	(%)	No.	(%)
Under 5	205	(0)	645	(2)	310	(1)	3	(0)	2	(1)	1,169	(1)
5-12	160	(0)	94	(0)	71	(0)	5	(1)	—		332	(0)
13-19	223	(0)	144	(0)	94	(0)	6	(1)	5	(3)	472	(0)
20-24	2,881	(3)	1,703	(5)	1,016	(5)	28	(3)	12	(6)	5,652	(4)
25-29	12,713	(15)	5,816	(16)	3,793	(17)	124	(14)	43	(22)	22,531	(16)
30-34	19,650	(23)	9,171	(25)	5,605	(25)	196	(22)	51	(26)	34,748	(24)
35-39	18,401	(22)	8,453	(23)	4,860	(22)	203	(22)	33	(17)	32,034	(22)
40-44	12,640	(15)	4,915	(13)	3,018	(14)	147	(16)	22	(11)	20,799	(14)
45-49	7,523	(9)	2,682	(7)	1,558	(7)	86	(9)	15	(8)	11,892	(8)
50-54	4,159	(5)	1,459	(4)	872	(4)	48	(5)	4	(2)	6,561	(5)
55-59	2,629	(3)	890	(2)	536	(2)	31	(3)	6	(3)	4,107	(3)
60-64	1,480	(2)	467	(1)	239	(1)	8	(1)	3	(2)	2,201	(2)
65 or older	1,320	(2)	290	(1)	155	(1)	26	(3)	1	(1)	1,797	(1)
Male subtotal	83,984	(100)	36,729	(100)	22,127	(100)	911	(100)	197	(100)	144,295	(100)

Females Age at diagnosis (years)	White, not Hispanic		Black, not Hispanic		Hispanic		Asian/Pacific Islander		American Indian/ Alaskan Native		Total[1]	
Under 5	195	(4)	619	(7)	287	(8)	1	(1)	4	(11)	1,107	(7)
5-12	42	(1)	81	(1)	51	(1)	3	(3)	—		178	(1)
13-19	42	(1)	89	(1)	24	(1)	1	(1)	1	(3)	157	(1)
20-24	288	(7)	508	(6)	259	(7)	4	(5)	5	(14)	1,068	(6)
25-29	778	(18)	1,563	(18)	742	(21)	8	(9)	4	(11)	3,103	(18)
30-34	942	(22)	2,312	(26)	857	(24)	17	(20)	10	(28)	4,147	(25)
35-39	648	(15)	1,807	(21)	619	(18)	11	(13)	5	(14)	3,098	(18)
40-44	371	(9)	851	(10)	330	(9)	16	(19)	2	(6)	1,572	(9)
45-49	192	(4)	374	(4)	147	(4)	8	(9)	2	(6)	726	(4)
50-54	145	(3)	219	(3)	90	(3)	5	(6)	1	(3)	460	(3)
55-59	164	(4)	134	(2)	51	(1)	3	(3)	—		354	(2)
60-64	155	(4)	84	(1)	27	(1)	6	(7)	1	(3)	273	(2)
65 or older	396	(9)	96	(1)	38	(1)	3	(3)	1	(3)	535	(3)
Female subtotal	4,358	(100)	8,737	(100)	3,522	(100)	86	(100)	36	(100)	16,778	(100)
Total	**88,342**		**45,466**		**25,649**		**997**		**233**		**161,073**	

[1] Includes 386 persons whose race/ethnicity is unknown.

Table 9. AIDS cases and annual rates[1] per 100,000 population, by race/ethnicity, age group, and sex, reported in 1990, United States

| Race/ethnicity | Adults/adolescents | | | | | | Children < 13 years old | | Total | |
| | Males | | Females | | Total | | | | | |
	No.	Rate	No.	Rate	No.	Rate	No.	Rate	No.	Rate
White, not Hispanic	20,943	27.4	1,236	1.5	22,179	14.0	163	0.5	22,342	11.7
Black, not Hispanic	10,263	92.4	2,539	20.0	12,802	53.8	384	5.2	13,186	42.3
Hispanic	6,026	71.9	1,069	12.6	7,095	42.0	227	3.6	7,322	31.6
Asian/Pacific Islander	238	9.4	19	0.7	257	4.8	3	0.2	260	3.8
American Indian/Alaskan Native	60	8.9	9	1.2	69	4.9	2	0.5	71	3.9
Total[2]	37,667	38.0	4,890	4.6	42,557	20.7	782	1.6	43,339	17.0

[1] Race/ethnicity annual rates are calculated using 1990 census projections. See technical notes.
[2] Includes 158 persons whose race/ethnicity is unknown.

Table 10. AIDS cases by year of diagnosis and definition category, diagnosed through December 1990, United States

| Definition category[1] | Year of diagnosis | | | | | | | | | | Cumulative total | |
| | Before 1987 | | 1987 | | 1988 | | 1989 | | 1990 | | | |
	No.	(%)	No.	(%)	No.	(%)	No.	(%)	No.	(%)	No.	(%)
Pre-1987 definition	37,239	(93)	21,908	(81)	23,264	(72)	24,388	(69)	17,154	(66)	123,953	(77)
1987 definition:[2]	2,680	(7)	5,152	(19)	9,208	(28)	11,158	(31)	8,922	(34)	37,120	(23)
Specific disease presumptively diagnosed	*1,434*		*2,773*		*5,173*		*6,369*		*5,432*		*21,181*	
Specific disease definitively diagnosed	*421*		*474*		*646*		*772*		*552*		*2,865*	
HIV encephalopathy	*249*		*697*		*1,124*		*1,287*		*908*		*4,265*	
HIV wasting syndrome	*576*		*1,208*		*2,265*		*2,730*		*2,030*		*8,809*	
Total	39,919	(100)	27,060	(100)	32,472	(100)	35,546	(100)	26,076	(100)	161,073	(100)

[1] Persons who meet the criteria for more than one definition category are classified in the definition category listed first.
[2] Persons who meet only the 1987 AIDS case definition and whose date of diagnosis is before September 1987 were diagnosed retrospectively.

Table 11.   AIDS-indicator diseases diagnosed in patients reported in 1990, by age group, United States

AIDS-indicator disease	Adults/adolescents		Children < 13 years old	
	No.	(%)[1]	No.	(%)[1]
Bacterial infections, multiple or recurrent	NA[2]		120	(15)
Candidiasis of bronchi, trachea, or lungs	1,004	(2)	33	(4)
Candidiasis of esophagus				
Definitive diagnosis	3,166	(7)	59	(8)
Presumptive diagnosis	2,473	(6)	44	(6)
Coccidioidomycosis, disseminated or extrapulmonary	110	(0)	0	(0)
Cryptococcosis, extrapulmonary	2,424	(6)	8	(1)
Cryptosporidiosis, chronic intestinal	777	(2)	15	(2)
Cytomegalovirus disease other than retinitis	1,597	(4)	46	(6)
Cytomegalovirus retinitis				
Definitive diagnosis	692	(2)	2	(0)
Presumptive diagnosis	591	(1)	4	(1)
HIV encephalopathy (dementia)	2,753	(6)	103	(13)
Herpes simplex, with esophagitis, pneumonitis, or				
chronic mucocutaneous ulcers	1,486	(3)	23	(3)
Histoplasmosis, disseminated or extrapulmonary	452	(1)	1	(0)
Isosporiasis, chronic intestinal	65	(0)	1	(0)
Kaposi's sarcoma				
Definitive diagnosis	3,772	(9)	1	(0)
Presumptive diagnosis	857	(2)	0	(0)
Lymphoid interstitial pneumonia and/or pulmonary lymphoid hyperplasia	NA[2]			
Definitive diagnosis			67	(9)
Presumptive diagnosis			91	(12)
Lymphoma, Burkitt's (or equivalent term)	289	(1)	11	(1)
Lymphoma, immunoblastic (or equivalent term)	882	(2)	5	(1)
Lymphoma, primary in brain	187	(0)	1	(0)
Mycobacterium avium or *M. kansasii*, disseminated or extrapulmonary				
Definitive diagnosis	1,847	(4)	22	(3)
Presumptive diagnosis	151	(0)	0	(0)
M. tuberculosis, disseminated or extrapulmonary				
Definitive diagnosis	1,009	(2)	4	(1)
Presumptive diagnosis	152	(0)	0	(0)
Mycobacterial disease, other, disseminated or extrapulmonary				
Definitive diagnosis	406	(1)	7	(1)
Presumptive diagnosis	230	(1)	4	(1)
Pneumocystis carinii pneumonia				
Definitive diagnosis	14,839	(35)	213	(27)
Presumptive diagnosis	5,978	(14)	74	(9)
Progressive multifocal leukoencephalopathy	297	(1)	1	(0)
Salmonella septicemia, recurrent	190	(0)	NA[3]	
Toxoplasmosis of brain				
Definitive diagnosis	850	(2)	2	(0)
Presumptive diagnosis	1,300	(3)	1	(0)
HIV wasting syndrome	7,187	(17)	124	(16)

[1] Percentages are based on 42,557 adult/adolescent and 782 pediatric cases reported to CDC in 1990. The sum of percentages is greater than 100. because some patients have more than one disease.

[2] Not applicable as indicator of AIDS in adults/adolescents.

[3] Tabulated above in "Bacterial infections, multiple or recurrent."

Table 12. AIDS cases, case-fatality rates, and deaths, by half-year and age group, through December 1990, United States

	Adults/adolescents			Children < 13 years old		
Half-year	Cases diagnosed during interval	Case-fatality rate	Deaths occurring during interval	Cases diagnosed during interval	Case-fatality rate	Deaths occurring during interval
Before 1981	77	81.8	30	6	66.7	1
1981 Jan.-June	92	93.5	38	8	62.5	2
July-Dec.	201	91.0	85	6	100.0	6
1982 Jan.-June	394	90.4	151	14	78.6	9
July-Dec.	686	88.8	283	15	80.0	5
1983 Jan.-June	1,262	92.2	517	32	93.8	13
July-Dec.	1,630	91.7	916	42	78.6	16
1984 Jan.-June	2,544	89.4	1,377	49	83.7	25
July-Dec.	3,338	90.1	1,920	62	72.6	24
1985 Jan.-June	4,822	89.2	2,754	94	74.5	44
July-Dec.	6,192	87.5	3,749	127	74.0	68
1986 Jan.-June	8,136	85.9	4,921	134	73.1	64
July-Dec.	9,778	83.1	6,262	178	66.9	84
1987 Jan.-June	12,594	82.4	7,282	219	62.1	113
July-Dec.	14,002	76.1	7,663	245	58.4	157
1988 Jan.-June	15,796	69.4	8,884	236	50.0	129
July-Dec.	16,122	62.8	10,099	318	45.3	151
1989 Jan.-June	17,728	52.5	11,330	309	42.7	154
July-Dec.	17,219	43.4	12,705	290	38.3	160
1990 Jan.-June	16,459	29.8	11,614	263	24.3	135
July-Dec.	9,215	16.2	6,620	139	18.0	78
Total[1]	**158,287**	**62.8**	**99,372**	**2,786**	**51.7**	**1,441**

[1]Death totals include 172 adults/adolescents and 3 children known to have died, but whose dates of death are unknown.

Table 13.   AIDS deaths by race/ethnicity, age at death, and sex, occurring in 1988 and 1989, and cumulative totals reported through December 1990, United States[1]

Race/ethnicity and age at death[2]	Males 1988	Males 1989	Males Cumulative total	Females 1988	Females 1989	Females Cumulative total	Both Sexes 1988	Both Sexes 1989	Both Sexes Cumulative total
White, not Hispanic									
Under 15	43	41	202	27	41	141	70	82	343
15-24	238	267	1,254	28	33	140	266	300	1,394
25-34	3,175	4,029	17,586	191	234	952	3,366	4,263	18,538
35-44	3,723	4,916	20,556	128	154	609	3,851	5,070	21,165
45-54	1,607	2,102	8,715	41	59	233	1,648	2,161	8,948
55 or older	873	1,012	4,481	131	107	581	1,004	1,119	5,062
All ages	9,659	12,367	52,869	546	628	2,659	10,205	12,995	55,528
Black, not Hispanic									
Under 15	70	70	366	72	77	369	142	147	735
15-24	197	191	904	58	57	279	255	248	1,183
25-34	1,768	2,049	9,016	479	577	2,344	2,247	2,626	11,360
35-44	1,738	2,335	8,803	345	456	1,673	2,083	2,791	10,476
45-54	573	723	2,878	76	123	389	649	846	3,267
55 or older	266	337	1,271	52	53	229	318	390	1,500
All ages	4,612	5,705	23,275	1,082	1,343	5,301	5,694	7,048	28,576
Hispanic									
Under 15	37	39	189	31	46	169	68	85	358
15-24	109	119	540	29	31	121	138	150	661
25-34	1,089	1,353	5,445	195	231	883	1,284	1,584	6,328
35-44	1,016	1,334	5,124	130	161	599	1,146	1,495	5,723
45-54	354	485	1,782	34	50	147	388	535	1,929
55 or older	147	192	692	14	24	77	161	216	769
All ages	2,752	3,522	13,800	433	543	2,005	3,185	4,065	15,805
Asian/Pacific Islander									
Under 15	2	—	7	1	1	2	3	1	9
15-24	3	4	14	1	—	2	4	4	16
25-34	33	39	156	3	4	14	36	43	170
35-44	44	61	217	4	7	20	48	68	237
45-54	17	27	96	4	2	10	21	29	106
55 or older	8	14	55	4	3	12	12	17	67
All ages	107	145	547	17	17	61	124	162	608
American Indian/Alaskan Native									
Under 15	—	1	2	—	—	1	—	1	3
15-24	3	2	10	—	—	1	3	2	11
25-34	7	10	48	1	1	9	8	11	57
35-44	4	11	35	—	3	5	4	14	40
45-54	3	4	17	—	1	2	3	5	19
55 or older	2	—	7	—	—	1	2	—	8
All ages	19	28	119	1	5	20	20	33	139
All racial/ethnic groups									
Under 15	152	151	767	131	166	683	283	317	1,450
15-24	551	583	2,728	116	121	544	667	704	3,272
25-34	6,079	7,491	32,287	869	1,048	4,208	6,948	8,539	36,495
35-44	6,541	8,677	34,800	607	783	2,910	7,148	9,460	37,710
45-54	2,559	3,346	13,507	155	235	781	2,714	3,581	14,288
55 or older	1,301	1,560	6,521	202	188	902	1,503	1,748	7,423
All ages	17,183	21,808	90,753	2,080	2,541	10,060	19,263	24,349	100,813

[1] Data tabulations for 1988 and 1989 are based on date of death occurence. Data for deaths occurring in 1990 are incomplete and not tabulated separately, but are included in the cumulative totals. Tabulations for 1988 and 1989 may increase as additional deaths are reported to the CDC.
[2] Data tabulated under "All ages" include 175 persons whose age at death is unknown. Data tabulated under "All racial/ethnic groups" include 157 persons whose race/ethnicity is unknown.

Table 14.   Adult/adolescent AIDS cases by single and multiple exposure categories, reported through December 1990, United States

	AIDS cases	
Exposure category	No.	(%)
Single mode of exposure		
Male homosexual/bisexual contact	90,407	(57)
Intravenous (IV) drug use (female and heterosexual male)	29,520	(19)
Hemophilia/coagulation disorder	855	(1)
Heterosexual contact	8,040	(5)
Receipt of blood transfusion, blood component, or tissue	3,684	(2)
Other/undetermined	5,696	(4)
Single mode of exposure subtotal	**138,202**	**(87)**
Multiple modes of exposure		
Male homosexual/bisexual contact; IV drug use	9,495	(6)
Male homosexual/bisexual contact; hemophilia	34	(0)
Male homosexual/bisexual contact; heterosexual contact	1,904	(1)
Male homosexual/bisexual contact; receipt of transfusion	1,670	(1)
IV drug use; hemophilia	42	(0)
IV drug use; heterosexual contact	3,905	(2)
IV drug use; receipt of transfusion	701	(0)
Hemophilia; heterosexual contact	9	(0)
Hemophilia; receipt of transfusion	509	(0)
Heterosexual contact; receipt of transfusion	400	(0)
Male homosexual/bisexual contact; IV drug use; hemophilia	8	(0)
Male homosexual/bisexual contact; IV drug use; heterosexual contact	749	(0)
Male homosexual/bisexual contact; IV drug use; receipt of transfusion	263	(0)
Male homosexual/bisexual contact; hemophilia; heterosexual contact	2	(0)
Male homosexual/bisexual contact; hemophilia; receipt of transfusion	17	(0)
Male homosexual/bisexual contact; heterosexual contact; receipt of transfusion	92	(0)
IV drug use; hemophilia; heterosexual contact	2	(0)
IV drug use; hemophilia; receipt of transfusion	19	(0)
IV drug use; heterosexual contact; receipt of transfusion	206	(0)
Hemophilia; heterosexual contact; receipt of transfusion	13	(0)
Male homosexual/bisexual contact; IV drug use; hemophilia; receipt of transfusion	7	(0)
Male homosexual/bisexual contact; IV drug use; heterosexual contact; receipt of transfusion	35	(0)
IV drug use; hemophilia; heterosexual contact; receipt of transfusion	3	(0)
Multiple modes of exposure subtotal	**20,085**	**(13)**
Total	**158,287**	**(100)**

Figure 6. Results of investigations of adult/adolescent AIDS cases with undetermined risk, reported through December 1990[1]

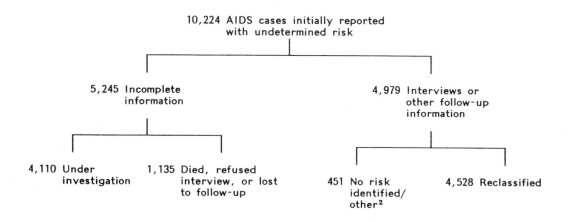

[1] Excludes 68 children under 13 years of age who have an undetermined risk: 60 children are under investigation and 8 have died, refused interview, or were lost to follow-up. An additional 108 children who were initially reported with an undetermined risk have been reclassified after investigation.

[2] **Health-care workers.** 3 of the 451 adults/adolescents are classified as "other" and are health-care workers who seroconverted to HIV and developed AIDS after occupational exposure to HIV-infected blood. For the remaining 448, the mode of exposure to HIV remains undetermined after investigation. 69 of these are health-care workers, 63 of whom responded to a standardized questionnaire. 36 (57%) reported needlesticks and/or mucous membrane exposures to blood and other body fluids of patients. None of the source patients was known to be infected with HIV at the time of the exposure and none of the health-care workers was evaluated at the time of the exposure to document seroconversion to HIV antibody. See *MMWR*, "Update: Acquired Immunodeficiency Syndrome and Human Immunodeficiency Virus Infection Among Health-Care Workers," (April 22, 1988)37:229-234,239.

Heterosexual transmission. 393 of the 448 patients who had no risk identified after follow-up responded to a standardized questionnaire; 126 (35%) of 359 persons responding to questions related to sexually transmitted disease gave a history of such disease and 84 (34%) of 247 interviewed men reported sexual contact with a prostitute. Some of these persons may represent unreported or unrecognized heterosexual transmission of HIV. See *MMWR*, "Update: Heterosexual Transmission of AIDS and HIV Infection — U.S.," (June 23, 1989) 38:423-424,429-434.

Technical notes

Surveillance and reporting of AIDS

All 50 states, the District of Columbia, U.S. dependencies and possessions, and independent nations in free association with the U.S.[1] report AIDS cases to CDC using a uniform case definition and case report form. The original definition was modified in 1985 (*MMWR* 1985;34:373-5) and again in 1987 (*MMWR* 1987;36 [suppl. no. 1S]:1S-15S). The revisions incorporated a broader range of AIDS-indicator diseases and conditions and used human immunodeficiency virus (HIV) diagnostic tests to improve the sensitivity and specificity of the definition. For persons with laboratory-confirmed HIV infection, the 1987 revision incorporated HIV encephalopathy, wasting syndrome, and other indicator diseases that are diagnosed presumptively (i.e., without confirmatory laboratory evidence of the opportunistic disease). AIDS cases that meet the criteria of both the pre-1987 and 1987 definitions are classified in the pre-1987 definition category. Compared with patients who meet the pre-1987 case definition, a higher proportion of patients who meet only the 1987 case definition were female, black, or Hispanic, or were intravenous drug users (*MMWR* 1989;38:229-36).

Each issue of this update includes information received and tabulated by CDC through the last day of the previous month. Data are tabulated by date of report to CDC unless otherwise noted. Data for U.S. dependencies and possessions and for associated independent nations are included in the totals.

Age group tabulations are based on the person's age at diagnosis of AIDS: adult/adolescent cases include persons 13 years of age and older; pediatric cases include children under 13 years of age. Age group tabulations in Table 13 (only included in the year-end edition) are based on age at death.

Metropolitan areas are defined as the Metropolitan Statistical Areas (MSA) for all areas except the 6 New England states. For these states, the New England County Metropolitan Areas (NECMA) are used. Metropolitan areas are named for a central city in the MSA or NECMA, may include several

---

[1]Included among the dependencies, possessions, and independent nations are Puerto Rico, the U.S. Virgin Islands, Guam, American Samoa, the Republic of Palau, the Republic of the Marshall Islands, the Commonwealth of the Northern Mariana Islands, and the Federated States of Micronesia. The latter 5 comprise the category "Pacific Islands, U.S." listed in Table 1.

cities and counties, and may cross state boundaries. For example, AIDS cases and annual rates presented for the District of Columbia in Table 1 include only persons residing within the geographic boundaries of the District. AIDS cases and annual rates for Washington, D.C., in Table 2 include persons residing within several counties in the metropolitan area. State or metropolitan area data tabulations are based on the person's residence at diagnosis of the first AIDS-indicator disease(s). The cities and counties which comprise each metropolitan area in Table 2 are listed in the Bureau of Census publication, "State and Metropolitan Area Data Book, 1986."

Data in this report are provisional. Fifty percent of patients are reported to CDC within 3 months of diagnosis. However, reporting delays vary widely and have been as long as several years for some cases. The median delay in reporting appears to have increased, from about 2 months in 1982 to about 3 months in 1988; however, recent analyses suggests that reporting delay may be decreasing.

Completeness of reporting of diagnosed cases to state and local health departments varies by geographic region and patient population; however, mortality studies suggest that 70 to 90 percent of HIV-related deaths in men 25 to 44 years old are identified through national surveillance of AIDS (*MMWR* 1989;38:561-3). In addition, multiple routes of exposure, opportunistic diseases diagnosed after the initial case report was submitted to CDC, and vital status may not be determined or reported for all cases. Caution should be used in interpreting case-fatality rates because reporting of deaths is known to be incomplete.

Exposure categories

For surveillance purposes, AIDS cases are counted only once in a hierarchy of exposure categories. Persons with more than one reported mode of exposure to HIV are classified in the exposure category listed first in the hierarchy, except for persons with a history of both homosexual/bisexual contact and intravenous drug use. They make up a separate exposure category.

"Homosexual/bisexual contact" cases include men who report sexual contact with other men. "Heterosexual contact" cases include persons who report either specific heterosexual contact with a person with, or at increased risk for, HIV infection (e.g., an intravenous drug user), or persons presumed to have acquired HIV infection through heterosexual contact because they were born in countries with a distinctive pattern of transmission termed "Pattern II" by the World Health Organization (*MMWR* 1988;37:286-8,293-5). Pattern II transmission is observed in areas of sub-Saharan Africa and in some Caribbean countries. In these countries, most of the reported cases occur in heterosexuals and the male-to-female ratio is approximately 1:1. Intravenous drug use and homosexual transmission either do not occur or occur at a low level.

"Undetermined" cases are persons with no reported history of exposure to HIV through any of the routes listed in the hierarchy of exposure categories. Undetermined cases include persons who are currently under investigation by local health department officials; persons whose exposure history is incomplete because of death, refusal to be interviewed, or loss to follow-up; and persons who were interviewed or for whom other follow-up information was available and no exposure mode was identified. Persons who have an exposure mode identified at the time of follow-up are reclassified into the appropriate exposure category.

Rates

Rates are on an annual basis per 100,000 population. The denominator for computing rates in Table 1 and Table 2 are extrapolations based on U.S. Bureau of Census data from the 1980 census and from 1988 post-census estimates. Each 12-month rate is the number of cases for a 12-month period divided by the 1989 or 1990 extrapolation, multiplied by 100,000.

The denominators for computing race-specific rates (Table 9, included only in the year-end edition) are based on 1990 census projections published in U.S. Bureau of Census publications, "Projections of the Population of the United States, by Age, Sex, and Race, 1988 to 2080," and "Projections of the Hispanic Population, 1983 to 2080." Race-specific rates are the number of cases reported for a particular race/ethnicity during the preceding 12-month period divided by the 1990 census projection for that race/ethnicity, multiplied by 100,000.

Case-fatality rates are on a semiannual basis by date of diagnosis. Each 6-month case-fatality rate is the number of fatal cases reported, divided by the number of total cases diagnosed in that period, multiplied by 100.

Trends in AIDS incidence

Tabulations of AIDS cases by date of report give a general description of AIDS cases, but analyses by date of diagnosis give a more accurate description of trends. Delays in reporting, however, can have a substantial impact on tabulated numbers of cases diagnosed in recent time periods. About half of all cases are reported within 3 months of diagnosis, but about 15% are reported more than 1 year after diagnosis. Delays are substantially longer for pediatric cases and for transfusion-associated cases in adults.

Figure 5 (included only in the year-end report) shows trends in AIDS incidence by month of diagnosis. The points on the plot show the estimated numbers of cases diagnosed, after adjusting for estimated reporting delays. The smooth curve is computed using the Lowess procedure (J.M. Chamber, W.S. Cleveland, B. Kleiner, and P.A. Tukey. *Graphical Methods for Data Analysis.* Duxbury Press, Boston, 1983, Chapter 4).

Reporting delays were estimated by a maximum likelihood statistical procedure for each HIV exposure category (J.M. Karon, O.J. Devine, and W.M. Morgan "Predicting AIDS incidence by extrapolating from recent trends." In: C. Castillo-Chavex, ed. *Mathematical and Statistical Approaches to AIDS Epidemiology. Lecture Notes in Biomathematics,* vol. 83, Springer Verlag, Berlin, 1989). The adjusted incidence used in Figure 5 is the sum of the adjusted incidences for each HIV exposure group.

The Lowess procedure makes no assumption about the overall trends in the data. A fitted value is computed for each month by weighted least squares regression using only the adjusted number of cases diagnosed during an interval about the month (in Figure 5, the 30% of months closest to the chosen month); the weights decrease for times further from the chosen month. The procedure assumes that incidence during the interval about each month is approximately a linear function of time. Lowess tends to produce a curve that is linear at each end, as observed in the figure; predictions of future numbers of cases should not be made by extrapolating the Lowess curve.

The Lowess curve should be considered a description of the overall trend in AIDS cases. This curve emphasizes that the rate of increase in incidence slowed during the middle of 1987. See *MMWR* 1990;39:81-86.

Name Index

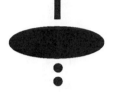

Subject Index

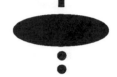